T0355123

Parenthood and
Mental Health

Parenthood and Mental Health

A Bridge between Infant and Adult Psychiatry

Sam Tyano

Professor Emeritus of Child and Adolescent Psychiatry,
Tel Aviv University, Sackler School of Medicine, Israel.
Vice President of the International Association of Child and
Adolescent Psychiatry and Allied Professions

Miri Keren

Head of the Infant Psychiatry Program, Tel Aviv University, School of Medicine, Israel. Director of Infant
Mental Health Unit, Geha Mental Health Center, Petach Tikvah. President Elect of the World Association
for Infant Mental Health

Helen Herrman

Professor of Psychiatry, Orygen Youth Health Research Centre, The University of Melbourne. Director,
World Health Organization Collaborating Centre in Mental Health, Melbourne. Secretary for Publications,
World Psychiatric Association

John Cox

Professor Emeritus, University of Gloucestershire, UK. Immediate Past Secretary General, World
Psychiatric Association

WILEY-BLACKWELL

A John Wiley & Sons, Ltd., Publication

Contents

     Sam Tyano and Miri Keren

     2.1   Introduction   23
     2.2   Continuity from intrauterine life to infancy   24
     2.3   The competent fetus and its receptive sensorial capacities   25
     2.4   Fetuses remember and therefore can learn . . .   26
     2.5   Fetuses can feel pain   26
     2.6   Fetal psychology: an emerging domain   27
     2.7   Conclusion: the fetus can no longer be thought as a 'witless tadpole'   28
     2.8   References   28

Challenging pregnancies

3   **Single parenthood: its impact on parenting the infant**   **31**
     Sam Tyano and Miri Keren

     3.1   Introduction   31
     3.2   Single-parent families come in a variety of profiles   32
     3.3   Single parenthood as risk factor for parental mental health   32
     3.4   Risk factors for mental health problems among single mothers 33
     3.5   Single-father families versus single-mother families   34
     3.6   Single custodial parenthood   34
     3.7   Psychological characteristics of single mothers by choice   35
     3.8   A double-edge risk situation: being a single parent of an
           infant at risk   35
     3.9   Clinical implications   36
     3.10 Summary   36
     3.11 References   37

4   **Surrogate mothers**   **39**
     Olga B.A. van den Akker

     4.1   Introduction   39
     4.2   Characteristics, motivations and experiences   43
     4.3   Attachment, bonding and pregnancy   44
     4.4   Relinquishing the baby and the social context   47
     4.5   Conclusion   48
     4.6   References   48

At-risk pregnancies

5   **The impact of stress in pregnancy on the fetus, the infant,**
     and the child   **51**
     Miri Keren

     5.1   Introduction   51
     5.2   Data from animal studies   52

Pathological parenting: from the infant's perspective

Concluding chapter

Foreword

After World War II, the newly created World Health Organization asked a British child psychiatrist to prepare a monograph on the mental health needs of children. The WHO was concerned about the large numbers of children who had been orphaned or experienced extended separations from their parents in the war. John Bowlby reviewed the world's literature and consulted with experts. His monograph, *Maternal Care and Mental Health* [1], appeared in 1951 and concluded that the quality of parental care which children receive in their earliest years is of vital importance for their future mental health. Specifically, he said, "... essential for mental health is that an infant and young child should experience a warm, intimate and continuous relationship with his mother (or mother substitute...) in which both find satisfaction and enjoyment (p. 13)."

Over the next several decades, Bowlby pursued his life's work of synthesizing a theory of attachment that elaborated these ideas on the importance of early experiences between young children and their parents. Bowlby's colleague, Mary Ainsworth, operationalized his theory by developing an observational method of assessing the young child's behavior with attachment figures. This groundbreaking work led to a large body of research that has extended and refined many of the ideas of attachment theory but, in the main, the accuracy of Bowlby's basic premises seems clear.

Indeed, Bowlby's emphasis on the importance of early experiences has implications well beyond attachment theory. Much of the excitement in contemporary developmental neuroscience is about attempts to describe the importance and effects of early experiences on human brain development. Moreover, the entire field of infant mental health rests on the premise that relationships between infants and caregivers are the most important developmental context affecting the child's social and emotional behavior. These relationships are the most important focus of assessment and the most important target of interventions.

Not all have found the emphasis on parenting meaningful. In 1998, Judith Harris published *The Nurture Assumption* [2], asserting that parents were not nearly as important for child outcomes as was generally believed. Instead, she asserted that genetic and peer influences were both underappreciated and far more important than parenting.

The intensity of the reaction to these assertions illustrates how far we have come in the 50 years since Bowlby published his monograph. In 1951, it was big news that parenting was considered vital for children's mental health. Fifty years later, Judith Harris provocatively staked out the contrarian position that parenting matters little. Although her selective review of the evidence and debatable conclusions have been strongly challenged, her thesis usefully invites us to reconsider our assumptions about parenting. Indeed, since her book was published, a great deal of research on the extraordinarily deleterious effects of children raised without parents has demonstrated the limitations of her basic thesis. This research redirects us to review what we know about parenting and its effects.

With that in mind, the present volume is timely and much needed. The editors of this book, Sam Tyano, Miri Keren, Helen Herrman, and John Cox, have assembled an outstanding group of international scholars who contributed to this comprehensive review of parenting in the prenatal, perinatal, and early infancy periods. Bridging a gap between infant and adult psychiatry, the volume considers in some depth normal parenting processes, risk factors for parenting, and a variety of special circumstances related to parenting under atypical conditions. Their developmental orientation reminds us that our emphasis on understanding infant trajectories ought to be accompanied by an understanding of parents' trajectories. For clinicians, the psychological origins of parenting, and the myriad factors that influence their development over time, are critically important topics. Investigators will find the reviews of special topics both interesting and stimulating with regard to questions that need to be addressed, and thus they can guide future research.

The sober assessment of children's mental health needs that followed the second World War and inspired Bowlby's illuminating vision has given way to even more complexities and challenges in the 21st century. Good enough parenting has never seemed more difficult nor more important. This volume promises to enhance our understanding of all that we know and all that we need to learn about this most vital human endeavor.

Charles H. Zeanah
January 2010

References

1. Bowlby, J. (1951) *Maternal Care and Mental Health*, The World Health Organization: Monograph Series, WHO Geneva.
2. Harris, J. R. (1998) *The Nurture Assumption: Why Children Turn Out the Way They Do* Bloomsbury Publishing PLC, London.

List of contributors

Adil Akram
Division of Mental Health
St George's University of London
Cranmer Terrace
London SW 17 ORE, UK

Massimo Ammaniti
Department of Dynamic and Clinical
    Psychology, Faculty of Psychology 1
University of Rome, 'Sapienza'
Via dei Marsi, 78
00185 Rome, Italy

Julio Arboleda-Flórez
Department of Psychiatry
Queen's University
Kingston ON K7L 3N6, Canada

Joanne Barton
North Staffordshire Combined
    Healthcare
NHS Trust Stoke-on-Trent
Staffordshire, UK

Thierry Baubet
Avicenne Hôpital, APHP, Paris 13 University
125, rue de Stalingrad
93009 Bobigny, (Seine-Saint Denis) France

Claire Baudry
École de psychologie
Université Laval
Québec, G1K 7P4, Canada

Annie Bernier
Département de psychologie
Université de Montreal (Québec)
Canada

Erika L. Bocknek
Dept. Pediatrics
LSU School of Medicine
Children's Hospital
200 Henry Clay Ave
New Orleans, LA 70118, USA

Marc H. Bornstein
Child and Family Research Program in
    Developmental Neuroscience
Eunice Kennedy Shriver National Institute of
    Child Health and Human Development
Suite 8030, 6705 Rockledge Drive
Bethesda MD 20892-7971, USA

Meena Cabral de Mello
Department of Child and Adolescent
    Health and Development
World Health Organization
22 Avenue Appia
Geneva, Switzerland

Prabha S. Chandra
Department of Psychiatry
National Institute of Mental Health and
    Neurosciences
Hosur Road
Bangalore 560029, India

Elise Charlemaine
Hôpital Port Royal
123, Boulevard de Port Royal
75104 Paris, France

Antoinette Corboz-Warnery
Centre d'Etude de la Famille
Site de Cery
1008 Prilly-Lausanne, Switzerland

John Cox
University of Gloucestershire
58 St Stephens Rd
Cheltenham GL51 3AE, UK

Ilana Crome
Coton House
St George's Hospital
South Staffordshire and Shropshire
Healthcare NHS Foundation Trust
Corporation Street
Stafford, ST 16 3SR, UK

Geetha Desai
Department of Psychiatry
National Institute of Mental Health
    and Neurosciences
Hosur Road
Bangalore 560029, India

Zivanit Ergaz
The Department of Anatomy and Cell
    Biology
The Institute of Medical Sciences,
    Faculty of Medicine
P.O.B. 12272, Jerusalem 91120, Israel

Jane Fisher
Centre for Women's Health, Gender and
    Society
Melbourne School of Population
    Health
University of Melbourne
Carlton, Victoria 3010, Australia

Sheehan D. Fisher
Department of Psychology
E11 Seashore Hall
The University of Iowa
Iowa City, IA 52242, USA

Hiram E. Fitzgerald
Psychology Kellogg Center
Michigan State University
East Lansing
MI 48824, USA

Elisabeth Fivaz-Depeursinge
Centre d'Etude de la Famille
Site de Cery
1008 Prilly-Lausanne, Switzerland

France Frascarolo
Centre d'Etude de la Famille
Site de Cery
1008 Prilly-Lausanne, Switzerland

Micheline Garel
INSERM
Epidemiological Research Unit on
    Perinatal and Women's Health
Villejuif, F-94807, France

Yvon Gauthier
Hôpital Sainte Justine
Department of Psychiatry
3175 Côte Ste Catherine
Montreal (Quebec) H3T 1C5, Canada

Catherine Grandsard
Université Paris VIII
Centre Georges Devereux
98 Bd de Sébastopol
75003 Paris, France

Antoine Guedeney
Hôpital Bichat Claude Bernard APHP
CMP Binet, 64 rue René Binet
75018 Paris, France

Carol Henshaw
Faculty of Health
Staffordshire University
Brindley Building
Leek Rd
Stoke on Trent, ST4 2DF, UK

Helen Herrman
ORYGEN Youth Health Research Centre
Centre for Youth Mental Health
The University of Melbourne
Parkville, Victoria, 3052, Australia

Kathryn Hollins
Perinatal and Parent-Infant Mental
    Health Service
Chelsea and Westminster Hospital
369 Fulham Road, London
SW10 9NH, UK

Sheila Hollins
Division of Mental Health
St George's University of London
Level 6 Hunter Wing
Cranmer Terrace
London, SW17 0RE, UK

Pälvi Kaukonen
Department of Child Psychiatry
Tampere University and University
    Hospital
Po Box 2000
33521 Tampere, Finland

Miri Keren
Tel Aviv University
Geha Mental Health Center
Helsinky str. 1.
P.O.B. 102
Petach Tikvah 49100, Israel

Simon Larose
Département d'études sur l'enseignement
    et l'apprentissage
Université Laval
Québec, G1K 7P4, Canada

Brigitte Martin
Programme de psychiatrie,
    neurodéveloppement et génétique
CHU Ste-Justine
3100 Ellendale
Montreal, QC H3S 1W3, Canada

James P. McHale
Department Psychology
University of South Florida
St. Petersburg
140 Seventh Ave. S.
St. Petersburg Fl 33701, USA

Barbara G. Melamed
School of Social and Behavioral Sciences
Mercy College
555 Broadway
Dobbs Ferry
New York 10522, USA

Sylvain Missonnier
L'Institut de Psychologie
Universite Paris Descartes
71, avenue Edouard Vaillant
92774 Boulogne Billancourt, France

Caroline Moisan
École de psychologie
Université Laval
Québec, G1K 7P4, Canada

Marie Rose Moro
Avicenne Hôpital, APHP, Paris 13
University
125, rue de Stalingrad
93009 Bobigny, (Seine-Saint Denis) France

Michael W. O'Hara
Department of Psychology
E11 Seashore Hall
The University of Iowa
Iowa City, IA 52242, USA

Asher Ornoy
Department of Anatomy and Cell Biology
The Institute of Medical Sciences,
    Faculty of Medicine
P.O.B. 12272, Jerusalem 91120, Israel

Howard J. Osofsky
Department Pediatrics
LSU School of Medicine
Children's Hospital
200 Henry Clay Ave
New Orleans, LA 70118, USA

Joy D. Osofsky
Department Pediatrics
LSU School of Medicine
Children's Hospital
200 Henry Clay Ave
New Orleans, LA 70118, USA

Campbell Paul
Royal Children's Hospital
Flemington Road
Parkville, Victoria, 3052
Melbourne, Australia

Kaija Puura
Department of Child Psychiatry
Tampere University and University Hospital
Po Box 2000
33521 Tampere, Finland

Atif Rahman
University of Liverpool
Child Mental Health Unit
Alder Hey Children's NHS
   Foundation Trust
Liverpool L12 2AP, UK

Joan Raphael-Leff
Academic Faculty for Psychoanalytic
   Research
UCL/Anna Freud Centre
London, UK

Dalila Rezzoug
Avicenne Hôpital, APHP, Paris 13
University
125, rue de Stalingrad
93009 Bobigny, (Seine-Saint Denis) France

Fanie Roy
École de psychologie
Université Laval
Québec, G1K 7P4, Canada

Veena A. Satyanarayana
Department of Psychiatry
Epidemiology and Prevention Research
   Group
Washington University School of Medicine
St Louis, USA

Myriam Szejer
Hôpital Antoine Béclère
157 rue de la Porte de Trivaux
92161 Clamart cedex, France

Martin St-André
Programme de psychiatrie,
   neurodéveloppement et génétique
CHU Saint-Justine
3100 Ellendale
Montreal, QC H3S 1W3, Canada

Olivier Taïeb
Avicenne Hôpital, APHP, Paris 13 University
125, rue de Stalingrad
93009 Bobigny, (Seine-Saint Denis) France

Renata Tambelli
Department of Dynamic and Clinical
   Psychology, Faculty of Psychology 1
University of Rome, 'Sapienza'
Via dei Marsi, 78
00185 Rome, Italy

George Tarabulsy
École de Psychologie
Pavillon Félix-Antoine-Savard, local 1210
Université Laval
Québec, G1K 7P4, Canada

Susana Tereno
Hôpital Bichat Claude Bernard APHP
CMP Binet, 64 rue René Binet
75018 Paris, France

Frances Thomson Salo
The Royal Children's Hospital
Flemington Road
Parkville
Victoria 3052, Australia

Mark Tomlinson
Department of Psychology
Stellenbosch University
Private Bag X1
Matieland, 7602, South Africa

Magdalen Toole
Child and Family Research Program in
    Developmental Neuroscience
Eunice Kennedy Shriver National Institute of
    Child Health and Human Development
Suite 8030, 6705 Rockledge Drive
Bethesda MD 20892-7971, USA

Sam Tyano
Tel-Aviv University, Sackler School of
    Medicine
P.O.B. 65352
Ramut Aviv Gimel, Israel

Olga B.A. van den Akker
School of Health & Social Sciences
Middlesex University
The Town Hall
The Burroughs
Hendon, London MW4 4BT, UK

Deborah Weatherston
Michigan Association for Infant Mental
    Health
13101 Allen Road
Southgate
Michigan 48195, USA

Jean-Victor P. Wittenberg
The Hospital for Sick Children
555 University Avenue
Toronto, Ontario, M5G 1X8,
Canada

Stella Woodward
Cardiff University Medical
    School
Heath Park
Cardiff
CF14 4XN, UK

Nathalie Zajde
Université Paris VIII
Centre Georges-Devereux
98 Bd de Sébastopol
75003, Paris, France

World Psychiatric Association *Evidence and Experience in Psychiatry* Series

Series Editor: Helen Herrman, WPA Secretary for Publications, University of Melbourne, Australia

The *Evidence & Experience in Psychiatry* series, launched in 1999, offers unique insights into both investigation and practice in mental health. Developed and commissioned by the World Psychiatric Association, the books address controversial issues in clinical psychiatry and integrate research evidence and clinical experience to provide a stimulating overview of the field.

Focused on common psychiatric disorders, each volume follows the same format: systematic review of the available research evidence followed by multiple commentaries written by clinicians of different orientations and from different countries. Each includes coverage of diagnosis, management, pharma and psycho- therapies, and social and economic issues. The series provides insights that will prove invaluable to psychiatrists, psychologists, mental health nurses and policy makers.

Depressive Disorders, 3e
Edited by Helen Herrman, Mario Maj and Norman Sartorius
ISBN: 9780470987209

Substance Abuse
Edited by Hamid Ghodse, Helen Herrman, Mario Maj and Norman Sartorius
ISBN: 9780470745106

Trauma and Mental Health: Resilience and Post-Traumatic Stress Disorders
Edited by Dan J Stein, Matthew J Friedman and Carlos Blanco
ISBN: 9780470688977

Schizophrenia 2e
Edited by Mario Maj, Norman Sartorius
ISBN: 9780470849644

Dementia 2e
Edited by Mario Maj, Norman Sartorius
ISBN: 9780470849637

Obsessive-Compulsive Disorders 2e
Edited by Mario Maj, Norman Sartorius, Ahmed Okasha, Joseph Zohar
ISBN: 9780470849668

Bipolar Disorders
Edited by Mario Maj, Hagop S Akiskal, Juan José López-Ibor, Norman Sartorius
ISBN: 9780471560371

Eating Disorders
Edited by Mario Maj, Kathrine Halmi, Juan José López-Ibor, Norman Sartorius
ISBN: 9780470848654

Phobias
Edited by Mario Maj, Hagop S Akiskal, Juan José López-Ibor, Ahmed Okasha
ISBN: 9780470858332

Personality Disorders
Edited by Mario Maj, Hagop S Akiskal, Juan E Mezzich
ISBN: 9780470090367

Somatoform Disorders
Edited by Mario Maj, Hagop S Akiskal, Juan E Mezzich, Ahmed Okasha
ISBN: 9780470016121

Other World Psychiatric Association titles

Series Editor (2005–): Helen Herrman, WPA Secretary for Publications, University of Melbourne, Australia

Special Populations

The Mental Health of Children and Adolescents: an area of global neglect
Edited by Helmut Remschmidt, Barry Nurcombe, Myron L. Belfer, Norman Sartorius and Ahmed Okasha
ISBN: 9780470512456

Contemporary Topics in Women's Mental Health: global perspectives in a changing society
Edited by Prabha S. Chandra, Helen Herrman, Marianne Kastrup, Marta Rondon, Unaiza Niaz, Ahmed Okasha, Jane Fisher
ISBN: 9780470754115

Families and Mental Disorders
Edited by Norman Sartorius, Julian Leff, Juan José López-Ibor, Mario Maj, Ahmed Okasha
ISBN: 9780470023822

Disasters and Mental Health
Edited by Juan José López-Ibor, George Christodoulou, Mario Maj, Norman Sartorius, Ahmed Okasha
ISBN: 9780470021231

Approaches to Practice and Research
Religion and Psychiatry: beyond boundaries
Edited by Peter J Verhagen, Herman M van Praag, Juan José López-Ibor, John Cox, Driss Moussaoui
ISBN: 9780470694718

Psychiatric Diagnosis: challenges and prospects
Edited by Ihsan M. Salloum and Juan E. Mezzich
ISBN: 9780470725696

Recovery in Mental Health: reshaping scientific and clinical responsibilities
By Michaela Amering and Margit Schmolke
ISBN: 9780470997963

Handbook of Service User Involvement in Mental Health Research
Edited by Jan Wallcraft, Beate Schrank and Michaela Amering
ISBN: 9780470997956

Psychiatrists and Traditional Healers: unwitting partners in global mental health
Edited by Mario Incayawar, Ronald Wintrob and Lise Bouchard
ISBN: 9780470516836

Psychiatric Diagnosis and Classification
Edited by Mario Maj, Wolfgang Gaebel, Juan José López-Ibor, Norman Sartorius
ISBN: 9780471496816

Psychiatry in Society
Edited by Norman Sartorius, Wolfgang Gaebel, Juan José López-Ibor, Mario Maj
ISBN: 9780471496823

Psychiatry as a Neuroscience
Edited by Juan José López-Ibor, Wolfgang Gaebel, Mario Maj, Norman Sartorius
ISBN: 9780471496564

Early Detection and Management of Mental Disorders
Edited by Mario Maj, Juan José López-Ibor, Norman Sartorius, Mitsumoto Sato, Ahmed Okasha
ISBN: 9780470010839

Also available in electronic editions only, through Wiley Online Library:

WPA Anthology of Italian Language Psychiatric Texts
WPA Anthology of Spanish Language Psychiatric Texts
WPA Anthology of French Language Psychiatric Texts

Introduction

Parenting is important to everybody, as the foundation of family life across cultures. Parenting is, in its essence, a domain where adult mental health meets with infant normal and abnormal development. Though the impact of the quality of parenting on a child's development is significant throughout the entire childhood and adolescence, we view pregnancy and the first year of life as a unique period. Indeed, the entry into parenthood has been described as a reorganization of the parent's psyche, that starts with pregnancy and culminates during the first year of parenting. We often see a very high motivation for change and learning during this period. From the other side of the umbilical cord, pregnancy is a time of risks and opportunities for the developing brain, and the first year of life is crucial in forming the first human significant interpersonal relationships.

Contingent to these perspectives, we have chosen pregnancy and first year of life as the focus of this book. We have tried to bring a comprehensive account of data that shows the points of encounter between adult and infant psychiatry, and to draw out clinical guidelines for prevention and treatment. Its target readers are all those whose profession faces them with physical and mental health of infants and their parents. In this book, we have tried to give equal focus on mothers, fathers and infants. The book focuses on developing a common evidence-based clinical understanding about the parenting of infants between different groups in the health and mental health professions including those concerned with adult and child mental health.

By nature of their work some professionals focus on the role of parents. Others overlook the prominence of this role in the life of a person who is mother or father of an infant or older child, especially when attention is focused on the person's personal distress and mental illness. This often leaves families with little support at critical times. We aim at providing a more holistic approach.

The book makes a unique contribution through expert coverage of several areas. It summarizes knowledge about normal and abnormal parenting from gestation to the first year of life, including a critical analysis of parenting, what it means to be a 'good-enough parent', and the relationship to infant, parent and family outcomes. It includes the psychiatric dimension by emphasizing the biological aspects of parenting, parental

Parenthood and Mental Health: A Bridge between Infant and Adult Psychiatry Sam Tyano, Miri Keren, Helen Herrman and John Cox
© 2010 John Wiley & Sons, Ltd.

psychopathology and infant's normal and abnormal development. It takes a period-related approach, looking at specific challenges that the twenty-first century brings to the universal, developmental task known as 'parenting', and assembles the academic and field experiences of authors from a wide variety of countries and cultures.

I.1   A historical overview: infants, parents, and parenting from ancient times to nowadays

Love for babies has probably existed for ever in all cultures. Still, when one reads descriptions of families through history [1], it becomes obvious that being an infant has not always been pleasurable, nor has the definition of the parental role always been as the main caretaker. One may see a parallel between views on what is 'good-enough parenting' in a number of countries and the history of Western civilizations.

In the ancient times, parents had many children, but family life was not organized around children's needs. In contrast, the modern Western family is organized in support of the children and their future. The turning point in valorizing and individualizing children happened in the eighteenth century (the Century of Lights).

Indeed, babies' fate was for a long time quite gloomy: only a few of them survived into childhood, since they either died from disease, or were abandoned at birth. Abandonment of babies at birth (especially girls), was a social norm induced by life constraints (poverty, hunger, sickness); although it was not a moral problem, it did create an emotional one, as described in some historical writings. Abandonment of babies became forbidden by law in the year 374 CE by the Christian emperors. Still in the fifteenth century, society perceived babies as screaming and dirty little creatures, and older children as annoyances that needed to be restricted through physical punishments.

The Church was the first to make the link between written culture (mostly religion at these times) and education, and therefore the first pedagogues were clerks. Children under the age of 7 years were not supposed to learn, nor to obey. In 1650, the Church decreed the age of 7 years as 'the age of reason', meaning also the age for potential sin. Education was to start only then. Before the age of 7, the Church perceives infants and toddlers as naïve and pure creatures, like the Virgin, between humans and God. Until the eighteenth century, the overall representation of the very young child is a negative one of a not-yet–developed human creature.

In parallel, during the years 1640 to 1720, a few church figures start to 'discover' that childhood is made up of different and unique stages, from infancy to adolescence. Infancy is defined from 0 to 2 years, the age at which the infant is breast-weaned, leaves the nursing servant and enters for the first time his or her biological family; until the age of 7years, boys and girls are with their mother and the servants, while nobody has specific expectations from them, besides making as little trouble as possible. At the age of 7, begins the 'third childhood', or the 'age of reason'. Boys and girls are separated, and parents are encouraged to send them to the Church for education. Adolescence, at 12 to14 years, is considered the end of childhood.

By the eighteenth century, philosophers had adopted this new approach and integrated it into the philosophy of the Century of the Lights that values reason, nature and legitimized search for individual happiness on earth. Children become valued and placed at the heart of the family; babies are desired, protected and loved, in spite of the terribly high mortality rate. Physical and moral education are most valued.

Parents' role in the care of their babies has changed also through human history and varies across cultures today. For centuries in Europe, infants were breastfed and cared for by expert servants. In ancient Sparta, the optimal 'nurse' was an expert woman who, instead of wrapping up the baby, would leave his or her body free to move, would teach him or her not to be picky about food, not to fear darkness or solitude, and not to cry aloud and burst into temper tantrums. Then, in the thirteenth century, the definition of good-enough nursing/ parenting care totally changed, based on what babies were thought to be capable of doing: babies 'limbs were perceived as fragile, therefore they needed to be held in a maillot; babies' eyes were thought to be too sensitive to sustain light, therefore babies were put to sleep in dark rooms; or babies were too fragile to take medications, therefore, if they were sick, the nursing servant should take it for them. The aristocratic society norm of having babies taken care by servants, started to be questioned; Recommendations for choosing a physically and mentally healthy servant nurse reflected the beginning of understanding of the impact of the environment on the infant: 'She should not be stupid, sad, or angry, her breath should smell good, and her breasts should not be too small nor too large' [1].

Fathers, in medieval times, were allowed to show tenderness and be involved in the child's education. At the end of the Middle Ages Joseph was considered as a model of fatherhood. From 1450, both Mary and Joseph are drawn as equally kneeling in front of the Child. David was pictured as crying at Absalom's death . . .

Until the eighteenth century, the role of the family in the socialization of the child is overall very marginal, while the community and the Church are the predominant influences. Then, with the change in the child's status, parents start planning their family size, while taking into consideration the significant investment each of their children has the right to. Family life becomes organized around the child's needs. Obviously, these major changes were slow and gradual, starting in the upper classes and spreading to the lower ones.

The nineteenth century is a difficult period for children, again because of the major changes societies face with the era of industrialization: children's salaries are indispensable to family survival. As a consequence, many children are exploited and maltreated and, in general, children's emotional needs are put aside, especially in the lower socioeconomical classes. Babies from poor families were either given to a nursing woman in villages (rate of mortality was one in three babies), to an old woman in the neighborhood for the whole day, or simply left alone in their bed while mothers were at the factory for 12 hours. In 1844, the first public nursery home for under-2-years-olds was opened in Paris, followed by others all around Europe. Needless to say that the quality of care in these nurseries was very low and the mortality rate very high (almost 50%!).

The turning point came towards the end of the nineteenth century, with the inauguration in several countries of elementary, obligatory and free school laws, together with a minimum age (for example 12 years) for factory work, and the limitation of work hours to 6 hours per day. The introduction of compulsory schooling implied a major change in the definition of who is responsible for the child: society, and not only parents, are in charge of the child's best interests, especially at times of conflict with the parents' interests. In 1849 in France, 10 years after the inauguration of the school law, a law against 'bad paternal behaviors' was announced. In parallel, the second half of the nineteenth century saw the beginning of punishment of pedophilia, sexual abuse and physical violence towards young children, and at the beginning of the twentieth century, judges began looking at the child as an individual with civil rights.

Indeed, the twentieth century was in many ways the century of the World Declaration of the Rights of the Child. Hopefully, the twenty-first will see the Babies' Rights Declaration, advocated by the World Association for Infant Mental Health.

I.2 Definition of some major concepts

For the sake of those readers who may not be familiar with concepts taken from the domain of child development, we clarify some of the concepts that figure throughout the book in the different chapters, specifically attachment, parenting and parenthood constellation.

Attachment, one of the concepts that illustrate the bridge between infant and adult psychiatry

Bowlby [2] argued for the existence of an innate drive to look for a protective figure while in distress: 'While attachment is at its most obvious in early childhood, it can be observed throughout the life cycle, especially in emergencies . . . Its biological function is protection . . . whatever our age is.' The age range of peak development is within 2 to 7 months, and distress is the trigger of activation of the attachment behaviors. Attachment behaviors are of two types:

- Signal behaviors (mainly crying and anticipatory arms rising), and

- Proximity-seeking to attachment figure (such as crawling, climbing on knees, and walking towards caregiver).

Based on these definitions, Ainsworth [3] has developed the well-known paradigm of the Strange Situation, where distress in the infant is triggered by separation from the caregiver, and attachment behaviors observed during the reunion.

Based on the analysis of the infant's attachment behaviors during the reunion, Ainsworth has defined the categories of secure attachment and insecure attachment. The latter includes two subtypes: resistant/ambivalent and avoidant. The securely attached infant reacts to the separation, greets the parent at reunion, looks for proximity, and returns to his or her baseline level of exploration and play.

For the insecure attachment group with the avoidant strategy of coping with distress, the effect is to dampen the attachment system down so that the infant appears indifferent to separation. This type of attachment is characteristic of infants who have internalized their caregiver as inefficient in their ability to calm them down while in distress (for instance, depressed or psychotic mothers). The resistant type of insecure attachment is the opposite, meaning the infant's attachment system is over-activated; the infant is very distressed by the separation but the parent's return does not calm him or her down. This pattern is typical of infants of unpredictable caregivers (such as parents with personality disorders). There is a fourth type, the disorganized attachment type, seen in clinical populations, especially where abuse and chaotic family functioning are common. The infant is distressed, but seems frightened by the caregiver, and therefore shows contradictory attachment behaviors.

The attachment system is in balance with the exploratory system: the more protected/ secure the child feels towards his or her caregiver, the more readily he or she will engage in exploration of the surroundings. The exploratory system is itself crucial for learning and curiosity development.

The securely attached child develops an internal schema of 'self-with-attachment figure' [4], and therefore is very much linked to the development of basic trust, one of the pivots of the quality of object relationships. Indeed, longitudinal studies [5] have shown that infants who were secure at 12 months were co-operative, popular, resilient and resourceful children at the age of 4.5 years; those who were avoidant at 12 months showed a lack of empathy, were hostile towards other children, and looked for the teacher's attention. Those who were resistant/ambivalent at 12 months were tense, impulsive, frustrated or passive and helpless. Finally, those who were disorganized at 12 months had severe behavior problems at the age of 4.5 years.

More recently, Fonagy [6] showed the link between adults' disorganized attachment representations , history of abuse in childhood and borderline personality disorder. He has summarized the common ground between psychoanalytic and attachment theories, and has gradually increased the general awareness of the relevance of attachment processes to the field of developmental psychology, especially in the development of borderline person- ality disorders. Many attachment researchers suggest looking at the adult classification of attachment as a continuum of structures for affect regulation: on one end, the dismissing type (equivalent to the avoidant type in the infant), whose structures suppress affect by using highly organized but rigid structures. At the other pole is the preoccupied (equivalent to the resistant/ambivalent type in the infant), whose structures 'hyperactivate' affective cues to caregivers.

Parenting

The impact of the parent's own attachment representations and her infant's seems very strong, when one looks at the amazing rate of 75% concordance between the infant's pattern of attachment to the parent, and the parent's attachment classification (measured by the Adult Attachment Interview [7]).

Still, some important aspects of parenting are independent of attachment security. Parents are supposed to do more than providing a haven of safety, a secure base for exploration, and a source of reassurance in times of distress: they need to provide ade- quately modulated stimulation, guidance, limits, structure, parent–child boundaries, pro- blem-solving strategies, and promoting the child's relationship with peers. A parent may be ineffective with regards to some of these roles, while she or he has been a secure base. Provision of a secure base is always important, because it has a survival value, but it is definitely not all that is meant by parenting. It is viewed by many authors as the whole of the representations, the affects and the behaviors of the parent with his/her child, even before this child was conceived.

Parenthood constellation

Winnicott [8] introduced the idea of 'maternal preoccupation' and defined it as 'Almost an illness' that a mother must experience and recover from, in order to create and sustain an environment that can meet the physical and psychological needs of the infant. This special state of heightened sensitivity is like a dissociative state that heightens the mother's ability to anticipate the infant's needs, and learn his or her unique signals.

Winnicott emphasized the crucial importance of such a stage for the infant's self-development (even before what we knew today about the impact of early interactive experiences on the brain development), and the developmental consequences for infants when mothers are unable to tolerate such a level of intense preoccupation. Too much preoccupation is detrimental because it does not leave room for other family members' needs (father, siblings and mother herself), is often linked with maternal obsessive fears of losing/not taking care well enough of the baby, and does not leave room for other care-takers, including the father. Too little maternal preoccupation can be observed in various clinical situations, such as post-partum depression, psychosis, severe narcissistic person-ality disorders where the mother's needs come first, and may lead to deprivation and maltreatment.

Stern [9] took the idea further, and wrote about the content of the maternal preoccupa-tion; four essential themes preoccupy her, as follows in the increased order of sophistication:

1 Will I be able to keep my baby alive and growing?

2 Will I be able to emotionally engage with my baby?

3 Will I be able to create the necessary support system for the baby?

4 Will I be able to transform my identity from 'daughter of' to 'mother of'?

Stern did not explicitly write about *paternal* preoccupation. Fathers and mothers displayed a similar time course of preoccupation, but its degree was less in mothers [10]. Actually, the more fathers are included in psychopathological developmental research, the more data we gather about their impact on their children's development. The First-Time Fathers study [11] has prospectively looked at the well-being of men during transition to parenthood, and their main finding was the lack of preparation for the impact of parenthood on their lives. We therefore definitely need to have fathers in mind whenever we promote preventive interventions, and this has been in our minds while planning for the structure of this book.

I.3 Structure of the book

Parenting begins in pregnancy, actually from the time of conception, and involves many conscious and unconscious processes. Recent studies have shown the significant impact of these processes on the fetus's development, and therefore the book starts with pregnancy.

The understanding of abnormal processes and pathological states is very much based on knowledge about normality. Therefore, the chapters are divided into normal and abnormal processes, during pregnancy as well as after birth and along the first year of life. Assessment and evidence-based treatments, psychological as well as pharmacotherapeutical are reviewed.

All along the chapters, risk and protective factors in the infant, the parents, and the environment are taken into consideration. Obviously, there is a great disparity in resources available around the world, and the interplay between risk and protective factors may lead to very different outcomes in various parts of the world.

The book fittingly concludes with a global perspective on good-enough parenting, which recognizes that, in times of political turbulence, terrorist atrocities, natural disasters and climate change, it is the parents and their infants who often suffer most; and that such suffering can be transmitted to the next generation.

For the editors, the production of this book has been a pivotal experience, and we would hope that our readers will be similarly inspired – and changed a little by the new knowledge in this field.

The Editors.

I.4 References

1. L'enfant et la Famille (2006) *Les collections de l'histoire*, **32**.
2. Bowlby, J. (1982) *Attachment and Loss: vol 1. Attachment*. Basic Books, New York. (Original work published 1969)
3. Ainsworth, M.D.S., Blehar, M., Waters, E. *et al.* (1978) *Patterns of Attachment*. Erlbaum, Hillsdale, NJ.
4. Stern, D. (1985) *The Interpersonal World of the Infant: A View from Psychoanalysis and Developmental Psychology*. New York, Basic Books.
5. Sroufe, L.A. (1988) The role of infant-caregiver attachment in development, in *Clinical Implications of Attachment* (eds J. Belsky and T. Nezworski), Basic Books, New York, pp. 70–94.
6. Fonagy, P., Steele, M., Steele, H. *et al.* (1995) Attachment, the reflective self, and borderline states: the predictive specifity of the Adult Attachment Interview and pathological emotional development, in *Attachment Theory: Social, Developmental, and Clinical Perspectives* (eds S. Goldberg, R. Muir and J. Kerr), Analytic Press, Hillsdale, NJ, pp. 233–79.
7. Hesse, E. (1999) Adult Attachment Interview, in *Handbook of Attachment* (eds J. Cassidy and P.R. Shaver), pp. 395–433.
8. Winnicott, D.W. (1956) Primary maternal preoccupation, in *Through Pediatrics to Psychoanalysis*. New York: International Universities Press, New York, pp. 300–5.
9. Stern, D. (1995) *The Motherhood Constellation*. Basic Books, New York.
10. Leckman, J., Feldman, R., Swain *et al.* (2004) Primary parental preoccupation: circuits, genes, and the crucial role of the environment. *Journal of Neural Transmission*, **111**, 753–71.

1

Mothers' and fathers' orientations: patterns of pregnancy, parenting and the bonding process

Joan Raphael-Leff

Academic Faculty for Psychoanalytic Research, UCL/Anna Freud Centre, London

1.1 Introduction

To begin at the very beginning: we were all conceived by union of male and female gametes. However, definitions of 'parents' vary geographically across the world, and at different historical periods.

Over the past decades, eternal facts of life altered dramatically. Due to efficient, female-based contraception methods, 12–20% of European women remain childfree-by-choice. For the first time in world history the death rate exceeds birth rate!

Western family formations now include single, multiple, same-sex, teenage and older parents, while in AIDS-ridden lower-income societies, oldest siblings serve as mother and/or father in child-headed families.

Thus, the concept 'parents' now comprises biological procreators, surrogates, foster and adoptive carers, and new kinship categories formed through reproductive technology as lone, virgin and post-menopausal mothers gestate genetically unrelated babies, asexually conceived by embryo, egg and/or sperm donation. Furthermore,

Parenthood and Mental Health: A Bridge between Infant and Adult Psychiatry   Sam Tyano, Miri Keren, Helen Herrman and John Cox
© 2010 John Wiley & Sons, Ltd

with the erosion of traditional customs and dispersed extended families, today's carers evolve parenting patterns shaped by their own subjective beliefs, emotional experience and unconscious desires.

Qualitative/quantitative research of parenting 'orientations' yields several findings[1]:

- In transitional societies, cultural heterogeneity, rapid urbanization and social mobility grant mothers and fathers more latitude, rendering parenting orientations a mixture of collective and personal expectations.

- However, the complex choices involved, and loss of supportive networks increase perinatal stress and anxiety, especially during the first postnatal year when internal conflicts and discordance between nurturing, domestic and work roles are most acute.

- Although it is the child who creates parents of people, bonding patterns are evident and measurable while anticipating parenting. Unless modified, such representations are predictive of parenting 'climate' and praxis.

- The nature of parenting practice is predictable antenatally from representations of self and baby. Infants born into different orientations come to differ significantly in attachment security, feeding and sleep patterns. Maternal orientation at 6 months discriminates among Secure and Insecure infants (predictive of the Strange Situation at one year).

- Mothers differ in responses to risk factors, timing of heightened anxiety and associated protective factors. Precipitants of disturbance vary according to orientation, largely attributable to discrepancies between subjective expectations and postnatal experience.

- Empirical evidence supports details of orientation theory. Replication in large community samples shows that different approaches to mothering cluster, validating clinical findings of underpinning beliefs. Multifarious pathways to work–family satisfaction and perinatal disorders indicate the benefits of subgroup identification.

- Large-scale research confirms psychoanalytic understanding that at times of transition (e.g. childbearing), unresolved/unprocessed issues are reactivated. Parental cognitive experience is accompanied by fantasies and revitalized memories which contribute to incongruous feelings being transferred into the new situation, potentially leading to distorted reactions to parenting and displaced responses to the baby.

---

[1] Parental orientations were initially formulated by the author on the basis of detailed thrice-weekly observations and longitudinal studies of mothers and fathers within a London community play-centre of 200 families, over an 8-year period, mapping parenting changes in successive cohorts beginning in 1977. This was augmented by focus-group discussions and pre-and postnatal in-depth interviews with purposively selected informants, at 18-month intervals. The findings from my small-scale qualitative studies engendered questionnaires which were subsequently applied by independent researchers in large-scale longitudinal-prospective projects additionally using measures with well-established reliability and validity, conducted with representative samples in various countries, including Israel, Belgium, Australia, Hong Kong, etc. [13, 4, 7, 17]. Understanding the subjective experience of moment-to-moment parenting activities and difficulties is enriched by psychoanalytically informed clinical work with individuals, couples, families and groups within a practice dedicated to issues of reproduction and early parenting over the past 35 years. Finally, to expand from the Eurocentric start-point, the author also conducts consultations, work discussion groups and supervision for midwives, mental health professionals and social service practitioners working with pregnant women, and/or teenage and older parents on six continents; and open-ended exploratory workshops (conducted through interpreters) with parents themselves in many countries, including the Azores, Argentina, Australia, Austria, Belgium, Canada, Chile, China, Crete, Czech Republic, Denmark, Egypt, England, Ethiopia, Finland, France, Greece, Guatemala, Holland, Hong Kong, India, Ireland, Israel, Italy, Japan, Latvia, New Zealand, Norway, Peru, Portugal, Romania, Russia, Scotland, South Africa, Spain, Sweden, Switzerland, Turkey, USA, West Indies, Venezuela.

- While consistent during a particular child's infancy, orientations often change in subsequent gestations, indicating these are neither traits nor personality types – and that parenting constitutes a life-long evolutionary process.

Germane to these findings two models are presented, depicting configurations of bonding with the imaginary baby during pregnancy, and emotional experience and beliefs which generates manifest parental behaviour postnatally.

1.2 Pregnancy and the 'placental paradigm'

Antenatal emotional experience primes postnatal interaction. Pregnancy is a blending of three intertwining systems: biological, psychological and social. The unconscious mind reflects these. An expectant mother's mental construction of the largely unknown fetus consists of her fantasies, wishes and projections, partaking of her imagined baby-self in the eyes of archaic carers, and her own particular mode of engagement with the procreative maternal body and its powers. If gestation is allowed to proceed, the baby growing within the pregnant woman is only viable as part of their symbiotic exchange. For approximately 280 days, floating in the amniotic sea, he or she swallows and excretes, depositing waste products for expulsion by the maternal system, and ingesting nutrients from the plasma filtrate of mother's diet and the hormonal transmissions of her emotional state.

Expectant mothers' subjective interpretations of this bidirectional connectedness are delineated as a *placental paradigm*, illustrating relational representations underpinning variations of antenatal bonding.

Table 1.1 indicates that many women experience flexible fantasies and healthy ambivalence during pregnancy. Ideas about the baby she harbours and herself as mother-to-be

Table 1.1 Placental paradigm

Maternal representations			
	Self-as-mother (archaic mother)	*Fantasy baby* (baby-self)	*Manifestation:*
Mixed representations			
1.	+/−	+/−	healthy ambivalence
Fixed representations:			
2.	+	+	idealization
3.	−	+	guilt/depression
4.	+	−	persecution
5.	−	−	anxiety
6.	+/−	+/−	obsession
7.	+/−	**0**	detachment

Note: Given myriad variations of individual and cross-cultural fantasies, an abstract notation is used – 'plus' signs to signify positive feelings and 'minus', negative ones.

Modified from J. Raphael-Leff, procreative process, placental paradigm and perinatal psychotherapy, *Journal of the American Psychoanalyic Association*, Female Psychology supplement, 1997, **44**, 373–99, which includes illustrative clinical examples.

vary in emotional timbre, richness and intensity, fluctuating during the course of an hour, let alone a day. This changeable process, allowing for playful 'practice'-bonding with the unborn baby, contrasts with 'fixed' representations. A woman's unwavering idea of her 'brilliant' pregnancy as perfect communion/fusion between munificent containing mother and 'special' baby is clearly romanticized. Unless she processes this idealized conviction before the birth, she is destined to be sorely disappointed in the ordinary baby she delivers and herself as merely a 'good-enough' mother. Similarly, a pregnant woman who feels insufficient or even full of toxic 'badness' may be consumed by guilt, seeing herself as incapable of nourishing her vulnerable baby. Minor symptoms, ultrasound deviations or complications seem to confirm her sense of failure. Postnatally, inevitable frustrations sadden her greatly, inducing guilt for betraying her desire to provide an idyllic infancy.

Conversely, another woman may experience herself as fine but for the parasite leaching her resources, an invader determined to maul her from within. When this sense of exploitation is overpowering, relief may be sought in an abortion. Persisting acrimonious representations augur badly for bonding with an infant who is envisaged as a demanding persecutor.

Suffering from low self-esteem, another troubled mother may feel that the critical baby inside knows her weaknesses and will expose her shortcomings once born. Nine months of incompatible connectedness can feel intolerable as apprehension erupts in severe panic attacks. Once again, abortion may seem to offer the only respite from chronic anxiety about damaging or being damaged by the baby inside her. If the pregnancy is sustained, this over-anxious conflicted mother feels compelled to constantly check on her baby, envisaged as dangerous and/or in mortal danger.

Pregnancy also weakens obsessional defences that aim to separate good from bad. Breakthrough intrusive thoughts of causing harm to the future baby include graphic visions of molesting or hurting the child, or herself. Fearing madness, these ideas from 'out of the blue' alarm perfectionists who consciously want to be excellent mothers, doing the best for their offspring.

While seeming far-fetched, such disturbances are extremely common. Confusion and tearfulness increase during the transition to parenthood. Domestic violence rises, boding badly for paternal bonding. Borderline tendencies to self-harm, risk-taking behaviours, dissociation and abusive enactments intensify. Numerous studies document poor antenatal clinic attendance, and adverse consequences of untreated depression, persecution, anxiety, post-traumatic stress disorder and childhood abuse, associated with self-neglect, unhealthy eating, smoking, alcohol or substance abuse affecting fetal growth, and resulting in low birth weight, preterm delivery and/or a hyper-reactive baby.

A final hazard is an expectant mother who behaves as if not pregnant, denying her condition or the importance of the changes to come. This portends badly for the future primary relationship, as emotional detachment leads to malattunement and neglect. Early maternal withdrawal is associated with hyper-vigilance in infants and borderline traits in older children.

Meanings she ascribes to their cord-linked interchange are coloured by circumstances of this conception, life events and her current view of maternity, affected by past experiences of being mothered, as well as her anticipation of future mothering.

Thus, no baby is immune to influences across the placental barrier. He or she already feeds on maternal aspirations and emotions, including her (seemingly universal) *primal anxieties* of formation, transformation and sustenance. One prospective study of 10,000 women found that true to folk beliefs, antenatal maternal anxiety indeed affects the offspring – through high cortisol levels, traceable biochemically and evident in behavioural problems even at age seven [1].

Antenatal disorders are commonly under-diagnosed. Strikingly, most treatment literature focuses on post-partum interventions despite prepartum antecedents of equal prevalence. Given the high rates of antenatal emotional disturbance, and great benefits of prophylactic treatment before the interactive process with the baby is affected, it is essential to identify troubled women during pregnancy. Perinatal staff are in a prime position to screen their clientele, and to refer pregnant women with bonding disorders.

Devised with this in mind, the placental paradigm can be easily taught to clinical practitioners (midwives, traditional birth attendants, nurses, obstetricians or paediatricians) as a simple evaluative chart requiring no knowledge of mental disorders but a capacity to listen in an empathic, non-judgemental way. Official guidelines (e.g. National Institute for Health and Clinical Excellence www.nice.org.uk, 45, 2007) advocate 'talking cures' over antidepressants or other medications while pregnant/breastfeeding. Contemporary psychoanalytic psychotherapists recognize pregnancy as a beneficial therapeutic period, aided by greater accessibility of unconscious material, rich fantasy, frequent and vivid dreams, introspective amenability to insight and high motivation to become a 'good' parent [2, 3].

1.3 The model of maternal orientations

This model, depicting parental beliefs and behaviours, interdigitates with the placental paradigm. The diverse orientations help clinicians understand women's subjective approaches to pregnancy, the baby, birth and motherhood, and how different challenges interact with each expectant mother's personal belief system, self-esteem and mental health.

The first of these orientations is that of the *Facilitator* who treats pregnancy as the culmination of her feminine experience. Throwing herself wholeheartedly into the process, she dons maternity clothes early, 'communes' with her baby, revelling in the special attention. She plans as natural a birth as possible, wishing to minimize the traumatic 'caesura' that will reunite her with her familiar baby (see Table 1.2).

This contrasts with the *Regulator* for whom pregnancy is an unavoidable means of getting a (unknown) baby. She resents being treated as an 'incubator', prey to comments by strangers. Childbirth is imagined as a dreaded, exhausting and painful event to be mitigated by medical intervention. Large studies find that Regulators have a higher rate of antenatal depression, anxiety symptoms and specific pregnancy-related fears. Their elevated incidence of elected Caesarean sections indicates preference for predictability and a way of bypassing the potentially humiliating experience of vaginal birth [4, 5, 6].

Facilitators, on the other hand, look forward excitedly to 'birthing'. Studies of expectations find that Facilitators anticipate more intrapartum feelings of fulfilment, marred by assisted delivery [7].

A third group is that of *Reciprocators* – expectant mothers (or fathers) able to tolerate uncertainty and mixed emotions, in themselves and the baby. They manage ambivalence as inevitable in all relationships, accepting occasional resentments as part of the complex experience of caring for a wordless, sleep-interrupting sentient infant, similar to them in having human emotions and needs, but different in being little, dependent and vulnerable.

Table 1.2   Facilitator and Regulator antenatal orientation[2]

Facilitator		Regulator
♀ uniquely privileged		♂ are privileged
Pregnancy enjoyable		'Necessary evil'
Dual identifications		Resists introspection
Natural birth	*labour/birth*	'Civilized' birth
Exciting		Humiliating
'mother'	*identity*	'Person'
Vocation	*mothering*	Skill
Mother and Baby	*primary unit*	Sexual couple

Other mothers are *Conflicted* – torn between an ideal of maternal perfection and rebellion against it. Preoccupied with painful feelings from childhood experiences and unresolved issues with her own mother, this woman feels trapped with a baby who seems not to recognize her. Confused and terrified of breached floodgates she experiences panic attacks. Her life becomes increasingly dominated by avoidant precautions to control intense anxiety, and envy of her baby's care. Meanwhile, the infant seen as needy but impossible to understand fails to thrive, often manifesting persistent crying, sleep or feeding problems, behavioural disruptions and disorganized attachment, both reflecting and contributing to interactive family symptomatology. Differences between these four groups are significant (p < .001) [6].

1.4 Mothering

Facilitators treat postnatal nurture as an extension of pregnancy – a 'fourth trimester' of sensually relishing the reunited baby. Enveloped in the maternal body, the infant rediscovers mother's voice, her wake/sleep rhythms, cadences of breathing and kinetic patterns of stillness and movement. Some experiences are new: the feel and fit of mother's fleshy contours, the taste of breast milk and odours of her breath, armpit, vaginal excretions, her bodily warmth, unmuffled immediacy and differing smooth silkiness/rough edges of her caress . . .

Feeling mothering is her vocation, the Facilitator mother adapts herself to her baby, convinced that only she, the biological mother primed by pregnancy, can fathom her infant's needs. Hence as exclusive carer, she maintains close bodily contact, treating every gurgle as a communication that must be responded to (Table 1.3).

By contrast, the Regulator believes that mothering is a 'learned skill', acquirable by others. Since to her neonates do not discriminate between people, she introduces co-carers early on, establishing a *routine* which reduces unpredictability, provides continuity between nurturers, and differentiates between 'valid' crying and ignorable 'noise'.

---

[2] These tables contrast two of the four orientations. Regarding the others, *Reciprocators* tend to remain open-minded, exploring perinatal experiences and negotiating each episode as it arises rather than holding a preconceived stance. *Conflicted* mothers oscillate between Facilitator and Regulator approaches (and conflicted fathers between a desire to participate fully and defended renunciation).

Table 1.3   Facilitators and Regulators – mothering

Facilitator		Regulator
Mother adapts	*praxis*	Baby adapts
'Baby knows'	*conviction*	'Experts know'
Gratification	*aim*	Socialization
Exclusive	*care*	Shared
Intuitive		'Right way'
Mother's presence	*security*	Routine
Communication	*crying*	'Real' vs. noise
Permissive; frequent	*feeding*	By schedule
Late	*weaning*	Early
Parents' bed	*sleep*	Own room
'Gift'	*feces*	'Mess'

Hence, proximity is not an issue. The main goal is to 'socialize' the asocial, presocial or even antisocial infant and regulate his or her desires. To this end the baby must adapt to the household regime.[3]

Apart from differences of adaptation and feeding, night-waking is elevated in Facilitator babies, associated with maternal separation anxiety. Sleep patterns differ most significantly at 11 months, but at two years Facilitators' babies are still requiring help in the night, as opposed to Regulators, many of whose babies (reportedly) are conditioned to sleep through from 5 weeks. Infants of Conflicted mothers take significantly longer to fall asleep [25 vs. 11 minutes] but sleep later [8].

The specificity of stressful precipitants for each group also makes sense of the inconsistent 'fractionated' findings in the *family-work-stress* literature. To maintain their self-esteem, Regulators need to engage meaningfully with adults outside the home, whereas Facilitators dread separation from the baby. Wishing to provide full-time exclusive care, they return to work reluctantly of economic necessity or job stipulations. Conversely, Regulators resent economic dependence, and the slow 'mommy-track' which penalizes career advancement and salary growth.

Reciprocator couples tend to be dual-career partners. If they can afford loss of earnings they work flexible hours or part-time, alternating in looking after the baby (prevalent in Scandinavian societies, which provide 12–18 months of parental leave at full pay). Otherwise, Reciprocators work from home or employ a helper.

Naturally, low earners are less able to afford either part-time paid jobs or personalized high-quality childminders, having to resort to available day-care. British surveys of the postnatal period indicate that across all social classes, income groups and educational levels (including lone women) 25% of mothers engage in full-time work, 25% stay at home and 50% work part-time [9].

---

[3] Professionals working with new mothers are of interest here because of their own concordance with the orientation model. For instance, a study of breastfeeding attitudes of health care professionals, found that some practitioners had a positive breastfeeding interest and a trust in the mother-child unit to manage breastfeeding as opposed to practitioners who regulate the mothers, instructing them how to organize their breastfeeding on a routine basis, instead of being sensitive to the child's needs [18].

The current recession is reshaping the financial roles of millions of mothers worldwide, who are becoming sole breadwinners, returning to work or taking on second jobs to compensate for partners' loss of earnings due to predominantly male employment cuts.

1.5 Postnatal disturbances

All primary carers of whatever sex and age find parenting difficult, especially in nuclear families. Being responsible at all times, attentive and attuned to the needs of someone else, is a daunting task. In addition to broken nights, dream-deprivation and exhaustion, birth mothers also contend with hormonal fluctuations and recovery from labour/birth. Breastfeeding mothers experience painful engorgement, frightening orgasmic contractions, cracked nipples or mastitis and sole accountability for the baby's growth. Teenage mothers experience conflicts between parenting demands and adolescent needs.

Not surprisingly, almost half of Westernized new mothers are distressed at some point over the first two postnatal years; 13–20% suffer clinical depression and 20–40% of disturbed mothers report compulsive thoughts or images of harming the child [10]. These preoccupations often remain secret, hidden and untreated. Although most are not acted upon, in severe disturbance, when delusional reasoning includes the baby, there is a serious risk of child abuse or infanticide.

Each mother or father is affected in his or her own way by the highly arousing emotional experience of nurturing a baby. Where new parents are concerned, my research has shown that a Facilitator mother experiences 'primary maternal preoccupation' (in Winnicott's phrase) before and during the months following childbirth. Her identity becomes primarily that of a mother. Holding a distinct mothering philosophy, she strives towards her maternal ideal of devotion, suspending her subjectivity by adapting to the baby, intuitively facilitating, holding and dedicating herself in unconscious identification with both maternal ideal and vicariously gratified baby-self. However, to sustain this orientation any negative feelings must be suppressed. These revert towards herself. Facilitating mothers feel devastated if unable to breastfeed. Desperation over minor lapses of maternal perfection induces irreparable guilt, remorse and anxious over-involvement. Self-reproach for 'ruining' the ideal may escalate to depression, hopelessness and, in extreme cases, even suicide.

Many other women have a different experience I term 'primary maternal persecution'. In-depth exploration of their subjective experience boils down to feeling trapped. If the sense of exploitation (Table 1.1: 4, 5, 7) persists, feeling undermined, and at the mercy of a potentially greedy/spiteful infant, hostility must be managed. Most Regulator mothers do this efficiently. More breastfeed today than in the past – health-education stresses both infantile immunity and maternal benefits of rapid return to pre-pregnancy shapeliness, with reduced risks of diabetes, heart disease, ovarian cancer and stroke.[4] Intake is regulated

---

[4] Breastfeeding rates, style and duration vary according to orientation. However these also reflect societal policies and local expectations: in Ethiopia (one of the poorest countries in the world) and Norway (one of the richest), breastfeeding approaches 100%, continuing for two-three years and one year respectively, whereas in Britain only 35% of babies are exclusively breastfed at one week! An Israeli study is currently testing the hypothesis that Facilitators show stronger *intrinsic* and Regulators *extrinsic* motivation to breastfeed, on the assumption that maternal orientation moderates the relationship between two developmental axes and this motivation. Facilitators' higher levels of need/lower anxiety regarding attachment vs Regulators' higher need/lower anxiety regarding individuation. Reciprocator mothers are deemed to have a higher need for both attachment and individuation and less anxiety than the Conflicted group, where two competing orientations of 'Facilitator' and 'Regulator' vie (Peleg).

by schedule, and feeding bottles are introduced early to ensure shared care. This allows the mother to replenish herself by spending time in an enriching social world, protecting her from risks of ruptured defences and/or surrendering to 'sentimentality'. However, if adult fulfilment is thwarted by obstacles, due to unemployment or her own inner conflicts, resentment accumulates. Unmitigated mothering of an infant saps her internal resources, threatening her self-discipline. Desperate to get away, she resorts to controlling the baby's sleep-patterns and abhorrent behaviors, but resents being perceived as coercive. Unconsciously the baby represents split-off dependent, ferocious and/or deprived aspects of herself. Persecuted by constant exposure to her repudiated weaknesses, internal pressure mounts to externalize old scenarios. If defensive detachment fails, punitiveness intensifies towards the baby, seen as cause of her problems,[5] (Table 1.4).

Table 1.4 Facilitators and Regulators – beliefs and fantasies

Facilitator		Regulator
Sociable/vulnerable	*newborn*	Pre/asocial. Tyrannical
Innate personality		Becomes person later
Recognizes mother		Undiscriminating
Communicative		Voracious
	Unconscious configuration	
Mother's ideal self	*baby*	Split off weakness
'Fusion'	*ideal*	Autonomy
Glorified	*internal mother*	Denigrated
	Emotional experience	
Primary maternal preoccupation		*Primary maternal persecution*
Insufficiency	*threats*	Competition
Idealization	*defences*	Control
Vicarious gratification		Dissociation/detachment
Fear of hating	*anxiety*	*Fear of loving*

Importantly, these different orientations towards mothering are already measurable during pregnancy and hence cannot be attributed to the baby's personality. The innovation is to treat postnatal distress not as a unified occurrence, but precipitated differentially in these groups by intrapsychic, socio-economic or cultural factors that conspire to prevent each woman from fulfilling her own maternal expectations. With greater involvement in childcare, about 25% of Western fathers also suffer postnatal distress, increasing to 40% if their partners are mentally ill (possibly due to assortative mating).

---

[5] Such responses are not rare. In various surveys, parents who admit to having smacked their baby, blame the child for doing something dangerous or 'naughty' or justify it as themselves 'letting off steam'. Recent research by the UK Office for National Statistics found that 88% of British people still think parents should have the right to physically discipline their young children despite massive anti-smacking campaigns, and a global initiative to prohibit it. The link between corporal punishment and fatal child abuse is evident in extinction of the latter in Sweden since the ban on physical chastisement was introduced in 1979. However, Sweden also has psychologists in every perinatal clinic and offers all parents 18 months of full economic and social support.

Disturbed parents are unresponsive, less attuned, inconsistent, ineffectual, and/or intrusive, rejecting or hostile, leading to cognitive and developmental deficits in the child, with threefold risk of developing emotional disorders. Chronic marital or socio-economic difficulties also affect parent–infant interaction. Babies of depressed mothers develop hypersensitive stress responses, with greater likelihood of depression in adulthood. Sons of postnatally depressed fathers are prone to conduct disorders, and children of angry parent/s have difficulties controlling their anger, self-soothing and/or understanding emotional states in themselves and others. In many places, therapeutic interventions are not readily accessible but supportive care from self-help groups or non-professionals may improve the quality of the primary relationship.[6]

Retriggering of the past is but one variable of parental perinatal distress. In addition, there are many psychosocial precipitants, of which an important factor is inability to live up to one's own ideal. Independent research confirms my early findings [6, 11, 12] that in each orientation, psychological strain, including perinatal depression, is related to *a discrepancy between personal expectations and fulfilling one's optimal form of mothering*. Statistical evidence reveals that Facilitators are tormented by disappointing birth-interventions. Regulators have increased independent risk during the first six weeks, suffering from a sense of reduced adult competence – confidence loss and self-reported inadequacy and dejection. Reciprocators are resilient. Even those who were distressed antenatally are statistically less likely to develop postnatal depression [6].

Acceptance of sad and angry feelings alongside joyous ones, and flexible reciprocity in meeting emotional needs of *both* parent and infant seems protective, unlike imbalanced emphasis on either baby or carer.

A Facilitator who fails to achieve her mothering ideal tends towards depression. Suffering agonies of self-blame and anxiety, she castigates herself for letting down the vulnerable baby as centre of the world. By contrast, a Regulator mother anticipates mothering 'rationally'. Horrified by her heightened emotions, she dreads becoming 'soppy', or scary. When persecutory feelings escalate, projective experiences of paranoia engender a need to escape or to impose further control. Contending with incompatible tendencies to extreme facilitation and simultaneous regulation, Conflicted mothers feel confusedly martyred or hostile, paralysed by phobias or helplessness (needing the infant's help), or become rejecting, punitive and/or intrusively autocratic.

Notably, *the orientation model is circular* rather than linear: half the circle – namely babies of Reciprocators and those of moderate Facilitators and Regulators – are found to be securely attached. The other half are insecure. Extreme Facilitator mothers tend to be enmeshed (babies ambivalent), extreme Regulator mothers dismissive (babies avoidant), while Conflictual orientations are preoccupied/inconsistent (babies disorganized) [13].

---

[6] In industrialized nations up to 20% of all mothers suffer from postnatal mental disorders, a figure that rises with poverty, discrimination and adversity. However, scarcity of professional resources means that in low and middle-income countries a high treatment gap exists between disorder and availability of therapeutic interventions, which may also be unevenly distributed and/or inefficient. The World Health Organization advocates a public health policy with 'task shifting' from specialists to training primary health-care workers to recognize distress and deliver cost-effective support and accessible care www.who.int/whr/2001/en. For an example of a randomized control trial of a home-based intervention to improve the quality of mother–infant relationship and attachment in a socio-economically deprived community in South Africa through lay community workers, see the *British Medical Journal* online www.bmj.com/cgi/content/full/338/apr14_2/b974.

1.6 Contagious arousal

Unremitting intimate contact with a newborn triggers formidable emotional forces. One of the first feminists to candidly disclose the arousal of long-buried feelings and her confused sense of maternal 'power and powerlessness' wrote in 1960: 'My children cause me the most exquisite ... suffering of ambivalence: the murderous alternation between bitter resentment and raw-edged nerves, and blissful gratification and tenderness' [14, p. 21].

The intensity of primary experience resides partly in evocations of the past: bittersweet dual identifications with the baby's neediness, as with one's own mother's protectiveness. A new parent's open receptivity to the infant's 'primitive' communications evokes his or her own implicit processes. Breaking down defences, the infant's helplessness unleashes unresolved 'power/powerlessness' conflicts in the carer, revitalized through *contagious arousal* (as I termed it). Archaic experience is also stirred up through sensual dealings with *primary substances:* the evocative smells and feel of amniotic fluid, lochia, colostrum, breast milk, as well as baby-poo, pee, vomit, navel and other excretions, all unique to infancy. I propose that these retrigger somatic sensations and subsymbolic preverbal memories from the adult's own infancy.

The focus and timing of a mother's or father's arousal reflect the weakest links of his or her infancy/early childhood (as the Conflicted group demonstrate vividly). Conversely, each orientation excels at different developmental phases – Facilitators' exquisite neonatal attunement; Regulators' encouragement of mobility; Reciprocators' negotiation of toddlers' choices ...

I suggest that perinatal distress is exacerbated by little previous contact with babies and lack of preparation for their emotional impact. Laying oneself open to comprehending preverbal emotions reactivates unprocessed feelings. Surprised by the fierce intensity of their elicited response, many mothers and fathers are deeply shocked by involuntary thoughts about neglecting, harming or even molesting the omnipresent infant.

In the West, the baby handed to parent/s to take home from hospital (with total responsibility for his or her welfare), is usually the first newborn they have ever seen. Furthermore, extended families are scattered. Unfriendly communities tender insufficient emotional and practical support, unrealistically increasing spousal-reliance. Most importantly, in many countries today people live in stratified societies which separate age-groups. Growing up within small isolated nuclear family units offers few opportunities to actively work through loss, grievances and early traumatic experience in the presence of a baby-sibling, -cousin or -neighbour, before caring for one's own infant. Facilitation and regulation (compensation/control) are defensive procedures to reduce the overwhelming aspects of contagious arousal.

In sum: the two-way systemic process of pregnancy continues postnatally. Parents are profoundly affected by emotional interchanges with their offspring, and conversely, a child's internal world is constituted intersubjectively with primary carers. Neuropsychological research reveals that the baby's brain itself is formed interactively, reflecting the degree of stimulation or deprivation, cultivation or pruning of neonatal synaptical connections. Using frame-by-frame microanalysis of filmed interactions, neonatal researchers (Beebe, Lyons-Ruth, Sander, Stern, Trevarthen, Tronick) demonstrate complex bi-directional patterns of mutual regulation and reciprocal influence between carers and infants.

Most importantly, the myth of perfect synchrony is dispelled. In ordinary dialogues between mothers and their babies, around half the communications are mismatched. However, the crucial element for infant mental health is not unadulterated harmony, but a reciprocal *meeting of minds*, and the capacity of both parent and infant to heal impingements and repair miscommunications collaboratively.

The ability to tolerate ambiguity and ambivalence without resorting to foreclosure, guilt or retaliation is something Reciprocators are good at. Aware of the baby's human *sameness* as well as *otherness* (being little, dependent and immature), their primary stance is one of empathy, curiosity and compassion (rather than identification or dis-identification). Although delineated many years before 'mentalization theory' was formulated [15], Reciprocators may be described as utilizing parenthood to enhance their capacity for 'reflective functioning'. Seeing the baby as a separate individual endowed with personal characteristics and changing mental states (feelings, intentions, beliefs, desires) enriches Reciprocators' interactive awareness and self-understanding.

1.7 Paternal orientations

Whereas male Reciprocators share care, striving to evolve a (preoedipal) relationship with the sentient baby, Participator fathers desire total involvement in the pregnancy and sole care of the infant. By contrast, alarmed by the emotional arousal intimate contact entails, Renouncer fathers wish to suspend their paternal role until the infant develops language. Conflicted fathers want both [16]. Clearly, in two-parent families, the interactive combinations of partners is crucial (Table 1.5).

Table 1.5 Parental permutations and precipitants of postnatal distress

Facilitator + Renouncer	**Regulator + Renouncer**
'Conventional' pattern	Dual-career pattern
Primary unit: mother+baby	Primary unit: sexual partners
Non-supportive partner→PND	Conservative partner→PND
Facilitator + Participator	**Regulator + Participator**
Division of care	Shared care
Competitive partner→PND	Role reversal

Note: PND = postnatal depression.

Stable partnerships mitigate psychogenic conflicts. However, Facilitators become distressed by competition over exclusive baby-care or spousal failure to safeguard on-demand breastfeeding against interruptions (by other children, economic needs or household chores). Conversely, Regulators abhor conservative non-egalitarian partners who insist they remain at home. In cultures of male machismo, 'liberated' women may be stigmatized, or subject to partner violence.

Finally, while consistent during the early years of a child's life, orientations often change with subsequent pregnancies, usually due to parental processing of affect. Influential *psychological* variables are the motive for this conception and degree of emotional support (even one confidante is protective). On a *socio-economic* level, issues include the mother's age, career/employment status, partner, number of children and age-gaps between them, social/economic pressures, cultural expectations and life events. *Physiological* complications of pregnancy, childbirth or baby, hormonal swings and sleep-deprivation all influence future decisions. However, the most important factor in determining a change of orientation is the *emotional experience* of parenting the previous child.

1.8 Conclusion

In Westernized countries, over the decades since the 1960s counter-culture, 'the pill', equal education and higher career expectations, many feminist mothers struggle desperately with *clashes between their own dramatically changed personal aspirations and those of the baby, unchanged since hunter–gatherer times.* This incongruity can lead to high discordance of needs between carer and infant, especially among professional women who wish to be 'good' mothers while pursuing career interests.

Most theoretical expositions depict mothers from the perspective of the child. However, qualitative studies focusing on maternal experience provide greater awareness of flesh-and-blood subjects with their own feelings and independent locus of agency, needs and desire. Nonetheless, painful issues of maternal resentment and anxiety remain under-theorized. In a cultural climate that promotes parenting as blissful, carers as well as mental health professionals are reluctant to acknowledge the depth of parental ambivalence. Accepting that responsiveness to an infant's affective communications inevitably evokes mixed feelings enables these to be voiced and processed rather than either inhibited (by Facilitators), split (by Regulators) or acted upon (by Conflicted parents).

Increased recognition of heterogeneous orientations and awareness of bi-directional psychodynamics engenders greater tolerance for the range of ways parents choose to relate. The emphasis is no longer on a 'correct' form, pathologizing deviations from conventional parenting, but rather helping each parent to develop flexibility and authentic enjoyment within the chosen mode of interaction he or she and this specific infant are comfortable with.

Given Western fragmentation of family and community networks, professionals now fill the gaps – offering developmental guidance and emotional support to both parent and child. And should the need arise, making timely referrals for rewarding perinatal or parent–infant psychotherapy.

1.9 References

1. O'Connor, T.G. *et al.* (2005) Perinatal anxiety predicts individual differences in cortisol in pre-adolescent children. *Biological Psychiatry*, **58**, 211–17.
2. Raphael-Leff, J. (1993) *Pregnancy – the Inside Story*. Karnac, London. 2nd edition, 2000.
3. Raphael-Leff, J. (2001) Climbing the walls: therapeutic intervention for post-partum disturbance, in *Spilt Milk: Perinatal Loss and Breakdown* (ed. J. Raphael-Leff), Routledge, London, pp. 60–81.
4. Raphael-Leff, J. (1985a) Facilitators and Regulators, Participators and Renouncers: mothers' and fathers' orientations towards pregnancy and parenthood. Journal of Psychosomatic Obstetrics and Gynaecology, **4**, 169–84.

5. Raphael-Leff, J. (1991) *Psychological Processes of Childbearing*, Anna Freud Centre, London. 4th edition, 2009.
6. Sharp, H. and Bramwell, R. (2004) An empirical evaluation of a psychoanalytic theory of mothering orientations: implications for the antenatal prediction of postnatal depression. *Journal of Reproductive and Infant Psychology*, **22**, 71–89.
7. Van Bussel, J.C.H., Spitz, B. and Demyttenaere, K. (2009) Depressive symptomatology in pregnant and postpartum women: an exploratory study of the role of maternal antenatal orientations. *Archives of Women's Mental Health*, **12**, 155–66.
8. Scher, A. and Blumberg, O. (2000) Night waking among 1-year olds: a study of maternal separation anxiety. *Child Care Health Development*, **26**, 323–34.
9. Hakim, C. *et al.* (2008) *Little Brittons: Financing Childcare Choice*, Policy Exchange, London.
10. Fairbrother, N. and Woody, S.R. (2008) New mothers' thoughts of harm related to the newborn. *Archives of Women's Mental Health*, **11**, 221–29.
11. Raphael-Leff, J. (1985b) Facilitators and Regulators: vulnerability to postnatal disturbance. *Journal of Psychosomatic Obstetrics and Gynaecology*, **4**, 151–68.
12. Raphael-Leff, J. (1986) Facilitators and Regulators: conscious and unconscious processes in pregnancy and early motherhood. *British Journal of Medical Psychology*, **59**, 43–55.
13. Scher, A. (2001) Facilitators and Regulators: maternal orientation as an antecedent of attachment security. *Journal of Reproductive and Infant Psychology*, **19**, 325–33.
14. Rich, A. (1976) *Of Woman Born – Motherhood as Experience and Institution*, Virago, London.
15. Fonagy, P. *et al.* (2002) *Affect Regulation, Mentalization, and the Development of the Self*, Other Press, New York.
16. Raphael-Leff, J. (2008) Participators, Reciprocators and Renouncers: paternal orientations in the 21st century. *Psycho-Analytic Psychotherapy in South Africa*, **16**, 61–85.
17. Van Bussel, J.C.H., Spitz, B. and Demyttenaere, K. (2008) Anxiety in pregnant and post-partum women: an exploratory study of the role of maternal orientations. Journal of Affective Disorders, **114**, 232–42.
18. Ekstrom, A., Matthiesen, A.S., Widstrom, A.M. and Nissen, E. (2005) Breastfeeding atti-tudes among counselling health professionals: development of an instrument to describe breastfeeding attitudes. *Scandinavian Journal of Public Health*, **33**, 353–58.

2
The competent fetus

Sam Tyano and Miri Keren

Tel-Aviv University, Sackler School of Medicine, Israel

Come into being
They met,
They desired me,
They united,
They secreted,
And I was created . . .
Who am I? What am I?
Do I feel? What?

2.1 Introduction

The domain of embryology studies deals with how and when human organs develop, from conception to birth. The field of fetal neurobehavioral development focuses on indicators of fetal behavior, and on the impact of external stimuli/events on the fetus. As stated in the Fels study of fetal behavior [1]: 'We must regard our interest in the problem of normal fetal behavior as a direct outgrowth of the widespread tendency within the past few years, to approach more closely the beginnings of human life in the hope of obtaining a picture of behavior as it emerges' [1, p. 1]. They were the first to view the fetal heart rate as a behavioral indicator. Already in 1935, they showed the movements of the human fetus in response to sound stimuli. In 1975, the chronological evolution of the maturation of the

Parenthood and Mental Health: A Bridge between Infant and Adult Psychiatry   Sam Tyano, Miri Keren, Helen Herrman and John Cox
© 2010 John Wiley & Sons, Ltd

various sensory systems during the gestational months was described [2], showing that the fetus has a neurophysiological apparatus, which, prior to any learning experience, readies it to perceive and to process sensory information, though in a diffuse and non-discriminative way. The notion of competencies of the fetus was then introduced.

Starting in the mid-1990s, descriptive studies of fetal neurobehavior, aimed at discovering the ontogeny of maturation prior to birth, have focused on five main indicators: fetal heart rate (FHR) and variability; behavioral state; qualitative motor patterns; activity level and the association between changes in FHR and fetal movement. Each of these is characteristic of the development of parasympathetic tone and modulation of sympathetic activation. With advancing gestation, fetuses display slower heart rate, increased heart variability, reduced but more vigorous motor behavior, coalescence of heart rate and movement patterns, emergence of distinct behavioral states, and increased cardiac responsiveness to stimulation. The gestational period between 28 and 32 weeks is a period of neurobehavioral transition [3].

2.2 Continuity from intrauterine life to infancy

Amazingly enough, long before science was able to study fetal neurobehavioral development, Freud [4] argued that intrauterine life and infancy are much more in continuity than the sharp break of delivery may make us think. The next study on fetal neurobehavioral development was published only close to 60 years later on the ontogeny of behavior neural regulation and demonstrated that there is *little neurobehavioral discontinuity* between the fetus and the neonate [5].

In the last 20 years, the increased survival rate of preterm infants and the reduction in the gestational age of viability have extensively increased our knowledge on the development of extrauterine functioning preterm babies [3, 6]. For instance, the link between high levels of motor activity *in utero* and difficult temperament after birth (unpredictability, poor adaptability, high level of activity) was demonstrated [6]. Higher fetal heart rate was associated with postnatal lower emotional tone, activity level and predictability. It is notable that contrary to previous studies [7, 8, 9], DiPietro and colleagues found no significant link between fetal heart rate *variability* and difficult temperament. Their explanation was that fetal heart rate variability is not a 'pure' characteristic of the fetus, because it is influenced by maternal factors, such as perceived stress or maternal age, in ways that other fetal measures are not. Taking into consideration the limitation of their study in that assessment of infant temperament was based strictly on maternal reports, the authors concluded that the various features of fetal neurobehavior provide the basis for individual differences in reactivity and regulation in infancy.

An additional set of data that show continuity from prenatal to postnatal life comes from gender studies. Several researches have brought substantial evidence for gender differences developing already *in utero*: preterm boys are at elevated risk for neonatal mortality and morbidity [10], male fetuses are more vulnerable to teratogenic risks and to hypoxia than females [11], or the finding that though boys weigh more at birth, a number of their systems tend to be less mature than the girls', including the respiratory and skeletal systems [12]. The finding of differences by gender in concentrations of an anti-inflammatory agent (Interleukin-1 receptor antagonist) in amniotic fluid indicates that it may be responsible for lower female perinatal risk [13]. These *in utero* gender differences in vulnerability may be of great significance when added to the findings of other gender difference studies in postnatal resilience. For instance, it has been shown that female patients show a better recovery rate from brain injuries than males [14].

Several studies have shown the significant impact of maternal emotions, especially stress and depression, on the fetus's level of activity and heart rate [6, 15, 16, 17]. Also, the impact of socio-economic status on all domains related to the fetus has been demonstrated [18]: fetuses of low socio-economic status mothers had lower heart variability and higher heart rate, moved less often and with less vigor, and exhibited less frequent synchronous periods of quiescence/activity. The authors concluded their article with the following remark: 'While the etiology of this socio-economic effect on the fetus observed in this study is not known, detection of associations between poverty and fetal maturation may have profound implications for child outcome' [18, p. 89] . The overall significance of these studies is that, already at the *in utero* stage, fetal development is influenced by a form of 'nurture' or parental influence that goes beyond the genetic, into the behavioral. In this sense one may argue that there is a continuum between prenatal and postnatal development.

2.3 The competent fetus and its receptive sensorial capacities

A paper entitled 'Story of the fetus, told by a neonate' [19], describing the evidence-based sensorial capacities of the fetus, implicitly has opened up the field of fetal psychology by 'putting words into the fetus's mouth'. Indeed, the use of the first-person pronoun, 'I', conveys the idea that a fetus is a subject with competencies:

Nine weeks old – I can burp and respond to loud noises.

Week 10 – I move my hands, Stretch, breathe in and out.

12 weeks – I can yawn, suck, swallow and taste the flavor of the liquid surrounding me.

At 24 weeks – I can feel the blood flow of my mother, hear the movement of her intestines and hear her voice which relaxes me.

My world – the womb – includes the placenta, umbilical cord, amniotic fluid and womb walls. The length of my umbilical cord is influenced by my movements . . . I already have an impact on my surroundings!

My placenta is very different from the one in the other wombs.

My mother's amniotic fluid is a world filled with chemical stimulations, smells, flavors and hormones. These characteristics influence me deeply. My amniotic liquid protects me from sudden movements that my mother makes, but whenever she or I move, I have many occasions to feel the walls of my womb with different parts of my body.

My mother's womb is never silent: I can hear a continuous background noise, I can hear my mother's blood pump, I can hear my mother's intestinal noises, I can hear high-frequency noises from the outside.

My mother's womb is dark. My heart reacts to light flashes. Seven and a half months after my parents have conceived me, I am physiologically ready to see, but I need the real world stimuli to start really seeing.

If my heart beat rate is slow while I hear voices or stories which are already known to me ... it is a sign that the familiar soothes me and leaves me with a feeling of confidence. Remember this because it is the same after I'm born.

If you introduce a drop of a bitter liquid into my amniotic fluid, I'll stop swallowing at once ... But if it is a sweet drop, I'll make twice the suction movements! When my mother does an amniocentesis test, I'll either approach or withdraw from the needle, even though my eyes are still closed at the time. I may even stop moving for two minutes, and slow down my heart rate [20].

2.4 Fetuses remember and therefore can learn . . .

Fetal memory has been studied *in utero* and after birth, through different techniques. An indirect proof of the existence of memory in the fetal brain *in utero* is habituation to vibro-acoustic stimulations, as measured by cardiac reactions [21], and it is present after about 32 weeks of gestation. The duration of fetal short-term memory is of at least 10 minutes while the duration of long-term memory is 24 hours. The period between 28 and 34 weeks is a transitional time for neurobehavioral development of the fetus [3, 22], and results from the linear increase of the parasympathetic influence on cardiac activity.

A special type of recurrent, naturalistic, auditory experience to which fetuses are exposed is their mother's voice. There is evidence that human newborns can discriminate between individual female voices and show strong preference for their mother's voice. Better yet, they even prefer to be told a story that was told to them during pregnancy [23]. In this study, preference was detected by the newborn's suction movements. It may be of interest to note, however, that human newborns do not show any preference for their father's voice over that of other males. A possible explanation of this finding is that the nature of the auditory stimulus is of different nature between the two parents, with the mother's voice acting as an 'inside-to-inside' stimulus, while the father's voice acting as an 'outside-to-inside' stimulus. Full-term fetuses can distinguish between mother's and a stranger's voice [21] and between musical tones [24]. In a follow-up study [25] that looked at the development of fetal perception of a music stimulus over gestational age, a pattern of maturation of music perception over the last trimester of pregnancy was demonstrated, using both movement and heart measures. Body movement responses were not observed until 35 weeks of gestational age, while heart rate response was seen already at 28 weeks of gestational age.

Finally, it was found that the preterm fetus (28–34 weeks of gestation) responds to a recording of an unfamiliar voice reciting a rhyme that had been recited by the mother twice-a day during the 28–34-week gestational period, in the same manner as the full-term fetus and the newborn infant [26]. Their findings support the thought that prenatal exposure to maternal speech is probably related to language acquisition, facilitated by the fetus's ability to remember and therefore to learn [27].

2.5 Fetuses can feel pain

The feeling of pain starts as an electric signal which runs through the spinal cord and from there to the thalamus where it finally reaches the cortex. The whole system is fully developed around the twenty-sixth week of pregnancy. EEG charts from weeks 30 to 35 reflect cortical activity that may be connected to the fetus's experiences [19].

2.6 Fetal psychology: an emerging domain

The cumulative data taken from the sensorial apparatus, as described above, show the importance of the receptive capacities that the fetus already possesses. Furthermore, the data-based evidence for the existence of some form of fetal memory, combined with the data about the impact of maternal stress, depression and anxiety on the fetus, raise a major issue for developmental psychopathologists and psychoanalysts, about the organization of a prenatal psychic core.

Lilley in 1972 [28] was the first to introduce the idea of the 'personality' of the fetus, describing him as an 'active passenger', who avoids pressing on the sharp regions of the womb, who can react violently to the needle of an amniocentesis, is sensitive to touch, showing preference for some tastes, and even capable of crying in the womb. Individual differences are expressed mainly by changes in body movements. Motion and emotion are tightly linked. For instance, Piontelli (1992) reported on a follow-up study of the movements of 11 fetuses, as observed in repeat ultrasound assessments throughout the pregnancy and the correlation that was found with their developmental and emotional course up to the age of four years. Numerous papers on fetus competencies [30, 31, 32] reflect the development of what has been named fetal psychology. It has been claimed that thumb-sucking is a pleasant pastime that can be observed from about nine weeks of gestational age [31]. Feelings may also be deduced from observations of thumb-sucking in conjunction with penile erections as early as 16 weeks of gestational age Furthermore, fetal emotions of fear, anger and hurt can be inferred from the infant's crying. The earliest audible cries and sounds from the fetal larynx have been recorded by ultrasound at 18 weeks of gestational age [33]. As Chamberlain writes [31, p. 109]: 'Emotions can be present without sound, but when the sound does come out, it is surely proof of an emotion within.' Increased fetal movement activity seems also to be an indirect indicator of emotions: fetuses of 28 panic-stricken mothers, during an earthquake, showed extreme hyperkinesia for two to eight hours [20]. Another notable result was found in a study that showed that fetuses become more agitated when their mothers' anxiety levels are heightened while waiting for routine ultrasound, as opposed to when mothers are waiting for amniocentesis [34].

Links between interpersonal difficulties along the course of life, and negative events *in utero*, such as rape, violent intercourse, rejection by father, death of a twin, drug-addicted mother or loss of a loved one, have been shown in a study [35].

Even more intriguing evidence for an unconscious struggle between the pregnant mother and her fetus, over the nutrients she provides, was recently described [36]. This theory has been gaining support in recent years, as scientists study the various ways pregnancy can go wrong. Meanwhile a fetus-produced protein has been identified in pre-eclampsia states. More specifically, the author argues that pre-eclampsia, that occurs in about 6% of pregnancies, is an extreme form of a 'strategy' used by all fetuses, by which fetuses raise the maternal blood pressure in order to drive more blood (more nutrients) into the low-pressure placenta. The maternal protective strategy then would be to shut down some of the genes in their own children.

2.7 Conclusion: the fetus can no longer be thought as a 'witless tadpole'

As we have seen in the information brought above, the human fetus possesses numerous competencies, some already fully developed well before birth. In addition, the fetus's pre-and postnatal development is significantly impacted by external as well as internal stimuli. The idea of parents communicating with their unborn baby (via talk, touch, etc.), the assumption of the existence of a psyche, and the enhancement of prenatal learning has become widespread. Guidelines for communicating with the mind of a fetus, have been suggested [31]:

> Gently put aside the traditional theories of learning and memory that impose severe restrictions on all human memory and automatically disqualify prenatal memory and learning. [31, p. 98]

> Scientific skepticism has long surrounded the senses of the baby in the womb. [31, p. 99]

> In addition to all their sensory radar, the womb babies you want to communicate with, have an emotional life which science always denied them. [31, p. 101]

> Life-threatening experiences seem to have high voltage imprints that tend to endure over time. [31, p. 102]

> Remember, babies are the ones with power to end the pregnancy and initiate labor. [31, p. 103]

> Babies that are anxious about being born, may often resist making the final turn from breech that will allow labor to proceed in a normal and comfortable way [31, p. 104]

Chamberlain concludes with:

> A baby who knows what is happening in the womb may be sending a stream of pertinent warnings, reassurances, or even directions to the mother and birth professionals, but what if no one is listening? [31, p. 105]

More evidence is needed to find out how these early sensorial competencies become integrated in the infant's experiences after birth. We need to be cautious to avoid imbuing the fetus's perceptions with affective adult significance on one hand, while also not underestimating its capacities on the other hand.

2.8 References

1. Sontag, L.W. and Richards, T.W. (1938) Studies in fetal behavior : I. Fetal heart rate as a behavioral indicator. *Monographs of the Society for Research in Child Development*, **3** (4), Serial No. 17.
2. Mistretta, C.M. and Bradley, R.M. (1975) Taste and swallowing in utero. *British Medical Bulletin*, **31**, 80–84.

3. DiPietro, J.A., Hodgson, D.M. and Johnson, T.R. (1996b) Fetal neurobehavioral development. *Child Development*, **67**, 2553–67.

4. Freud, S. (1926) Inhibitions, Symptoms and Anxiety. SE.20, 138.

5. Prechtl, H.F. (1984) Continuity and change in early neural development, in *Continuity of Neural Functions from Prenatal to Postnatal Life*, Clinics in Developmental Medicine **94** (ed. H.F. Prechtl), Lippincott, Philadelphia, pp. 1–15.

6. DiPietro, J.A., Hodgson, D.M. and Costigan, K.A. (1996a) Fetal antecedents of infant temperament. *Child Development*, **67**, 2568–83.

7. DeGangi, G.A., DiPietro, J.A., Greenspan, S.I. *et al.* (1991) Psychophysiological characteristics of the regulatory disordered infant. *Infant Behavior and Development*, **14**, 37–50.

8. Fox, N.A. (1989) Psychophysiological correlates of emotional reactivity during the first year of life. *Developmental Psychology*, **25**, 364–72.

9. Porges, S.W., Doussard-Roosevelt, J. and Maiti, J. (1994) Vagal tone and the physiological regulation of emotion. *Monographs of the Society for Research in Child Development*, **59**, 167–88.

10. McGregor, J., Leff, M., Orleans, M. and Baron, A. (1992) Fetal gender differences in preterm birth: findings in a North American cohort. *American Journal of Perinatology*, **9**, 43–48.

11. Spinillo, A., Capuzzo, E., Nicola, S. *et al.* (1994) Interaction between fetal gender and risk factors for fetal growth retardation. *American Journal of Obstetrics and Gynecology*, **171**, 1273–77.

12. Khoury, M., Marks, J., McCarty, B. *et al.* (1985) Factors affecting the sex differential in neonatal mortality: the role of respiratory distress syndrome. *American Journal of Obstetrics and Gynecology*, **151**, 777–82.

13. Romero, R., Gomez, R. and Cotton, D. (1994) The natural pnterleukin-1 receptor antagonist in the fetal maternal, and amniotic fluid compartments: the effect of gestational age, fetal gender, and intrauterine infection. *American Journal of Obstetrics and Gynecology*, **171**, 912–21.

14. Groswasser, Z., Cohen, M. and Keren, O. (1998) Female TBI patients recover better then males. *Brain Injury*, **12**, 805–8.

15. Van der Bergh, B.R.H., Mulder, E.J.R. and Prechtl, H.F.R. (1989a) The effect of (induced) maternal emotions on fetal behavior: a controlled study. *Early Human Development*, **19**, 9–19.

16. Weinstock, M. (1997) Does prenatal stress impair coping and regulation of hypothalamic-pituitary-adrenal axis? *Neuroscience and Behavioral Reviews*, **21**, 1–10.

17. Dieter, J.N.I., Field, T., Hernandez-Reif, M. *et al.* (2001) Maternal depression and increased fetal activity. *Journal of Obstetrics and Gynecology*, **21**, 468–73.

18. Pressman, E. and DiPietro, J.A. (1998) Fetal neurobehavioral development: associations with socioeconomic class and fetal sex. *Developmental Psychobiology*, **33**, 79–91.

19. DeCasper, A.J. (1990) Histoire de fetus par un nouveau-ne. *Progres en neonatologie*, **10**, 168–73.

20. Ianniruberto, A. and Tajani, E. (1981) Ultrasonographic study of fetal movements. *Seminars in Perinatology*, **5**, 175–81.

21. Kisilevski, B.S., Hains, S.M.J., Lee, K. *et al.* (2003) Effects of experience on fetal voice recognition. *Psychological Science*, **14**, 220–24.

22. Groome, L., Loizou, P. and Hoff, C. (1999) High vagal tone is associated with more efficient regulation of homeostasis in low-risk human fetuses. *Developmental Psychology*, **35**, 24–34.

23. DeCasper, A.J. and Prescott, P.A. (1984) Human newborns' perception of male voices: preference, discrimination, and reinforcing value. *Developmental Psychobiology*, **17**, 481–91.

24. Lecanuet, J.P., Granier-Deferre, C., Jacquet, A.Y. *et al.* (2000) Fetal discrimination of low-pitched musical notes. *Developmental Psychobiology*, **36**, 29–39.

25. Kisilevski, B.S., Hains, S.M.J., Jacquet, A.Y. *et al.* (2004) Maturation of fetal responses to music. *Developmental Science*, **7**, 550–59.

26. Krueger, C., Holdich-Davis, D. Quint, S. *et al.* (2004) Recurring auditory experience in the 28 to 34 week-old fetus. *Infant Behavior Development*, **27**, 537–43.

27. Busnell, M.C., Granier-Deferre, C. and Lecanuet, J.P. (1992) Fetal audition. *Annals of the New York Academy of Sciences*, **662**, 118–34.

28. Lilley, A.W. (1972) The foetus as a personality. *Australia and New Zealand Journal of Psychiatry*, **6**, 99–105.

29. Piontelli, A. (1992) *From Fetus to Child: an Observational and Psychoanalytic Study.* Tavistock/Routledge, New York.

30. Chamberlain, D.B. (1989) Babies remember pain. *Pre Perinatal Psychology Journal*, **3**, 297–310.

31. Chamberlain, D.B. (1998) Prenatal receptivity and intelligence. *Journal of Prenatal Perinatal Psychology and Health*, **12**, 95–117.

32. Chamberlain, D.B. (2003) Communicating with the mind of a prenate: guidelines for parents and birth professionals. *Journal of Prenatal Perinatal Psychology and Health*, **18**, 95–108.

33. Ramon, Y. and Cajal, C.L. (1996) Description of human fetal laryngeal functions: phonation. *Early Human Development*, **45**, 63–72.

34. Rossi, N., Avveduti, P., Rizzo, N. *et al.* (1989) Maternal stress and fetal motor behavior: a preliminary report. *Pre Perinatal Psychology Journal*, **3**, 311–18.

35. Gaubert, E. (2001) *De **mémoire** de foetus.* Le Souffle d'Or, Barret-sur Meouge.

36. Haig, D. (2006) Self imposed silence: parental antagonism and the evolution of x-chromosome inactivation. *Evolution*, **60**, 440–47.

3

Single parenthood: its impact on parenting the infant

Sam Tyano and Miri Keren

Tel-Aviv University, Sackler School of Medicine, Israel

Clinical vignette

A 35-year-old pregnant woman is referred to our Infant Mental Health Unit by the community nurse because of panic attacks. She is a single mother of a 2½-year-old girl and is six months pregnant. She is a well-educated, energetic and self-sufficient woman, who maintains that 'Psychology is for the weak'. She has no insight regarding the reasons for her panic attacks. When asked how she became a single mother, she answers: 'My girl has a father, but I don't want any connection with him, he doesn't even know of her existence. It was a meaningless and short relationship. I wonder myself . . . what attracted me to him . . . Anyway, I don't want any more complications with fathers at this time and this pregnancy comes from the sperm bank!. During the session, it turns out that the trigger for the panic attacks was a severe flu she had: 'I suddenly realized that I'm going to become responsible for two children . . . what if anything happens to me . . .?' She realized that being a single mother by choice may actually, carry a price . . . and so she panicked.

3.1 Introduction

The societal change in the definition of the concept of a family is reflected in the increasing frequency and legitimization of single parenthood both among women and among men.

Parenthood and Mental Health: A Bridge between Infant and Adult Psychiatry   Sam Tyano, Miri Keren, Helen Herrman and John Cox
© 2010 John Wiley & Sons, Ltd

Fathers do develop primary parental preoccupation [1], are able to take care of their infants and babies do develop secure attachments to them (refuting the psychoanalytic-based primacy of the mother–infant relationship). In parallel, the majority of mothers, nowadays, go out to work, and fathers are much more involved in the upbringing of their children, than in the past. Last but not least, the impressive advances in procreative technologies play a predominant factor in facilitating single-parent pregnancies. Some have written about the day when the woman's womb will not be needed anymore [2] . . .

Two main categories of single-parent families need to be differentiated: those who decide to have a child, unrelated to any romantic relationship ('single parenthood by choice'), and those who become single parents after not having found a good-enough partner for life, as opposed to the first group who deliberately give up the idea of partnership.

Technologies allow both groups of individuals to become parents. Still, these two groups reflect very different psychological attitudes: Single motherhood by choice minimizes the role of the father in the child's future development, as opposed to single parenthood 'by life events' for those who would have preferred to conceive and raise the child in the context of a romantic relationship.

3.2 Single-parent families come in a variety of profiles

The experience of growing up in a single-parent family varies, depending on three major factors: the nature of the family (divorced, widowed or unmarried), the parent's age and life experiences (teenaged single mothers versus older mothers), and the family context. Consequently, the term 'single-parent family' cannot, in itself, explain or predict a particular child's outcome; one has to consider the specific circumstances of his or her single-parent family and how it came to be as such. In addition, for many parents, single parenthood is a transitional status. Whether a single-parent experience starts early or late in a child's life may lead to very different outcomes.

Among single-parent families, the most significant demographic change is the increase in single-parent families where the parent never married – from approximately 6% in 1970 to 37% in 1997 [3]. This change is due, at least in part, to the sociological phenomenon whereby affluent and well-educated women started having children without getting married. This is particularly prominent among women in their thirties.

Even more remarkable is the phenomenon of never-married single-father families, the incidence of which has increased by 59% from 1990 to 1997. In the USA, almost 20% of single-parent families are headed by fathers [3], namely, nearly one in five children living in a single-parent home lives with the father. Most of these fathers became single parents as a result of divorce, separation or out-of-wedlock birth. Consequently, this is a very significant population to be aware of, in our clinical practice as well as in our research designs.

3.3 Single parenthood as risk factor for parental mental health

Common mental disorders (anxiety, depression and substance abuse disorder) have been found to be significantly more frequent among single mothers than among partnered mothers [4, 5, 6]; 45% of single mothers were found to have experienced a common mental disorder in the previous 12 months, as compared with 23.6% of partnered mothers [4].

Post-partum depression among single mothers

In a two-year prospective study, single mothers were found to be twice more likely to experience the onset of depression as married mothers [7]. In a meta-analysis of 84 studies published in the 1990s [8], single motherhood was one of the 13 significant predictors of post-partum depression. In another study [9], 31 out of 41 women who were suffering depression at 28 weeks pre-partum were single or legally unmarried, and 17 out of the 18 women who continued to have depression at six weeks post-partum were single as well. Similarly, five out of seven women who suffered depression only in the post-partum period were single. More specifically, it was found [10] that negative thinking is an important factor in the development of depressive symptoms among single mothers. As a symptom, negative thinking may present a target for more efficient intervention than the general target of reducing chronic stress.

3.4   Risk factors for mental health problems among single mothers

Various studies have attempted to explain the higher prevalence of mental health problems among single mothers, by looking at various risk factors.

1 *Financial hardship* has been found to be the primary mediating variable, while employment, social support, number of children, and pre-existing mental health problems made only modest to negligible contributions [11]. When financial hardship was present in both groups, partner status made no significant difference in depressive symptomatology – single as well as partnered mothers were depressed [5]. In contrast, when there was no financial hardship, single mothers were significantly more depressed than partnered ones. A more recent study [12] supported these findings, showing that nearly twice as many single mothers experienced moderate to severe mental disability as compared with partnered mothers. The joint effect of financial hardship and social support accounts for most of the predictive power of the socio-demographic variables. Overall, it seems that, given the significance of financial hardship as an explanatory factor for mental health problems, an important implication for social policy would be to implement financial management interventions.

2 *Social support* is both a risk and a protective factor. Lack of social support during a crisis has been associated with increased risk for depression [13]. Its presence protects against the negative effects of stress and disadvantage [14]. Antenatal mental health of single mothers was compared to partnered women's with poor partner relationship [15] and an increased risk of antenatal depression was observed in the latter. Thus, previous history of depression and current emotional problems, rather than single-mother status, were significant risk factors for antenatal depression. Also, what makes the difference, at least before giving birth, is partner support and not merely the presence of a partner.

3 *Maternal young age* Adolescent pregnancies, 79% of which result in single parenthood [16], are the most disadvantaged of the single-parent group, because they are impacted by several risk factors: the young women are likely to have poor schooling and poor scholastic achievements, and they tend to be isolated and financially poor. With the birth of the child, the adolescent mother's social isolation increases and her chance of becoming self-sufficient is reduced (the topic of teenage pregnancies, with its unique psychological challenges, is discussed in depth in Chapter 7).

These are probably the underlying factors for the reported high risk for antenatal and post-partum depression in adolescent, single mothers. Antenatal depression has been linked to negative response to pregnancy and financial difficulties, which may explain the finding that pregnant teenagers are at the highest risk [17]. Adolescent mothers are also at the highest risk for developing postnatal depression – 48% of adolescent mothers experience depressive symptoms [18], as compared to 13% of adult mothers [19]. In-depth description of the themes that characterize these adolescent mothers may make one think of the metaphor of 'being hit by a nor'easter storm' [20].

3.5 Single-father families versus single-mother families

As noted above, we are still entrenched in the stereotypical assumption that only women create single-parent families. This is probably the reason for our inability to find any epidemiological studies about single-father families. The data that we found relates to small, select samples of volunteers. Most single fathers are divorced, while among single mothers the distribution between 'never-married' and 'divorced' is about equal. When compared to divorced single mothers, single fathers' financial status is better [21], but when compared to married fathers, single fathers' income tends to be lower.

This demographic data has significance for the child's outcome according to a study [22] that showed how a single parent's parenting behavior is affected by both satisfaction at work and economic status, both of which are higher for single fathers than for single mothers. The higher economic status and higher level of education are mediating factors that impact on overall psychological well-being, which has been found higher among single fathers than among single mothers [21, 22].

Custodial fathers are different, as a group, from custodial mothers, in several characteristics: they are often older, better-educated, earn better incomes and receive more offers of support but are less likely to take them [23].

3.6 Single custodial parenthood

Divorced parents are still the largest group of single parents [3]. Economically, they are also the most prosperous of all single parents; in particular, the fathers. In most countries the majority of divorced parents with custody are mothers. Still, the increasing divorce rates, combined with the changing roles of fathers in the upbringing of their children, have led to a growing number of fathers willing to take on and win custody of their children in the courts [3]. Resolving the emotional experiences involved in separation and divorce often takes months, even years. During this time the custodial parent's adjustment, well-being and economic status are very much affected. Not surprisingly, parents are more irritable and unresponsive in their interactions with their children during that time [24]. The first two years after divorce are the most difficult [25]. Within two years, most custodial parents feel happier and function better than prior to the divorce.

The custodial parent, be it the mother or the father, needs to adjust to an additional role: mothers, in addition to being homemakers, become the financial supporter, and fathers must become homemakers in addition to being the financial supporter. In a study of 626 divorced single mothers and 100 divorced single fathers who are their children's custodians, satisfaction with the new role was the strongest predictor of depression or lack thereof, in both groups [26].

3.7 Psychological characteristics of single mothers by choice

As illustrated in the clinical vignette above, single mothers by choice are a special group who deliberately decide to rear their child without a partner. As opposed to the other groups of single parents, these women have a fairly homogenous demographic profile: they tend to be in their middle to upper thirties, come from upper-middle-class socio-economic status, are financially secure and well-educated, and hold high-level positions at work [27]. In addition to frequently holding feminist views, single mothers by choice are usually motivated by their biological clock (their thirty-fifth or fortieth birthday being a hallmark of the biological clock). The decision to become a single mother is often the result of a long and difficult process [27].

In our experience, the psychological profile of these women is less homogenous than their demographic one. There are those who deliberately decide 'not to bother with men' and display a derogatory attitude towards them. They are self-sufficient, and often have good social support. Another group includes women who have deficits in social and interpersonal skills, are isolated, experience financial hardships, and create an almost symbiotic relationship with their infant.

3.8 A double-edge risk situation: being a single parent of an infant at risk

The transactional model of normal and abnormal development presumes that the child's socio-emotional outcome depends on the dynamic transactions between risk and protective factors in the child as well as in the parent and in their environment along the time axis [28]. The highest risk situation is whenever significant risk factors are present in both the parent and the infant and our role, as clinicians, is to detect them early, so we can implement target-oriented interventions, aimed at changing the child's, the parent's or the environmental risk factors. For instance, parenthood of children born with chronic illness is especially challenging. When it is added to single parenthood that carries its own risk factors, the result may become overwhelming and dangerous for both the parent's mental well-being and for the child's overall development.

On the other side of the equation, single-mother pregnancies, and especially teenage pregnancies, are a risk factor for delivering small for gestational age (SGA) infants – as compared with married-women pregnancies – and for reduced inter-pregnancy interval that is, in itself, an additional risk factor [29]. Poverty, also more frequent among single mothers, is an additional risk factor for low birth weight, more than the effect of racial and ethnic factors [30]. Smallness for gestational age is, in itself, a risk factor for the infant's physical development, and more specifically for feeding problems. This, in turn, often leads to parent–infant relation disorders. Being a single parent to a temperamentally difficult infant is another common example where risk factors in the parent and in the infant are in dynamic interplay, and have a severely detrimental impact on the emotional well-being and development of both parties.

Another quickly growing group of single parents and infants at risk is the group of adoptive single parents. Children with pre-adoption adversity (such as traumatic early relationships, deprivation, loss, separations and instability) show more problems overall (including post-traumatic stress disorders; attachment disorders, depression, attention deficits disorders, learning disorders, oppositional defiant disorder, autistic spectrum disorders) than those without histories of extreme deprivation [31]. Understandably, it is quite stressful for parents to care for infants presenting multiple difficulties, and even more so for single parents, especially when parental risk factors, as described above, are present.

3.9 Clinical implications

Based on the literature review, single parenthood is definitely a challenge for good-enough parenting. Obviously, many single parents function perfectly well, but our task as clinicians is to detect those who are at risk as early as possible. Knowing the mediating parental risk factors – such as young maternal age, depression, anxiety, poor education, poor social support and financial hardship – should help with planning psychosocial interventions, starting already in pregnancy. We hereby wish to emphasize the need for detecting the dyads where risk factors are present not only in the parent but also in the infant. Community health nurses and pediatricians have a special role to play in this early detection process, since they are those who meet the infant with his or her single parent early in the first year of life. They should subsequently consult with mental health professionals, in order to diagnose the parent and the infant, and to tailor an intervention program for them. Single-parent self-support groups have become quite common, but the dyads at the highest risk tend not to seek help, and therefore have to be reached through other means.

3.10 Summary

There is no prototype of single-parent families, because each family type is characterized by different circumstances. Divorced custodial mothers and fathers face similar challenges in their parental tasks. Single motherhood appears to be a strong risk factor in negative social, behavioral and emotional outcomes for children. One may argue that this is due to the absence of a male parent but this explanation has been refuted by long-term developmental outcome studies of children born to lesbian couples, where no difference was found between those children and children of heterosexual couples with regard to gender development, self-esteem, emotional well-being and social development [32]. In contrast, there is strong evidence to suggest that negative outcomes are the result of the very young age, educational and economic disadvantages and social isolation that often accompany single motherhood. When these disadvantages are not present with single motherhood, neither are the negative outcomes [33].

Consequently, early detection and intervention should be targeted to these specific risk factors among single mothers, with the aim of minimizing the risk for poor socio-emotional outcome in their infants.

3.11 References

1. Leckman, J.F., Feldman, R., Swain, J.E. *et al.* (2004) Primary parental preoccupation: circuits, genes, and the crucial role of the environment. *Journal of Neural Transmission*, **111**, 753–71.
2. Atlan, H. *L'utérus artificiel* (The artificial womb) (2005) Paris, Payot.
3. Weinraub, M., Horvath, D.L. and Gringlas, M.B. (2002) Single parenthood, in *Handbook of Parenting, Being and Becoming a Parent*, Vol. 3 (ed. M.H. Bornstein), Lawrence Erlbaum Associates, Mahwah, New Jersey, pp. 109–40.
4. Butterworth, P. (2004) The prevalence of psychiatric disorders among lone mothers: association with physical and sexual violence. *British Journal of Psychiatry*, **184**, 21–27.
5. Wang, J.L. (2004) The difference between single and married mothers in the 12 month prevalence of major depressive syndrome, associated factors and mental health service utilization. *Social Psychiatry and Psychiatric Epidemiology*, **39**, 26–32.
6. Targosz, S., Bebbington, P., Lewis, G. *et al.* (2003) Lone mothers, social exclusion and depression. *Psychological Medicine*, **33**, 715–22.
7. Brown, G.W. and Moran, P.M. (1997) Single mothers, poverty and depression. *Psychological Medicine*, **27**, 21–33.
8. Beck, C.T. (2001) Predictors of postpartum depression: an update. *Nursing Research*, **50**, 275–85.
9. Wissart, J., Parshad, O. and Kulkarni, S. (2005) Prevalence of pre- and postpartum depression in Jamaican women. *BioMedicine Central Pregnancy and Childbirth*, **5**, 1–5.
10. Peden, A.R., Rayens, M.K., Hall, L.A. *et al.* (2004). Negative thinking and the mental health of low-income single mothers. *Journal of Nursing Scholarship*, **36**, 337–44.
11. Hope, S., Power, C. and Rodgers, B. (1999) Does financial hardship account for elevated psychological distress in lone mothers? *Social Science Medicine*, **49**, 1637–49.
12. Crosier, T., Butterworth, P., Rodgers, B. (2007) Mental health problems among single and partnered mothers: the role of financial hardship and social support. *Social Psychiatry and Psychiatric Epidemiology*, **42**, 6–13.
13. Brown, G.W., Andrews, B., Harris, T.O. *et al.* (1986) Social support, self-esteem, and depression. *Psychological Medicine*, **16**, 813–31.
14. Harris, T., Brown, G.W. and Robinson, R. (1999) Befriending as an intervention for chronic depression among women in an inner city. 2: role of fresh-start experiences and baseline psychosocial factors in remission from depression. *British Journal of Psychiatry*, **174**, 225–32.
15. Bilstza, J.L.C., Tang, M., Meyer, D. *et al.* (2008) Single motherhood versus poor partner relationship: outcomes for antenatal mental health. *Australian and New Zealand Journal of Psychiatry*, **42**, 56–65.
16. Ventura, S., Curtin, S. and Mathews, T. (2000) Teenage births in the United States: national and state trends, 1990–96, in *National Vital Statistics System*, Hyataville, Maryland, National Center for Health Statistics.
17. Kitamura, T., Yoshida, K., Okano, T. *et al.* (2006) Multicenter prospective study of perinatal depression in Japan: incidence and correlates of antenatal and postnatal depression. *Archives of Women's Mental Health*, **9**, 121–30.

18. Deal, L. and Holt, V. (1998) Young maternal age and depressive symptoms: results from the 1988 National Maternal and Infant Health Survey. *American Journal of Public Health*, **88**, 266–70.

19. O'Hara, M. and Swain, A. (1996) Rates and risks of postpartum depression: a meta-analysis. *International Review of Psychiatry*, **8**, 37–54.

20. Clemmens, D.A. (2002) Adolescent mothers' depression after the birth of their babies: weathering the storm. *Adolescence*, **37**, 551–65.

21. Amato, P.R. (2000) Diversity within single-parent families, in *Handbook of Family Diversity* (eds D.H. Demo, K.R. Allen and M.A. Fine), Oxford University Press, New York, pp. 149–72.

22. Christoffersen, M.N. (1998) Growing up with dad: a comparison of children aged 3-5 years old living with their mothers or fathers. *Childhood: a Global Journal of Child Research*, **5**, 41–54.

23. Greif, G.L. (1995) Single fathers with custody following separation and divorce, in *Single-Parents Families: Diversity, Myths, and Realities* (eds S.M. Hanson, M.L. Heims, D. Julian and M.B. Sussman), Hawthorne, New York.

24. Thiriot, T.L. and Buckner, E.T. (1991) Multiple predictors of satisfactory post-divorce adjustment of single custodial parents. *Journal of Divorce and Remarriage*, **17**, 27–48.

25. Hetherington, E.M., Bridges, M. and Insabella, G.M. (1998) What matters? What does not? Five perspectives on the association between marital transitions and children's adjustment. *American Psychologist*, **53**, 167–84.

26. Hill, L.C. and Hilton, J.M. (2000) Changes in roles following divorce: comparison of factors contributing to depression in custodial single mothers and custodial single fathers. *Journal of Divorce and Remarriage*, **29**, 23–53.

27. Bock, J.D. (2000) Doing the right thing? Single mothers by choice and the struggle for legitimacy. *Gender and Society*, **14**, 62–86.

28. Sameroff, A.J. and Fiese, B. (2000) Models of development and developmental risk. In *Handbook of Infant Mental Health* (ed. C.H. Zeanah Jr), The Guilford Press, New York, pp. 3–19.

29. Auger, N., Daniel, M., Platt, R.W. *et al.* (2008) The joint influence of marital status, inter-pregnancy interval, and neighborhood on small for gestational age birth: a retrospective cohort study. *BMC Pregnancy and Childbirth*, **8**, 7.

30. Reichman, N.E., Hamilton, E.R., Hummer, R.A. *et al.* (2008) Racial and ethnic disparities in low birthweight among urban unmarried mothers. *Maternal and Child Health Journal*, **12**, 204–15.

31. Costello, E. (2005) Complementary and alternative therapies: considerations for families after international adoption. *Pediatrics Clinics of North America*, **52**, 1463–78.

32. Fitzgerald, B. (1999) Children of lesbian and gay parents. *Marriage and Family Review*, **29**, 57–75.

33. Golombok, S. (2000) *Parenting: What Really Counts?* Routledge, London.

4
Surrogate mothers

Olga B.A. van den Akker
Middlesex University, London, UK

Clinical vignette

A 42-year-old mother of three children with low educational and occupational achievements has presented to her general practitioner with symptoms of anxiety and depression relating to her last pregnancy. She is unable to disclose the reasons for her symptoms, and does not reveal she has been a surrogate mother some seven years previously until she meets with the psychiatrist. During the psychiatric consultation she reveals that her husband is the only person in her immediate family who has been aware of the surrogate pregnancy. He was in favor of her doing this for an infertile couple in return for reasonable expenses approximating £10,000. However, because they both felt they would be judged by others around them, they had agreed to keep this a secret from everyone. Upon delivery of the baby, the mother came home alone to their other children and claimed she had suffered a neonatal death. She now believes the decision to hide the surrogate arrangement was the wrong thing to do, and fears the consequences if the truth came out. Her anxiety about the implications of the sympathy she (wrongly) received led to the prolonged depression.

4.1 Introduction

Surrogate mother arrangements can take place between two women within one country or state, or across borders, which is often referred to derogatorily as 'reproductive tourism'. In some countries (including the USA and India) surrogates can be paid, whereas in other countries (including the UK and Canada) payment is illegal, although reasonable expenses

Parenthood and Mental Health: A Bridge between Infant and Adult Psychiatry Sam Tyano, Miri Keren, Helen Herrman and John Cox
© 2010 John Wiley & Sons, Ltd

are allowed. Germany, Italy and France are among the countries that do not legally recognize surrogacy at all. In practice, in countries where altruistic surrogacy is carried out, the amounts paid for reasonable expenses may be more than the fees paid to a surrogate mother in, for example, India. Furthermore, no legislation can entirely prevent surrogates from carrying babies for other people for social reasons, and no legislation can control for people travelling to other countries to bypass restrictions (such as single embryo transfers), to secure an economically less costly arrangement, or as a commodity.

Surrogacy, although already perceived as unorthodox, can also help homosexual couples and single men to create families. In some US states, gay men can commission a surrogate mother to help create a family for them and they can use the couple's or donor sperm, using insemination or embryo transfer respectively. Clinical practice also varies in line with social and economic changes, with the relatively non-invasive (donor) insemination resulting in a genetic surrogacy arrangement, initially predominating over the much more invasive, time-consuming and expensive gestational surrogacy arrangement, involving embryo transfer.

There are two types of surrogacy: genetic and gestational surrogacy, which are different in a number of meaningful ways as shown in Figure 4.1. In *genetic surrogacy*, the surrogate

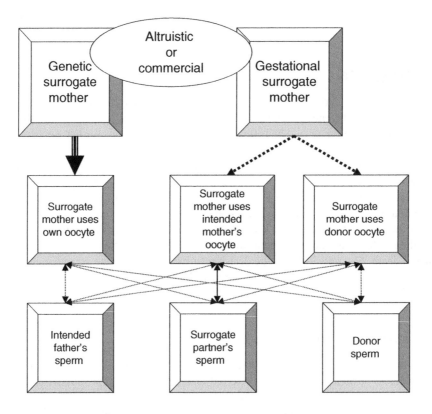

Note: Broken lines indicate distance of genetic origins which are likely to be anonymous and untraceable. Closed lines refer to closer genetic origins of the surrogate infant to the intended and therefore social parents.

Figure 4.1 Showing different genetic combinations of the fetus in genetic and gestational surrogate practices

uses her own gametes and relinquishes, in effect, a child that is genetically related to her, just like any other children she may carry naturally as her own. The genetic surrogate children will come to know that their genetic surrogate mother conceived and carried them to term and then relinquished them following delivery to a couple who may have invested the father's but not the mother's gametes. Her own (other non-surrogate) children too will know that their mother relinquished their half sibling(s) within a purposeful arrangement, as will the grandparents and extended family and social network.

Gestational surrogacy is more complex, not only in its procedure as it requires embryo transfer, but also bio-psychosocially. Here, the surrogate carries a genetically unrelated baby conceived *in vitro* in a clinic usually with the intended mother's oocyte and the intended father's sperm, although entirely donated gametes or embryos are also used, as shown in Figure 4.1. Relinquishment of the gestational surrogate baby therefore is different for a surrogate, as this child does not carry the surrogate's genes. In law, however, legal motherhood is determined either by gestation or by genetic link (for examples see later in this chapter).

The opposite meaning of genetic and gestational terminology applies to the intended or commissioning mother. Here, the genetic surrogate's baby does not carry the intended mother's genes, whereas the gestational surrogate's baby can (and usually does) have the intended mother's genetic make-up. These genetic link differences determine the clinical and commissioning economic costs involved in the arrangement and the psychological affinity associated with genes, although issues of gestation, delivery and breastfeeding are present for both.

Figure 4.2 shows the complexity of the potential identity of a commissioned *surrogate baby*. The surrogate is responsible for nurturing and relinquishing a surrogate baby, which may be fully genetically related to the surrogate, the commissioning couple, or be made up of gametes donated by unknown people from a number of different countries. Upon relinquishment, the surrogate passes on the care of this genetically diverse infant to the individual or couple commissioning the baby. The baby may have no traceable genetic or gestational origin (as shown in scenario's below the line in Figure 4.2), since even some surrogate arrangements are carried out anonymously. It is unclear who is responsible for these infants should the intended couple not want to pursue the original commission.

It is estimated that approximately one in seven couples experience infertility, and in the Western world an estimated 1.4% of all births are the result of infertility treatments. Of these, only a relatively small proportion use surrogacy to overcome their infertility. Success rates for surrogacy are similar to *in vitro* fertilization (IVF) success rates and in the UK it is estimated that every year some 50 surrogate infants are processed through a system determining eligibility for Parental Orders for registration with the commissioning couple. As pointed out above, this is because under some laws, e.g. UK Section 27 of the 1990 Human Fertilization and Embryology Act, the surrogate is the legal mother of the infant regardless of her genetic contribution. Similarly, under Section 28 of the same Act, her husband (if she has one) is the legal father of the infant. Under Section 30 of the Act, a married commissioning couple can apply for a Parental Order, not dissimilar to regulations in place for adoptions.

In India, a recent media article reported one surrogate baby was born every 48 hours to foreign couples. Indian surrogate babies can leave the country as the gestational surrogate mother is not considered by law to be the legal mother of the child. However, foreign couples (e.g. UK residents) could have difficulty gaining the child's

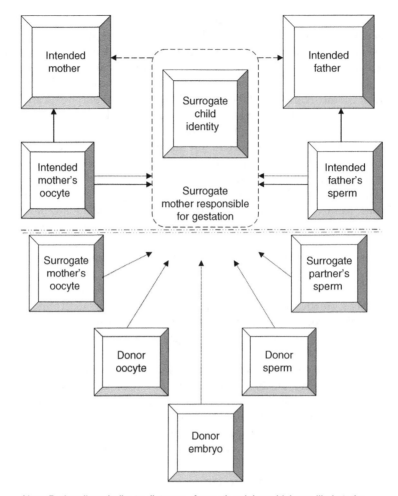

Note: Broken lines indicate distance of genetic origins which are likely to be anonymous and untraceable. Closed lines refer to closer genetic origins of the surrogate infant to the intended and therefore social parents.

Figure 4.2 The potentially complex genetic nature of a commissioned surrogate baby

entry on a British passport, because the commissioning mother (couple) is not recognized in the UK as the legal mother (parents) of the infant, even if she (they) contributed (all the) genes. Should the Indian surrogate use her own ova, the commissioning couple will have to legally adopt the baby. Across the world, once adoptions or Parental Orders have been agreed, birth certificates will record the commissioning or adoptive parents as the legal parents of the child. Current debates are focused on a drive to accurately reflect genetic descent on birth certificates, be that through adoptions, gamete or embryo donation or surrogacy.

The increasing availability of infertility services has increased the demand for these services and consequently increased the numbers of births resulting from technological interventions and third-party reproduction – including surrogate births. The increase in surrogate babies born demands that the babies' and their mothers' welfare is investigated and followed over a period of time. Although a limited amount of research has been published in the scientific literature, further longer-term research is needed using larger samples to monitor the long-term outcome of all parties involved in surrogate motherhood: the intended mothers, fathers, babies and surrogate mothers and their families. The type of surrogacy used is also likely to have a differential effect on the wider social network of both surrogate and intended mothers in the short and long term. Research on surrogate and commissioning fathers is very rare. One detailed case report published 13 years since the baby's birth indicated good adjustment to fatherhood of a surrogate baby gestated by a sister-to-sister arrangement using the intended mother's ova and donor sperm [1].

4.2 Characteristics, motivations and experiences

Early research questioned the psychological characteristics of surrogate mothers, because the practice was perceived as highly controversial. Franks [2] studied the psychological functioning of a small group of US surrogates and reported minor psychopathology. Later studies, for example [3,4], confirmed no psychopathology was evident in the surrogate mothers they studied. Helena Ragone's [5] US research and some UK studies have reported that surrogate mothers are altruistically motivated to bear this gift for another couple and that psychopathology does not feature in these women. There have also been suggestions that surrogates participate in these arrangements to compensate for previous (usually though not equivocally reproductive) losses [6], suggesting this may indicate a potential vulnerability.

Research has also focused on other characteristics, in attempts to determine if surrogates were drawn to arrangements for socio-demographic or commodity reasons. Socio-economic status and education tend to be lower in surrogates than their commissioning counterparts [7,4]. However, most surrogates report altruism as the motivation although some report financial incentives are additional important factors. Surrogates seem to enjoy pregnancy and childbirth and report feeling fulfilled. For example, self-worth and self-confidence may be increased. The development of intense friendships with the commissioning parents – particularly the commissioning mothers – has added value to the surrogate arrangements for surrogates. Relinquishment of the baby is generally reported as a happy event for most surrogates, although some report feeling relief when it was all over. The happiness with their extraordinary achievement is coupled with sadness following the relinquishment of the baby for a proportion of the women as reported in American and European studies.

As is shown in Figures 4.1 and 4.2, the surrogate motherhood experience separates the genetic from the gestational and both from the social components of parenthood. The surrogate mother is responsible for the biological/gestational environment, for the genetic environment in genetic surrogacy and for the delivery. The intended mother becomes responsible for the infant's postnatal nurturing and rearing, although she might have contributed the genetic component in gestational surrogacy. The importance of the interactions between genetic and environmental factors in shaping a large part of an individual's identity has been researched extensively by geneticists and psychologists and has informed progress in nature versus nurture debates. Infertile couples commissioning a baby through surrogacy prefer to maintain a genetic link with the resultant offspring, and have often been cited as choosing gestational surrogacy over adoption precisely to maintain a genetic link. Even couples opting for genetic surrogacy say that they prefer to have a partial male genetic link, over no link at all – the same reason why this is popular with homosexual couples. Those couples unable to have any genetic link, but who opt to use surrogacy to overcome their involuntary childlessness, do so in order to have a child from infancy because, unlike adoption, it is rare to be able to adopt a newborn infant in the twenty-first century, at least for white Western couples.

Disclosure of genetic origin in adoption, gamete and embryo donation and disclosure of gestation as well as genetic origins in surrogacy have been extensively debated across the world over many decades. Issues of disclosure are important because children have a right to access medical information that can be crucial to survival (e.g. prevention of the expression of predispositions to certain diseases, opting for early screening or initiating appropriate lifestyle changes minimizing genetic risk). Having information of otherwise unknown factors in (not genetically related) offspring subjected to a surrogate mother's perinatal environment could impact on a mother or health-care professional's ability to interpret the infant's state of health accurately. Arrangements carried out with donated gametes or embryos, particularly if these are anonymous and not traceable, therefore not only threaten the infant's right to find out its genetic origins to form an identity as it grows into adolescence, but it also leaves a gap in knowledge of his or her medical information and is therefore not in the best interests of the child.

4.3 Attachment, bonding and pregnancy

Surrogate motherhood is unique because the surrogate mother is exposed to the pregnancy and delivery and therefore has the opportunity to go through all the usual stages associated with prenatal attachments prior to delivery and immediately following delivery [8]. A commissioning mother on the other hand does not carry the baby and therefore misses out on the ability to bond and form attachments with the baby in the prenatal period. She may be unable to bond with the infant because she has not gone through the gradual fetal development. Research and theory on traditional childbearing practice has shown that attachment to the fetus begins in pregnancy and that this carries on in the majority of cases to the baby following delivery. Following delivery the bonding process becomes strengthened by nurturing and caring behaviors including breastfeeding. These continuing nurturing behaviours also tend to be absent in intended mothers, who rarely breastfeed.

However, research on traditional pregnant women also reports that many factors, including maternal age and attitudes towards the pregnancy, can influence prenatal attachment. Few studies have assessed attachment in people treated for infertility and even less research has considered attachment issues in surrogate or intended mothers. However, the research which has been carried out on surrogate mothers has shown that surrogates tend to develop a sense of detachment and ambivalence towards the surrogate fetus during pregnancy, in attempts to lessen the impact of relinquishment [8–10]. Information provided by surrogate agencies on successful practices discourages attachment or bonding between the surrogate and the fetus. It is expected that if a surrogate is not attached to the fetus it will be easier to give the baby away following delivery. Paradoxically, ensuring a successful relinquishment (which is completely contrary to usual practice), ensures a successful outcome. The intentional detachment from the fetus is therefore encouraged for both genetic and gestational surrogate mothers.

Numerous court cases and legal wrangles have followed a few instances where surrogates changed their minds and kept the baby. The legal ownership of the baby is usually with the surrogate; hence the pregnancy for both the surrogate and the commissioning mother is filled with uncertainty. Similarly, if a commissioning mother allows herself to attach to the fetus during the surrogate pregnancy she puts herself at emotional risk (in potential non-relinquishment). The huge disappointment and pain evident in media reports of non-relinquishment if the surrogate changes her mind about keeping the baby is there for all to see. However, the consequences of the ensuing disputes about who cares for the child when it grows up are not known. There are no studies of the welfare of the surrogate mother and surrogate baby (or the intended parent[s]) where the surrogate reneged on the arrangement.

Research on bonding in the recipient mothers has also been carried out. Bonding in intended mothers may be compromised by the lack of biological connectedness. For example, a recipient mother in adoption or commissioning mother in surrogacy will not have opportunities for gestational attachment, delivery, bonding through breastfeeding and they may lack the genetic link compared to mothers who do have the gestational, delivery and breastfeeding opportunities and the genetic link. However, as far as the author is aware, no specific practical/informational help is provided for commissioning intended mothers (and fathers) to encourage them to develop positive attachments to the fetus while within a surrogate's uterus. Most clinics do encourage the presence of the intended couple in the delivery room so that the bonding process can begin right at the start of the infant's entry into the world. However, this is not possible in countries where anonymous surrogacy is practised, or if the intended couple lives too far from the surrogate to be present in time during delivery.

In addition to high-risk obstetric complications (including multiple failed pregnancy attempts and miscarriages, ectopic pregnancies and ovarian hyper-stimulation), stress or anxiety in pregnancy could have detrimental effects on the health and well-being of the surrogate and the fetus. Reame and Parker [11] investigated stress in surrogates. They reported increased levels of stress in surrogates towards the end of pregnancy, during labour, delivery and at relinquishment. High levels of anxiety in pregnant surrogates can lead to adverse perinatal outcomes and are therefore of clinical importance. In the only prospective longitudinal study of surrogate and intended mothers reported so far, no adverse psychological effects for genetic versus gestational surrogacy were found in surrogate mothers or in intended mothers [10]. A genetic link with a baby on its own therefore does not appear to have a differential effect on psychological functioning during the surrogate arrangement. Surrogate mothers were detached from the fetus during pregnancy and they did not show the often reported increase in anxiety during pregnancy and no increases in depression up to six months post delivery [10].

In the same study, differences in state of anxiety were found during the pre-pregnancy period, in late pregnancy and at six months post delivery, with pre-pregnancy state of anxiety higher in intended mothers going through gestational surrogacy. These intended mothers used their own embryos for transfer to the surrogate mothers. It is possible that they felt they had invested most into the arrangement. In the final stages of pregnancy, intended mothers were significantly more anxious than surrogate mothers. This is likely to reflect their increasing concerns for the health and well-being of the fetuses, which, in the case of gestational intended mothers, are genetically theirs. A genetic link and being an intended mother therefore does differentiate anxiety from other groups. Interestingly, anxiety in commissioning mothers waiting for the birth of the surrogate baby may be advantageous for subsequent attachment and bonding, as it may be indicative of notable parental concern.

Raised anxiety was still evident in gestational commissioning mothers at six months post delivery, possibly reflecting characteristics of women undergoing fertility treatment who experience some additional problems in adjustment to motherhood [12]. This could be a cause for concern in relation to later parent–child interactions. These issues need to be explored in future research following intended mothers over a longer time period as discussed in a review of assisted conception family functioning [13]. A number of significant differences in attitudes toward the fetus between surrogate and intended mothers have also been reported during the course of the pregnancy. In the first trimester, intended mothers report significantly more positive attitudes about the baby than surrogate mothers. Surrogates explained they were trying to distance themselves emotionally from the fetus.

In the second trimester, intended mothers rated significantly more negative attitudes towards the pregnancy and the baby, and they were also more worried about the baby's health and well-being. This may have been an attempt on the part of the intended mothers to distance themselves from the fetus as the pregnancy viability was now more certain but the relinquishment less certain. Also, the surrogate would have started to show the visible signs of pregnancy, a much-wished-for event in the never successfully pregnant intended mothers. In the final term of pregnancy, intended mothers (particularly the ones using embryo transfer via gestational surrogacy) were still significantly more worried about the baby's health and well-being and more negative about the pregnancy. The intended mothers' responses were confusing but could be explained as showing concerns coupled with feelings of excitement towards the impending birth, which may be an attempt to form a bond or attachment with the fetus.

The surrogates in the same longitudinal prospective study [10] did not report experiencing many feelings about the baby, dissociating themselves from possible attachment. According to attachment theory, attachment in pregnancy transfers to attachment to the baby following delivery. By not developing attachments in pregnancy, surrogates may be coping effectively with relatively detached feelings towards the baby following delivery, and so minimizing feelings of loss at relinquishment. These results mimic those reported by others [9] who showed that surrogates are less attached to the fetus, and this was also confirmed in retrospective studies of surrogate mothers [7,14].

The in-depth prospective study [10] has provided longitudinal data showing that detachment in surrogate mothers is reported early on and throughout the pregnancy, with little variation post delivery. No differences in the experience of the blues or postnatal depression (PND) were reported, although some surrogates reported experiencing PND. None of the recipient intended mothers reported experiencing the maternity blues or PND. Unfortunately, the sample was too small to make meaningful statements about this. However, surrogate and intended mothers provide ideal research participants for separating the genetic and biological and social aspects of motherhood, which may all or individually contribute to negative affective states in the first year post delivery.

4.4 Relinquishing the baby and the social context

Surrogate motherhood is theoretically interesting because it separates sex, conception, gestation and, in half the cases, a genetic link from subsequent parenthood. Parenthood is traditionally and preferentially defined in biological rather than social terms [12]. This historic preference is likely to contribute to the popular use of treatments which mimic natural parenthood, where there is a genetic, gestational or neonatal link. Research on the effects of genetic and gestational differences in families has shown that most new parents want to be considered the real parents of the baby even if the baby resulted from donated gametes, embryos or surrogacy, and despite not taking part in the biological, gestational or genetic aspects of the creation of the baby.

The deviation from traditional parenthood in assisted parenthood and surrogacy are likely to have an effect on the couples involved. In surrogate motherhood a surrogate goes cognitively against the norm (dissonance versus consonance) and may therefore be stigmatized. For example, a non-relinquishing surrogate may not have reconciled the difference between her cognitions (traditional beliefs of gestating and keeping a baby; consonant) and her actions (of gestating and relinquishing a baby), which are dissonant to her belief systems [4,5,15]. The normative values are fuelled by the media, which generally report on controversial surrogate arrangements. Cognitive dissonance is an unbalanced and uncomfortable state, and people generally strive for consonance. Thus, surrogates cognitively restructure their feelings to match their behaviors [8], and many therefore report that surrogacy is a positive (for the intended couple) rather than negative (for themselves) arrangement, see for example [1]. Nevertheless, society does not necessarily agree.

Although the short-term welfare of surrogates appears to be relatively problem-free, little longitudinal research is available on the long-term well-being of the surrogate mother who has relinquished her surrogate babies. Research on the well-being of any non-surrogate children of surrogate mothers is non-existent. It is possible that some surrogates are too young and too impressionable to fully understand the short- or long-term consequences of entering a surrogate arrangement, and that a surrogate's own children are concerned about being relinquished if they do not behave as required. Regret and coercion have been reported in a few surrogate mothers [12]. However, there are reports of positive long-term functioning of the surrogate mother, the surrogate child and the intended family [1,4,8], and the popular press has reported on the 'addictive qualities' some surrogates associate with their participation in repeated surrogate arrangements.

The relationships which are known to develop between surrogate and intended mothers in open arrangements tend to be intense. In the UK, surrogate and intended couples frequently attend embryo transfers together. They meet up for antenatal visits and discuss the developments, growth rates and expected delivery date. There have been concerns that the newly developed relationships between surrogates and intended mothers may affect their usual sources of social support and their marital relationships, which in turn could affect their moods. These concerns are important for surrogates because, following a successful arrangement, they are left alone without a baby and without the attentions they received during pregnancy. Genetic surrogates are particularly prone to being isolated following delivery and relinquishment of the baby. They do not benefit from the same clinical involvements as gestational surrogates, which could lead to a significantly worse psychological outcome in genetic surrogates [7,4].

The development of supportive extended family relationships is also important for positive social functioning. A limited amount of research exists reporting on details of specific family interactions between commissioning parents, their genetically related or unrelated child(ren) and the grandparents and extended family (for a review see [13]). In one of the authors' studies, social support received from important people in the surrogates' lives were reported as lacking whereas intended mothers maintained good social support with family and friends throughout the process. The parents, friends and family of genetic surrogates (those using their own oocytes) were less supportive pre-pregnancy and parents were significantly less supportive in the first trimester of pregnancy. It is possible that they may have found it more difficult to accept the fact that the genetically related offspring would not become part of their family and social network. Moreover, many surrogates are outside stable relationships [7,8]. Their post-delivery support is also weaker than that reported for commissioning mothers. In clinical practice, surrogates could be less supported emotionally and socially following their departure to a home without the baby they carried for nine months. Counselling should be offered to surrogates to monitor their longer-term welfare, and to support them. Social support acts as a buffer for psychological health, and shortcomings in social support need to be addressed as part of the clinical care offered.

4.5 Conclusion

Surrogate motherhood is unusual and relatively problem-free but has the potential to have traumatic consequences for the surrogate, the intended couple and the surrogate baby, child or adult. Most surrogate pregnancies fare well and few complications have been reported in research studies. However, long-term follow-up of surrogates who experienced complications of pregnancy or miscarriages needs to be carried out to ensure they are well supported. In successful surrogacy arrangements, surrogates relinquish the baby at or soon after delivery. Relinquishing a baby, although reported as a joyous experience, also leaves surrogates filled with sadness. Research into the surrogate's own children and her extended family who lose a genetically related or unrelated infant needs to be explored. The health, well-being and family functioning of commissioning mothers and fathers are under-researched. Although no problems with attachment have been reported to date, no long-term follow-up has been carried out determining the quality of family functioning of commissioning couples and their extended family who gained a genetically related or unrelated infant.

4.6 References

1. Kirkman, M. and Kirkman, A. (2002) Sister to sister gestational surrogacy 13 years on: a narrative of parenthood. *Journal of Reproductive and Infant Psychology*, **20** (3), 135–147.
2. Franks, D. (1981) Psychiatric evaluation of women in a surrogate mother program. *American Journal of Psychiatry*, **138**, 1378–79.
3. Hanafin, H. (1984) Surrogate mothers: an exploratory study. Department of Psychology, Los Angeles, California School of Professional Psychology PhD Dissertation.

4. van den Akker, O.B.A. (2003) Genetic and gestational surrogate mothers' experience of surrogacy. *Journal of Reproductive and Infant Psychology*, **21**, (2), 145–61.
5. Ragone, H. (1994) *Surrogate Motherhood: Conception in the Heart*. Westview Press, Colorado, USA.
6. Kanefield, L. (1999) The reparative motive in surrogate mothers. *Adoption Quarterly*, **2** (4), 5–19.
7. Blyth, E (1994) I wanted to be interesting. I wanted to be able to say 'I've done something interesting with my life'. Interviews with surrogate mothers in Britain. *Journal of Reproductive and Infant Psychology*, **12** (3), 189–98.
8. van den Akker, O.B.A. (2005) A longitudinal pre pregnancy to post delivery comparison of genetic and gestational surrogate and intended mothers: confidence and gynecology. *Journal of Psychosomatic Obstetrics and Gynecology*, **26** (4), 277–84.
9. Fisher, S. and Gilman, I. (1991) Surrogate motherhood: attachment, attitudes and social support. *Psychiatry*, **54**, 13–20.
10. van den Akker, O.B.A. (2007a) Psychological trait and state characteristics, social support and attitudes to the surrogate pregnancy and baby. *Human Reproduction*, **22** (8), 2287–95.
11. Reame, N. and Parker, J. (1990) Surrogate parenting: clinical features in 44 cases. *American Journal of Obstetrics and Gynecology*, **162**, 1220–25.
12. van den Akker, O.B.A. (2007b) Psychosocial aspects of surrogate motherhood. *Human Reproduction Update*, **13** (1), 53–62.
13. Segev, J. and van den Akker, O.B.A. (2006) A review of ART family functioning. Invited paper for *Clinical Effectiveness in Nursing*, **9S2**; e162–e170.
14. van den Akker, O.B.A. (2000) The importance of a genetic link in mothers commissioning a surrogate baby in the UK. *Human Reproduction*, **15** (8), 110–17.
15. Snowden, C. (1994) What makes a mother? Interviews with women involved in egg donation and surrogacy. *Birth*, **21**, 77–84.

5

The impact of stress in pregnancy on the fetus, the infant, and the child

Miri Keren

Tel-Aviv University, Sackler School of Medicine, Geha Mental Health Center Israel

5.1 Introduction

Already in 1926, Freud [1] wrote that 'Intrauterine life and infancy are much more in continuity than the sharp break of delivery make us think'. Recent studies [2, 3] have provided convincing support for the importance of human fetal experience in determining developmental patterns, and for the proposal that many illnesses begin in fetal life.

The concept of *programming* [4] is defined as a process by which a stimulus or an insult during a critical developmental period has a long-lasting or permanent influence. Different organs are sensitive to environmental influences at different times, depending on their rate of cell division. Critical periods are defined by epochs of rapid cell division within an organ.

Glucocorticoids seem to be the main factor in programming the fetal brain and behavior [5], since they are necessary for normal maturation of most regions of the central nervous system. Cortisol may impede formation of neural connections, and reduce neural plasticity. Among the brain structures, the hippocampus has the highest levels of corticosteroid receptors and is thus highly vulnerable to excess levels of glucocorticoids, which may lead to depletion of hippocampal pyramidal neurons, and persistent reduction in the number of hippocampal glucocorticoid receptors.

Parenthood and Mental Health: A Bridge between Infant and Adult Psychiatry Sam Tyano, Miri Keren, Helen Herrman and John Cox
© 2010 John Wiley & Sons, Ltd

The hippocampus also regulates the hypothalamic–pituitary–adrenal (HPA) axis, the function of which changes dramatically during pregnancy with the production and release of CRH (corticotropin-releasing hormone) from the placenta, which triggers the release of CRH, ACTH (adrenocorticotrophin hormone), and cortisol in the fetus as well as in the mother. Sustained elevations of glucocorticoids, such as cortisol in stressful situations, can have deleterious consequences for brain structure and function. Evolution has produced a physiological system where fetal exposure to circulating maternal cortisol is moderated by oxidation of the cortisol to its inactive form by placental 11 beta-hydrosteroid dehydro-genase type 2. Still, 10–20% of active maternal cortisol passes through the placenta, and fetal cortisol levels are significantly correlated with maternal levels.

Consequently, in parallel to the increasing knowledge about the influences of various factors on the developing fetal brain, the issue of the impact of maternal stress on the fetus has become very relevant for adult as well as for child mental health clinicians.

5.2   Data from animal studies

Impact on postnatal behavior

Experimental prenatal stress in rats and monkeys has been shown to induce behavioral changes in their offspring [6]: decreased coping behavior, increased fear of novelty, decreased hippocampal benzodiazepine receptor production, decreased binding capacity of hippocampal glucocorticoid steroid receptors [7] and resulting impact on memory, and delay in developmental milestones.

Impact on postnatal glucose metabolism

In another study, prenatal stress was shown to induce intrauterine growth restriction [8] and lead to glucose intolerance and perturbed feeding behavior in the aged rat. Rat fetuses from stressed rat mothers showed reduced body weight in males and in females, as well as reduced adrenal and pancreas weight in males. Plasma glucose and CORT levels were also significantly reduced [7]. The oral glucose tolerance test showed an increase of plasma glucose and insulin levels. When they were 24 months old, prenatally stressed rats had no alteration in their body or organ weights; however, they exhibited hyperglycemia under basal conditions and after a glucose load, whereas insulinemia was not affected. Maternal stress therefore could program Type II diabetes mellitus. Still, this finding should not be extrapolated to humans without evidence.

5.3   Human studies of the impact of maternal stress on offspring

Definitions of stress during pregnancy

The definition of a stressful event during pregnancy is obviously much more complicated in humans than in rats. First, one needs to take into account the *pregnancy-related anxiety*, i.e. the anxiety inherent to the state of pregnancy (mainly health issues, usually focused on her fetus, but also around herself, and around the fear of delivery itself), to which each woman relates in various ways, depending on her defense mechanisms, own maternal representations, self-image and marital relationship. For the purpose of catching these individual differences, a pregnancy-related anxiety questionnaire has been recently developed [9].

In addition, *life hassles and extraordinary events* may superimpose upon the basal pregnancy-related anxiety level. Again, the definition of what is a stressor for an individual pregnant woman may be quite difficult, because of the pre-pregnancy different levels of resilience and vulnerability. The Prenatal Emotional Stress Index [10] has been developed with these issues in mind.

Another issue is *the timing and the chronicity of the stressor*. 247 women with singleton full-term pregnancies were studied [11, 12], and evaluated on their psychological state (anxiety, depression and perceived stress) and saliva cortisol at three points, the eighteenth, twenty-fourth and thirtieth weeks of gestation. At eight weeks post-partum, the infant's temperament was assessed. Endogenous maternal stress hormones during the *third trimester* of pregnancy (30–32 weeks) *only*, predicted *impaired cortisol regulation, behavioral inhibition and fearfulness in response to novelty* in their infants (very similar to findings in animal studies). It is of note that the effect of prenatal maternal cortisol and depression on infant temperament remained significant after controlling for post-partum maternal depression. In contrast, another study [13] found that women who were in the *first trimester* of pregnancy at the time of the World Trade Center bombing in New York delivered infants significantly earlier than women at later stages of pregnancy. According to the authors, the impact of the stressful event on the fetus depends on whether it occurs before or after the placenta produces the enzyme 11 beta-hydrosteroid dehydrogenase, which converts noxious cortisone to benign cortisone. This is probably not the only mediating factor, since in a sample of pregnant women exposed to earthquake, the same result of earlier delivery was found, but when the exposure occurred during the *second trimester* [14]. One of the possible explanations would be that the time of onset of the production of the enzyme is only one factor among others, such as the intensity of its expression. An eventual support for this hypothesis comes from a study [15] that found that the expression of the enzyme is dramatically reduced in the last period of pregnancy, allowing glucocorticoids to interact with their receptor systems and to influence brain development.

Furthermore, the impact of stressful event may impact on different developmental functions, at different periods of the pregnancy. For example, 58 pregnant women exposed to an ice storm in 1998 and their offspring were studied for two years [16]. The more severe the level of prenatal stress exposure, the poorer was the toddler's *language* ability, *regardless of the timing* of the event. The *cognitive* functioning was worse when the stressor occurred in the *first two trimesters*, especially in the *earliest* period [15].

These findings altogether suggest significant complexity. A precise definition of the nature of the measured stress is therefore crucial to the interpretation of the findings. For instance, is there a different impact of *endogenous individual* stress compared with *exogenous, collective* stress (such as war, natural disaster)? Not less important is the *chronicity* of the stressor. To our best knowledge, there is no comparative study of the impact of chronic stress and acute stress during pregnancy on the fetus and the child's later development.

The definition of endogenous stress is also complex. When 166 pregnant women with high and low anxiety during the second trimester were studied [17], the high-anxiety group had high scores on depression and anger, and raised prenatal norepinephrine and low dopamine levels. High scores on depression and anger were found both pre- and postnatally. The authors concluded that *maternal stress, anxiety and depression may be confounded, and that postnatal anxiety and depression* must be controlled in follow-up studies on the impact of stress from pregnancy to childhood.

Multifetal pregnancy reduction and stress

For women who have experienced the well-documented stresses of infertility, a multifetal pregnancy presents a profound irony: for one potential child, they need to 'kill' another. It would therefore be expected that they develop some emotional distress.

When 91 women between 1.3 and 4.5 years after multifetal pregnancy reduction were interviewed [18], 70% of them recalled a period of mourning after the procedure that lasted an average of three months; *37% of the women reported an anniversary reaction* to the reduction; none was experiencing severe depressive symptoms.

Although multifetal pregnancy reduction is a distressing event, when pregnancy outcome is delivery, it has no significant impact on the mother's mood and psychiatric status [19]. The rate of major depression disorder was the same in mothers who had undergone reduction of a fetus and those who underwent a regular pregnancy. Most of them experienced the infertility as a much more stressful event than the reduction.

Impact of maternal prenatal stress and anxiety on the fetus and newborn

Heart rate

Fetuses of depressed women (N = 57) had higher basal heart rates than fetuses of women with anxiety disorders and those of healthy, low-anxiety women [20].

Weight and alertness

Prenatal cortisol has been found as a significant predictor of prematurity [21], and among 131 pregnant women, prenatal maternal cortisol level, highly correlated with depression and anxiety, was *one of* the contributing variables for fetal activity (as coded during the ultrasound session at 20–28 weeks) and fetal weight [22]. Cortisol level was related to prematurity, and norepinephrine was to birth weight. The mothers with depressive symptoms exhibited a profile of higher prenatal cortisol levels and lower dopamine and serotonin levels. Their infants were born with low birth weight, and low dopamine and serotonin and high cortisol, mimicking their mothers. They also exhibited relatively greater right frontal asymmetry and lower vagal tone. On the Brazelton test, they showed lower scores for optimal habituation, orientation, motor, range of state, and autonomic stability. Among low- and high-anxiety groups of pregnant women, the newborns of the high-anxiety group were more likely to be born under 2500 grams than the controls (34% versus 12%), spent more time in deep sleep and less time in quiet and active alert states, and showed less optimal performance on the Brazelton test [17].

Impact of maternal prenatal stress on the infant

Temperament

When 70 healthy pregnant women were interviewed [23], they showed a significant positive relationship between high levels of maternal state and trait anxiety in late pregnancy and maternal *reports* of difficult temperament of the infant at ten weeks and seven months.

The design was improved in a later study [9] by using observational measures of temperament as defined by difficultness, adaptability and attention regulation (N = 170 mothers and full-term babies, low risk factors sample). Levels of perceived stress were associated with more problems in the infant's adaptation to new situations and unfamiliar persons, and to more crying. This link was much stronger at eight months than at three months, and this may be related to the infant's developmental stage of increased sensibility to unfamiliarity. Motor and mental development at eight months was affected by a high level of stress in pregnancy and were correlated with IQ score in later childhood [24].

Interesting links between infant temperament and maternal stress have been shown [25]: maternal cortisol levels during *the third* trimester of pregnancy predict maternal *report* of increased negative reactivity (startle, or distress in response to novel and surprising stimuli as measured by the fear subscale of the Infant Behavior Questionaire [IBQ] during infancy). Levels measured earlier in pregnancy did not correlate.

Smoking during the first period of pregnancy is a major confounding factor that is associated with temperament and behavior [26]. While controlling for that variable, a significant, though weak, relation between maternal prenatal stress and toddler temperament and problem behavior at 27 months was found in their 119 pregnant women sample with overall low amount of stress and psychosocial risk factors.

Long-term impact of maternal prenatal stress on offspring development

The Avon longitudinal study [27, 28, 29] from pregnancy to ten years (N = 6493) showed that children whose mothers experienced high levels of anxiety (*though mostly not clinical*) in late pregnancy exhibited higher rates of mothers' *report* of emotional/behavioral problems (*though mostly not in the clinical range*) at four years and at six years, and predicted individual differences in cortisol at age ten years. In a more recent study [30], of 636 mother–child pairs from month 4 of pregnancy to age of ten years, found that prenatal exposure to maternal anxiety and depression, together with *poor support in pregnancy*, predicted *clinical* childhood anxiety and depression at age ten, independently of the effect of postnatal maternal depression.

5.4 Discussion

The findings described above have strengthened the notion that prenatal stress has a significant, but not linear, nor necessarily clinical, effect on the development of the fetus, the newborn and the child. Still, the underlying mechanisms of the association between prenatal stress and infant development are unknown. One of the hypothesized pathways of prenatal maternal stress, from pregnancy to adulthood, based on the above data, is the following. Maternal stress during pregnancy leads, in the fetus, to an alteration in programming and development of the HPA axis and the limbic system. This in turn would, in the child and adult, lead to dysregulation of the HPA and/or alteration in limbic functions, with possible long-term outcomes of anxiety, depression, memory impairment and sensitization to post-traumatic stress disorder. The *risk* factor of poor support during pregnancy is very important to remember, since its association with childhood problems in the clinical range has been shown (above). To our best knowledge, *protective* factors have not been systematically studied; for instance, is there a link between the level of pregnancy-related anxiety and stress in pregnancy in the mother and her general attitude towards her baby?

In spite of the well-documented links between maternal prenatal stress and/or anxiety and offspring behavioral, emotional and cognitive outcomes, one may advocate caution in the interpretation of the findings. First, it is not yet clear whether the programming mechanism demonstrated in animals applies to humans, because too few studies have directly assessed the infant's HPA axis function. In most cases, neither the maternal stress/anxiety level during pregnancy, nor the children's behavior difficulties, was in the clinical range. In addition, although prenatal and postnatal development is essentially continuous, analysis of outcome must include consideration of alterations in mother–infant interactions, which have major influences on development and subsequent functions of the HPA axis.

5.5 Conclusion: implications for social health policy

The main clinical implication of knowing that prenatal maternal stress may have a long-term impact on the child's mental health is the need to detect clinical levels of stress, anxiety and depression early in pregnancy. Obviously, universal prevention is unrealistic; therefore the preventive effort should be selective, targeted to women at risk for significantly stressful pregnancies. Exogenous as well as endogenous sources of stress should be identified. One may categorize stressful pregnancies as follows:

- Conflicted pregnancies (unplanned, untimely, acute ambivalence).

- Emotional sensitization (post-infertility pregnancy [IVF, etc.], family history of perinatal complications, maternal borderline disorders/psychiatric history).

- Complicated pregnancies (physical illness of mother, lack of emotional support, socio-economic factors and adverse life events).

Exogenous sources of stress are numerous and diverse. Chronic violent conflict and war are a common example, but surprisingly enough, pregnancy outcomes in these stressful environments have been poorly studied.

In many ways, the decision to give pregnancies a priority in preventive medicine and research is a society-dependent value. Some countries do, many others don't. The more scientific data we can gather on the impact of external factors on fetal brain development, the stronger will be the advocacy for early detection and intervention.

5.6 References

1. Freud, S. (1926) *Inhibitions, Symptoms and Anxiety*. SE. 20, 138.
2. Barker, D.J. (1998) In utero programming of chronic disease. *Clinical Science*, **95**, 115–28.
3. Gluckman, P.D. and Hanson, M.A. (2004) Living with the past: evolution, development and patterns of disease. *Science*, **305**, 1733–36.
4. Nathanielsz, P.W. (1999) *Life in the Womb: the Origin of Health and Disease*. Promethean, Ithaca, NY.
5. Owen, D., Andrews, M.H. and Matthews, S.G. (2005) Maternal adversity, glucocorticoids and programming of neuroendocrine function and behavior, *Neuroscience Biobehavior Review*, **29**, 209–26.
6. Weinstock, M. (2005) The potential influence of maternal stress hormones on development and mental health of the offspring. *Brain Behavior Immunology*, **19**, 296–308.
7. Koehl, M., Darnaudery, M. Dulluc, J. *et al.* (1999) Prenatal stress alters circadian activity of hypothalamo-pituitary-adrenal axis and hippocampal corticosteroid receptors in adult rats of both gender, *Journal of Neurobiology*, **40**, 302–15.
8. Lesage, J., Del-Favero, F., Leonhardt, M. *et al.* (2004) *Journal of Endocrinology*, **181**, 291–96
9. Huizink, A.C., Robles de Medina, P.G., Mulder, E.J.H. *et al.* (2002) Psychological measures of prenatal stress as predictors of infant temperament. *Journal of American Academy of Child and Adolescent Psychiatry*, **41**, 1078–85.
10. Mohler, E., Parzer, P., Brunner, R. *et al.* (2006) Emotional stress in pregnancy predicts human infant reactivity. *Early Human Development*, **82**, 731–37.
11. Davis, E.P., Glynn, L.M., Dunkel-Schetter, C. *et al.* (2005) Maternal plasma corticotropin-releasing hormone levels during pregnancy are associated with infant temperament *Developmental Neuroscience*, **27**, 299–305.
12. Davis, E.P., Glynn, L.M., Dunkel-Schetter, C. *et al.* (2007) Prenatal exposure to maternal depression and cortisol influences infant temperament. *Journal of American Academy of Child Adolescent Psychiatry*, **46**, 737–46.
13. Lederman, S.A., Rauh, V., Weiss, L. *et al.* (2004) The effects of the World Trade Center event on birth outcomes among term deliveries at three Lower Manhattan hospitals. *Environmental Health Perspectives*, **112**, (2004) 1772–78.
14. Glynn, L.M., Wadhwa, P.D., Dunkel-Schetter, C. *et al* (2001) When stress happens matter: effects of earthquake timing on stress responsivity in pregnancy. *American Journal of Obstetrics and Gynecology*, **184**, 637–42.
15. Diaz, R., Brown, R.W. and Seckl, J.R. (1998) Distinct ontogeny of glucocorticoid and mineralcorticoid receptor and 11beta-hydroxysteroid dehydrogenase types I and IImRNA in the fetal rat brain suggest a complex control of glucocorticoid actions. *Journal of Neuroscience*, **18**, 2570–80.
16. Laplante, D.P., Barr, R.G., Brunet, A. *et al.* (2004) Stress during pregnancy affects general intellectual and language functioning in human toddlers. *Pediatric Research*, **56**, 400–10.
17. Field, T., Diego, M., Hernandez-Reif, M. *et al.* (2003) Pregnancy anxiety and comorbid depression an danger effects on the fetus and neonate. *Depression and Anxiety*, **17**, 140–51.
18. Schriner-Engel, P., Walther, V.N., Mindes, J. *et al.* (1995) First-trimester multifetal pregnancy reduction: acute and persistent psychological reactions. *American Journal of Obstetrics and Gynecology*, **172**, 541–47.

19. McKinney, M., Downey, J. and Timor-Tritsch, I. (1995) The psychological effects of multi-fetal pregnancy reduction. *Fertility and Sterility*, **64**, 51–61.

20. Monk, C., Sloan, R.P., Myers, M.M. *et al.* (2004). Fetal heart rate reactivity differs by women's psychiatric status: an early marker for developmental risk? *Journal of American Academy of Child and Adolescent Psychiatry*, **43**, 283–90.

21. Field, T., Diego, M., Hernandez-Reif, M. *et al.* (2004) Prenatal depression effects on the fetus and the newborn. *Infant Behavior and Development*, **27**, 216–29.

22. Field, T., Hernandez-Reif, M., Diego, M. *et al.* (2006) Prenatal cortisol, prematurity and low birthweight. *Infant Behavior and Development*, **29**, 268–75.

23. Van den Bergh, B. (1990) The influence of maternal emotions during pregnancy on fetal and neonatal behavior. *Pre- and Perinatal Psychology Journal*, **5**, 119–30.

24. Huizink, A.C., Robles de Medina, P.G., Mulder, E.J.H. *et al.* (2003) Stress during pregnancy is associated with developmental outcome in infancy. *Journal of Child Psychology and Psychiatry*, **44**, 810–18.

25. Davis, E.P., Glynn, L.M., Dunkel-Schetter, C. *et al.* (2007) Prenatal exposure to maternal depression and cortisol influences infant temperament. *Journal of American Academy of Child and Adolescent Psychiatry*, **46**, 737–46.

26. Gutteling, B.M., de Weerth, C., Willemsen-Swinkels, S.H.N. *et al.* (2005). The effects of prenatal stress on temperament and problem behavior of 27 months-old toddlers. *European Child and Adolescent Psychiatry*, **14**, 41–51.

27. O'Connor, T.G., Heron, J., Glover, V. and the ALSPAC Study Team. (2002) Antenatal anxiety predicts child behavioral/emotional problems independently of postnatal depression. *Journal of American Academy of Child and Adolescent Psychiatry*, **41**, 1470–77.

28. O'Connor, T.G., Heron, J., Golding, J. *et al.* (2003) Maternal antenatal anxiety and behavioral/emotional problems in children: a test of a programming hypothesis. *Journal of Child Psychology and Psychiatry*, **44**, 1025–36.

29. O'Connor, T.G., Ben-Shlomo, Y., Heron, J. *et al.* (2005) Prenatal anxiety predicts individual differences in cortisol in pre-adolescent children. *Biological Psychiatry*, **58**, 211–17.

30. Leech, S.L., Larkby, C.A., Day, R. *et al.* (2006) Predictors and correlates of high levels of depression and anxiety symptoms among children at age 10. *Journal of American Academy of Child and Adolescent Psychiatry*, **45**, 223–30.

6

Unintended pregnancies

Myriam Szejer

Maternity Ward, Antoine Béclère Hospital, Clamart, France

6.1 Introduction

In the animal kingdom, one fact is constant: life calls for more life, and reproduction is an injunction inherent to humans as it is to all living beings. These are the physiological bases behind the definition of the desire for a child. For humans however, in contradistinction to animals but perhaps not for very long, reproduction takes place for the most part sexually. Now, this is what disrupts reproduction, because we are speaking of mammals subject subdued to the order of language. Some reproduce with difficulty, with sterility troubling and threatening. Moreover, sterility is present from the very start: in the Bible it is written that Sarah and Rachel did not manage to give a child to Abraham and Jacob. We can only define the desire for a child based on the failure to bring it about. This may take on different forms: infertility or a pregnancy that imposes itself when it is not wanted.

6.2 The insistence of desire

Today, the desire for a child has to emerge within a culture of planned births ordered by the programming of life and death. This is why the ambivalence inherent in all desire leads to the production of parapraxes responding to a push from the unconscious at the origin of all kinds of inhibitions and transgressions. Among the most widespread we find errors in contraception and its failure. These include forgetting to take the pill and conceptions after the IUD or IUS expiry date. Such errors lead in some cases to termination of pregnancy [1].

Parenthood and Mental Health: A Bridge between Infant and Adult Psychiatry   Sam Tyano, Miri Keren, Helen Herrman and John Cox
© 2010 John Wiley & Sons, Ltd

For teenagers, sexual education lays the accent principally upon contraception, risk of pregnancy and protection against contamination by sexually transmitted diseases. Thus, a culture of the fear of conception is replacing a preparation for reasoned parenthood. This is one of the reasons why in our times we are seeing an upsurge in unintended pregnancies in young people. When the prohibition against having children is so constrictive, the only way left for desire to express itself is to proceed via parapraxis, or even the *passage à l'acte*. Contraceptive errors or stopping contraception temporarily are the most widespread forms of this. They are underwritten by various psychological contexts. The need for self-affirmation in immature young girls, redress following mistreatment, or else pregnancy in the place of an anxiolytic drug are frequent. Sometimes it is a matter of calls for help which one must not forget to interpret. We also come across pregnancies from affective short-comings in which the identification with the child or with an ideal childhood leave behind the imaginary for the real production of a scenario with reparatory properties. The result is more often than not disappointing because these pregnancies are taken up in the inexorable circuit of unconscious repetition.

The irruption of sexual life in young people often happens without words. They tend to retreat into a silence whose wordless outcome may be a pregnancy. First sexual relations are taking place at an ever younger age. The absence of contraceptive is extremely widespread, leading to pregnancies that follow first-time intercourse and which are only revealed very late on, frequently giving rise to traumatic personal and family dramas centered on problems of termination of pregnancy or of the giving up of the child at birth. The morning-after pill and chemical terminations have greatly improved things, but the desire for a child still makes its way through too often. These days, there are very few families who show themselves to be willing to welcome the child of a pregnant adolescent and offer help. It is rather termination of pregnancy, separation from their family or their child, or mother-and-baby hostels that are offered to them. Today, society considers that a woman has to establish herself in life, stabilize her affective life, finish her studies, and set herself up professionally before dreaming of having a child. The ideal time for reproduction is short, and infertility is being encountered more and more. In this context, one would not be surprised to see the fall in birth rates lamented in our industrialized societies. Desire is not so easily tamed.

Since time immemorial so-called 'undesirable' pregnancies have been produced by humans, regardless of their age, just as some have always sought to cancel out pregnancies that seemed too out of place, whether the termination was legal or not, forbidden by religion or not, according to the era or the country [2]. Numerous circumstances governing these pregnancies may be mentioned. The narcissistic reassurance of women with regard to their femininity or even their fertility can lead to pregnancies whose outcome is often abortion or even giving-up the child at birth. The legalization of contraception and then of abortion have certainly improved the way these cases are taken care of, but it hasn't stopped them existing, with their rate remaining stable in most countries where this holds true.

A large number of embryos are conceived at the outset without ever giving rise to living children. Most often they are representatives of poorly resolved Oedipal conflicts in women for whom the access to genitality seems to be thwarted by the difficulty of integrating sexual difference and the recognition of the man in his otherness and complementarity. The child is then often, from the point of view of the unconscious, the fantasmatic incestuous child of the father, a status which does not always authorize the possibility of birth. The fetus then embodies a representation that is only tenable in the register of repression. In such cases, these pregnancies are not seen through to the end and their termination is inevitable. These aborted children remain no less symbolically inscribed and might emerge again in the form of remembrance ('he would have been such and such an age today', and so on) [3], a trace of the mourning that could not be done, vouching for the reality of the desire for a child that produced the event.

Any pregnancy carries meaning in a woman's history, including cases of accidental pregnancy. They arise at moments of psychological crisis and allow for a rejigging of investments in which it is a question of rearranging the places of daughter and mother, of child and adult in the psyche. Moving house, long trips abroad, any destabilizing life situation can offer up circumstances that favor parapraxes responsible for contraceptive failures [4].

Sometimes sterility is linked to the same kind of problem, except that the child who cannot be conceived is not an Oedipal child but a baby made with her mother and paradoxically destined to separate from her or to take her place. For these women, Freudian penis envy represented by the desire for a child is the expression of a refusal of the feminine as a partner to the masculine [5]. In this context, the rejigging sparked off by analytic work or simply provoked by a gynecologist's medical words, or even words from an administrative authority in the case of a request for adoption, can trigger a process and allow for a spontaneous pregnancy, which is always puzzling for couples who were not expecting it. It has happened that spontaneous pregnancies also arise in sterile couples who are being treated medically, and then they decide to terminate. These situations, which fortunately are rare, perturb the medical teams who are often ill at ease with the rambling maze of their patients' unconscious. Such situations underline the complexity of these stakes and the obstacles to mastery and fertility in human beings [6].

Unintended pregnancies are not the prerogative of women. It can happen that men find themselves confronted with the conception of a child that at first they did not want. Sexual desire can blur the stakes of risk-taking. A defective speech-bond in the couple or false or scanty information given to the partner about the mode of contraception can lead to pregnancy. For some, of obsessional temperament, this will be the opportunity to become conscious of their desire for a child. Facing the man with the fait accompli is a way frequently used by women to convince an overly hesitant partner. Such men might even sustain the discourse, saying that they did not want the child; these women have understood that this is the only way for such men to authorize themselves to become a father. The men might demand a termination, but at the risk of the couple's relationship because women take such coercion very badly. It may be that they choose to keep the child, possibly without the father. It is rarer, but possible, to see a father assume on his own the child his partner has brought into the world. We won't go into the development of affective, social and unconscious mechanisms of paternity here; we shall deliberately limit ourselves to those of maternity.

A popular but misguided belief holds that breastfeeding can have a contraceptive effect. A number of brothers and sisters of a newborn who was still at the mother's breast have been conceived in this way. Not wanting to know anything about this biological reality whose information is nevertheless systematically conveyed by the obstetric team has enabled the birth of numerous children in close succession, children whose mother would not have deliberately authorized their conception, but in whom one may ascertain the existence of a very real desire.

The surprise child that stems from before the return of the menstrual cycle is very often the one who allows for the expression of a resistance to weaning. Modern society, which has legalized contraception, finds it hard to accept prolonged breastfeeding. For some mothers, the only solution that enables them to get round the question of weaning will be to replace the newborn they are being asked to separate from with another. The new baby will come to take his place and will thus enable the risk of seeing the mother's anxiety over lack to be put to one side, an anxiety provisionally distanced by the pregnancies and breastfeeding.

The different scenarios from the history of couples and their difficulties in becoming parents are very numerous. Nevertheless, the question of time imposes upon the woman at a certain point in her life the encounter with the real of her body that will no longer be able to wait for the decision to procreate. On this point, the mastery of contraception has made things very complex for some women. The decision to stop it is sometimes much more difficult than the whims of fertility that let the unconscious attend to its business. This is a bit like in the old days, when the child used to arrive more or less when it wanted. Today, you no longer fall pregnant, you decide to get pregnant. It happens that women make up their minds too late and find themselves utterly astonished when confronted with the medical verdict. They had been led to believe that everything could be mastered, in reaction to generations of women that preceded them who submitted to the constraint of having to bring children into the world in an imposed way. Without contesting the social progress acquired by sexual liberation, from contraception to abortion, difficulties of a different order are rearing their heads today. These difficulties bear on the way sexual desire, the desire for a child and their vagaries are taken account of in a society that claims an ever more operational mastery.

Thus it can happen that women who think they are menopausal are surprised to realize they are very much pregnant even though they were persuaded that there was no risk of falling pregnant. These are often women who have made a new life and for whom the investment in the new partner has triggered a hormonal upheaval following the reactivation of metaphorical libidinal stakes from their past: a new man, a new child. Others, faced with the unforeseen event of 'a little one' on its way find themselves disturbed in the investments that they directing towards their grandchildren. The time of grandmothers is no longer the time of mothers. Big families having become rare these days, the discovery of a late unforeseen pregnancy can be an upheaval, whereas prior to contraception it was frequent in families with many siblings. Young women old enough to procreate most often take a dim view of their mothers resuming the maternal function, the implicit rule being: to each her turn in the order of generations.

Clinical vignette

A woman aged 49 went to a medical consultation because she felt nauseous. When she was diagnosed pregnant, she crumbled psychologically, so strong was the shock faced with this unexpected pregnancy. The medical team, doubtless taken up by the patient's imaginary, likewise considered the event to be a catastrophe. Psychological support had to be brought in immediately. This allowed this woman to realize that the child was not a tragic transgression, that she had made a new life for herself, and that a mother's relatively advanced age was perhaps not an obstacle to a child's life to the extent that his adult half-brothers and half-sisters could look after him if ever he were to lose his parents. They were consulted and accepted the new family situation with pleasure. The parturient woman found her lust for life again; the pregnancy and the birth went by without a hitch (she was very appreciative of the progress in obstetrics over the last 30 years). After the turmoil of the first moments of gestation, the child was welcomed by its mother as a gift from life.

6.3 Abortion

In some contexts, whether they be psychological in disturbed women, socio-economic in poor families, or political in some countries where contraception and/or termination of pregnancy are outlawed, abortion can become commonplace and serve as a means of contraception when it becomes repetitive, disregarding the health of the person concerned. Everything transpires as if desire were insisting in spite of any logical reasoning. These women are poorly supported by the family planning centers because their repetitive behavior signals for them the powerlessness of the system faced with the persistence of the symptom when it is not being heard in a symbolic dimension.

6.4 Rape, incest and denials of pregnancy

Pregnancy following a rape will be treated differently according to the victim's history. Where some become attached to the child as something from this violence that allows them to stay alive and make amends; others will only see in the baby the figure of the rapist. The baby will constantly recall the trauma. These women will envisage an abortion or, if the pregnancy has gone too far, giving up child, emblematic of the drama, whose memory they will never stop trying to distance by not taking the risk of seeing, in the expression of the baby's genes, the traits of the aggressor. When such children are given up, it is with the goal of allowing them to grow up in a family where the phantom of the aggressor will not be summoned in the parents' looks.

During the violence of war in the former Yugoslavia, a program of rapes was perpetrated. There were pregnancies arising from these rapes. Some of these women came to France. We observed that, depending on their history, they would choose abortion or, if the legal limit-date had been exceeded or their religious orientation prohibited the operation, to give up the child at birth. Nevertheless, a minority decided to keep their child, stating that it was not the child's fault and calling upon a maternal sentiment that came to fend off the horrors they had lived through, allowing for the exorcising of the unconscious guilt that is linked to any sexual abuse.

We may compare these situations to those of pregnancies that are the outcome of incestuous relationships. In this case, the problem is rendered even more complex by the modification in filiation this entails. The figure of the aggressor is superimposed onto that of a father or brother. While being faced with the transgression of the fundamental laws that structure our society, these women are taken up in a double discourse, often supported by the silence of a mother who implicitly imposes a feeling of guilt on them for what they have been submitted to. This is why a large number of them never lodge a complaint. They cannot betray the family bond even if its definition has been scorned. Children who are the product of these crimes will have to get by with the difficulty, even the impossibility, of thinking of themselves in their right place in society.

Whether it is a matter for rape or incest, the consequences on the victims will remain in part irreducible and may become manifest through one symptom or another throughout their existence.

Pedophilia can produce pregnancies in young, barely pubescent girls, and one may wonder what status it will take on in their psyche. Their level of maturity does not allow them to think through these pregnancies and they might take refuge behind a repression using the negation of their emotions. It is difficult to anticipate what form the symptomatic return will take later on.

The denial of pregnancy, which consists in getting to the end of the gestation period without consciously knowing that one is pregnant, has been estimated as occurring for one out of every 1500 births [7]. One may observe a high representation in that population of women who suffer from psychological disorders. One must distinguish carefully between denial and negation. In the latter case, repression is incomplete and only bears on a part of the representation and the feelings linked to it. Negation is much more frequent than denial, which allows the mother to either mask her ambivalence towards the child or to protect it from hostile feelings that come from her or those around her. Birth can bring with it relief and allow the mother–baby bond to develop. More often than not, the child is warmly welcomed; often however the child might be given up due to the socio-economic, psychiatric or family situation.

Clinical vignette

A woman, mother of three, comes to A & E for acute abdominal pain. She is in fact in labor. The child is born, to the great astonishment of its mother, who had already seen three pregnancies through to the end. The father is summoned and the couple decide to give the child up. The mother explains to the psychologist that she does not want to bring another child into a family where the husband is seriously alcoholic and violent. Not wanting to add the misfortune of a fourth child to that of the first three, the denial had functioned to save its life. If this mother had been aware of her pregnancy, she would have quite reasonably felt the duty to terminate in spite of a desire for a child being well and truly present but repressed on account of the necessities of the context it arose in.

6.5 Pregnancy and mental illness

Finally, psychiatric patients suffering from serious and chronic psychotic states, such as schizophrenia, delusional states and serious neuroses, may not realize they are pregnant. For them, the reality of their body has no link to their perceptions and their mental representation. The diagnosis is made late on in the pregnancy, which takes a long while to become visible. For these women, the real is their delusions and hallucinations, and not their body which they perceive in a disturbed way. Moreover they are rarely sick and feel very little pain. These are the same women who burn or scar themselves to try to gain access to their sensations. The perceptions of pregnancy are not felt or interpreted as such.

Some births following a denial or a psychiatric pathology can lead to infanticide. These are pregnancies that unfold in silence. They are unthinkable, as much for the women themselves as for their partner, family and society, which let themselves be contaminated by the denial and do not suspect that a child might be developing. These babies, not managing to inscribe their otherness in their mother's psyche, are killed by the mothers, with neither emotion nor guilt. The child is not an other, and pregnancy does not exist for them. These stories often make headline news. Babies' bodies are sometimes found deep-frozen, buried or hidden, and provoke widespread indignation and incomprehension. Denial, a well-known pathology for obstetric services, fascinates and triggers the public's incomprehension when it is followed by infanticide committed by women who appear, but only appear, to be of sane mind [8].

6.6 Conclusion

All out-of-place pregnancies have always posed a problem for society because they upset human order. Though we are tending towards an evolution in which procreation is becoming increasingly dissociated from sexuality, even today children are still being conceived without their mothers being aware of it. We can see that the question of unintended pregnancy is not limited to forgetting to take the pill but covers multiple situations which, though they can be categorized, still have to be approached case by case in accordance with each pregnancy's history, so as to be able to propose the best-adapted accompaniment.

A certain number of children are born of these unintended gestations. Might one say, somewhat provocatively, based on the analytic definition of desire considered as being exclusively unconscious, that there only exist children who are desired? Numerous patients report however in analysis that they were not desired. Some thereby justify psychological and physical abuse they feel they have been subjected to. Others lay the emphasis on their capacities of personal resilience; they situate this de-narcissizing aspect of their history as the motor of their success. Thus they come to legitimize their birth and move on.

The children who arise from involuntary pregnancies are for the most part warmly welcomed, a baby's capacity for seduction being immense. They may be pampered to make up for their parents' guilt at not having consciously wanted them. It sometimes happens that some are impeded in their development. Either because of parental over-investment – because stuffing a child full of food is not necessarily an act of love, and parental over-investment can put the child in an affective prison he will never escape from – or through all the forms of abuse that shape their psyche, sometimes in a way that is irreversible.

If their intelligence is preserved, some will call upon perverse adaptive defense mechanisms that may lead them to marginalization and delinquency [9]. Depending on the history each pregnancy will take root in, the child will confront its destiny with a handicap of varying weight. Its development will depend principally on the quality of the parents' affective adjustment and the support of the social and family circle that will welcome the child and accompany its development.

6.7 References

1. Fourez, M. (2004) L'enfant du désir, in *Paroles de femmes, paroles de mères* (ed. M. Fourez), Editions L'Harmattan, Paris, pp. 156–69.
2. Szejer, M. (1994) *Ces neuf mois-là*, Robert Laffont editeur, Paris.

3. Lambrichs, L. (1993) *Journal d'hannah*. Editions La différence, Paris.

4. Bachelot, A. (2002) Aspects psychologiques de la grossesse non prévue, in *De la contraception à l'avortement, sociologie des grossesses non prévues. Questions en Santé Publique* (eds N. Bajos and M. Ferrand), Éditions de l'INSERM, Paris, pp. 79–109.

5. Faure Pragier, S. (2004) *Les bébés de l'inconscient*. PUF éditions, Paris.

6. Chatel, M. (1998) *Malaise dans la procreation*. Albin Michel éditions, Paris.

7. Dayan, J. (2010) Le déni de grossesse, in *La naissance* (eds. R Frydman and M.Szejer), éditions Albin Michel, Paris.

8. Daligand. L. (2010) L'infanticide, in *La naissance* (eds. R Frydman and M.Szejer), éditions Albin Michel, Paris.

9. Szejer, M. (2009) *Si les bébés pouvaient parler*. éditions Bayard, Paris.

7

Clinical challenges of adolescent motherhood

George M. Tarabulsy,[1] Annie Bernier,[2] Simon Larose,[3] Fanie Roy,[1] Caroline Moisan[1] and Claire Baudry[1,*]

[1]École de psychologie, Université Laval, Canada
[2]Département de psychologie, Université de Montréal, Québec, Canada
[3]Département d'études sur l'enseignement et l'apprentissage, Université Laval, Canada

7.1 Introduction

In most Western nations, there was a time in the last 50 years when it was not unusual for young women before the age of 20 to bear children. This is no longer the case. One of the major trends over the last few decades has been for women to choose to delay having children. Presently, in Canada, the mean maternal age for a first child hovers around 29 years and the situation is very much the same for many Western nations. As might be expected, the infants of adolescent mothers make up a small minority of births every year in developed nations. For example, in Canada, the adolescent fertility rate for every 1000 women is 14, it is 15 in Australia, 9 in Finland, and 8 in France. At 26 and 41 for every 1000 women in the United Kingdom and the United States respectively, the fertility rate of adolescent women is substantially higher in these countries [1]. Worldwide, however, there is great variability in these rates, as can be observed in Table 7.1, and the implications of

*The authors would like to thank the Social Sciences and Humanities Research Council of Canada, and the Fonds québécois de recherche sur la société et al culture for funding.

Table 7.1 Adolescent fertility observed in different countries

Argentina	62
Australia	15
Brazil	56
Canada	14
China	5
Columbia	96
Dominican Republic	98
Egypt	27
Finland	9
France	8
Nigeria	126
Slovakia	21
Thailand	46
United Kingdom	26
United States	41
Zambia	146

Source: Data taken from World Health Organization (2009). *World Health Statistics*. World Health Organization Press, Geneva.

young motherhood are necessarily different across cultures and national contexts. In most cases, however, they are considered as vulnerable.

Even though their numbers are small in absolute terms in Western culture, adolescent mother–infant dyads are considered to be at high psychosocial risk. Risk for the mother is often defined in terms of the limited academic and occupational opportunities that emerge after the birth of a first child, and in the quality of relationships that adolescent mothers engage in after the birth of their child. It is also defined on the basis of the general environment that provides the context for the mother–child relationship, as well as different maternal psychological factors that characterize young mothers. Adolescent mothers report greater levels of poverty and isolation, anxiety, depression and substance abuse [2]. Care for these young women often comes at high human and social cost. For infants of teen mothers, risk often materializes in terms of their over-representation in different public sectors. Researchers have demonstrated that the children of adolescent mothers in the United States are widely over-represented in specialized educational services, in the use of health care, in child welfare services and in different legal categories (delinquency, incarceration). The human concerns and social cost linked to adolescent motherhood have led researchers, clinicians and public health officials to devote considerable attention to this phenomenon. Clearly, not all young mothers are at risk and not all infants of young mothers are destined to problems in development and much has been said about overstating this risk [3]. Risk is defined in terms of statistical likelihood and, from a clinical perspective, remains a hypothesis that requires validation with each specific individual.

But the risk is there, and several research groups have documented it on several levels. The goal of this chapter is threefold. First, we will highlight some of the challenges that adolescent mothers and their infants face during both the prenatal and postnatal periods. These challenges include biological, psychological and social dimensions. Second, we will highlight how these factors are related to one of the important motors of infant development: mother–infant interaction and the establishment of the attachment relationship. We will make the point that the relation between problematic biology and contexts and infant cognitive and socio-emotional development may be mediated by the processes involved in the establishment of early attachment relationships. In the third section, we will describe approaches to prevention and intervention that have proven useful in addressing some of these challenges and in breaking the mediation between risk and child development.

7.2   Early challenges faced by young mothers

As a social and psychological phenomenon, adolescent motherhood constitutes a confirmation of both social selection and social influence theories of human development. Social selection theories suggest that the risk of early motherhood, for mothers and infants, actually precedes pregnancy. Social influence theories suggest that adolescents who become mothers increase the level of risk to which they expose themselves and their infants by engaging in a developmental path that involves fewer positive developmental opportunities in personal, social, educational and professional spheres [3]. Within this perspective, there is also the notion that pregnancy and motherhood in adolescence may be the beginning of new developmental paths, where the probability of positive outcome is lower than prior to the pregnancy. Here, early motherhood actually adds to the level of risk the dyad is already exposed to. Both the social selection and social influence positions have received empirical support and, as such, it is important to view the developmental challenges of young motherhood in the context of a continuously evolving ecological context that precedes pregnancy, extends beyond birth, but for which decisive changes take place with the onset of pregnancy and infant birth.

Biological risk and fetal programming

The biological challenges of pregnant adolescents are numerous. Adolescent mothers have often not completed their physical maturation processes such that their own biological development may compete with the fetus for resources. As well, they are more likely to engage in problematic nutritional behaviors, smoking, and drug and alcohol use, than mothers in low-risk contexts. Adolescents make less use of medical services during their pregnancy. They more frequently encounter complications during the prenatal and perinatal period [3] and pregnant teens report greater levels of prenatal stress [4]. Increasingly, researchers have pointed towards such prenatal factors as contributing to infant neonatal health and early development through processes linked to fetal programming [4, 5]. The fetal programming hypothesis suggests that atypical intrauterine environments, caused by problematic nutrition, the consumption of toxic substances or by high levels of parental stress, may cause the fetus's neurological and endocrinological systems to develop in ways that are adapted to their current environment, but that alter its ability to adapt to subsequent, postnatal environments. Recent work by Keenan [4] and O'Connor [5] demonstrate that such processes may be particularly salient for adolescent mothers.

Keenan has shown an association between indices of psychological distress during pregnancy and a number of basic neonatal health outcomes. That these indices of neonatal health were gathered at birth precludes postnatal factors as confounding results. O'Connor has shown that prenatal stress predicts different aspects of postnatal socio-emotional development, even after controlling for postnatal levels of stress. Parallel findings have been observed for smoking, and drug and alcohol use, where even small doses consumed during pregnancy have been linked to emotional regulation and cognitive development. Such findings underline the notion that a major challenge during the prenatal period is to address basic biological risk and fetal health [4, 5]. However, this class of risk factors does not occur independently of the pregnant or parenting teen's developmental ecology. In particular, it has been shown that problematic health behavior is linked to the social ecology that provides the context for the mother–infant dyad.

Social challenges

Parents draw on different forms of social support during the transition to parenthood. In low-risk circumstances, the most helpful support for mothers comes from the partner, usually the biological father of the infant. Other members of the social network are involved in providing support to new mothers and fathers, most notably members of the extended family and friends. Support processes seem to be similar in the high-risk contexts of adolescent mothers. Milan and her colleagues [6] found that patterns of emotional distress in pregnant or parenting adolescent girls over the course of 18 months were directly linked to levels of partner support. However, some of the results in this study also raise important questions. For example, teen mothers reporting high levels of relationship conflict were at greatest risk for emotional distress, most of this conflict taking place with the partner. Other studies have made similar observations regarding partner support: Spieker and Bensley [7] showed that support provided by fathers was unrelated to infant attachment security, a result also found by Tarabulsy and colleagues [8], who even showed a negative association between paternal support and attachment security. Spieker and Bensley and others have suggested that partner support was perhaps more important for maternal emotional well-being, but caregiving was under the greater influence of the support provided by the adolescent mother's own mother.

Relatedly, in a large study of high-risk families, Jaffee and colleagues [3] were able to document that the presence of fathers in the family may be a risk factor for behavior problems, if fathers showed high levels of antisocial behavior. Thus, while some have found that the presence of fathers helps mothers' overall adjustment [6], results have not been nearly as consistent as in the low-risk literature, and there is the suggestion that, sometimes, the presence of fathers may prove to be problematic for parenting and child development in high-risk contexts. These studies suggest that adolescent mothers draw on their support network somewhat differently than low-risk mothers, perhaps depending on non-partner support to a greater degree, more often calling on their own parents and extended families. This suggestion may take on added significance when one considers the relative instability of many adolescent mother–father relationships, and the risk that such relationships pose for conflict and sometimes violence [3, 7, 8]. In many cases, the father of the child often is not a teenager and is sometimes many years older than the mother [8]. This difference, and the possibility that the father may have adjustment problems [3] at a developmentally meaningful time for the mother, may contribute to exacerbating the difficulties that high-risk motherhood already presents [3, 8]. Similar suggestions have been made regarding the potential recourse to friends as support. In effect, while social support is clearly viewed as a positive characteristic of the developmental ecology, and fathers have the potential of being helpful to mothers, there is question as to whether young mothers' networks and marital relationships are objectively helpful, or whether they possess the same, high-risk characteristics as the young mothers themselves [6, 7, 8, 9].

Representational challenges

The biological and social support features of adolescent mothers may be derived from, and contribute to, different aspects of their cognitive representations of relationships. The study of mothers' general representations of relationships has been undertaken from different perspectives: parental attitudes, expectations about relationships, internal working models, attachment state of mind, interpersonal models or relational schemas. Presently, we will focus on findings derived from attachment research that have addressed attachment state of mind relative to the young mother's own parents or towards her child. Attachment research has provided numerous insights into the workings of relationship representations of parents and children. Furthermore, in much the same way that the Bowlby-inspired theory drew from different perspectives in psychiatry, psychology and the biological sciences, the development of attachment theory – especially in the area of cognitive representations – has received contributions from many different theoretical and methodological paradigms. This framework will be helpful in understanding how general relationship representations are involved in the manner in which young mothers structure the early interactive environments of their infants.

This research has revealed at least three noteworthy aspects of adolescent mothers' general relationship representations: First, young mothers often report traumatic experiences related to abuse or loss. Bailey and colleagues [9] showed that between 35% and 37% of adolescent mothers in their sample reported experiencing either maltreatment or loss as children, a result that had been documented in other reports. To the degree that these experiences are not cognitively integrated, researchers suggest that young mothers remain 'Unresolved with respect to trauma or loss' in their attachment state of mind. When discussing traumatizing events, these young mothers will show signs of confusion or disorientation, and will have difficulty situating events in time or regulating emotions. Much research has shown that an unresolved state of mind predates many different psychological syndromes, including depression, anxiety disorders, borderline personality disorder and substance abuse. This is an important concern in that these mental health problems are highly prevalent in populations of adolescent mothers, sometimes two or more times more so than in low-risk circumstances [3, 6]. Unresolved states of mind are also related to problems in the development of relationships. Bailey and colleagues describe a process by which traumatic experiences (especially those related to maltreatment), structure memories of events to prevent highly negatively charged emotions from impinging on consciousness. Such defensive processes may be helpful to regulate the negative affect derived from these memories, but they prevent the individual from coping with the contexts that elicit these memories, and from integrating present circumstances with past events. Sometimes, the eliciting events involve interactions with parents, and the young mother's emotions and behavior in such circumstances will draw on early attachment experiences characterized by trauma, thus hindering cognitive integration of trauma. When the eliciting events are interactions with her own infant, such lack of resolution will set a problematic relationship framework for the dyad and problematic maternal responses to infant behavior. If traumatic experiences were frequent or chronic, integrating them will prove even more difficult [9].

Second, high-risk environments may foster relationship representations linked to hostility or helplessness. Even in the absence of traumatic events, the high-risk environments that provided the context for young mothers' development may have been characterized by chronically high levels of relationship insensitivity or hostility, leading mothers to become vigilant toward their social environment. Such vigilance may be viewed as adaptive in the immediate high-risk context in that it may help individuals predict and avoid problematic interactions, or mobilize their own hostility to respond in a way that is coherent with immediate demands. It is also possible that during their childhood, when confronted with regularly dysfunctional interactions, the attempts of young mothers to change them were met with repeated failure. Such failure by children may lead to perceptions of helplessness and compliance towards others in different social settings. Again, there may be an adaptive function to an attitude of helplessness in a dysfunctional environment: attempts to change the content of relationships and interactions being repeatedly unfruitful, an individual may perceive themselves as unable to exert any control in such settings, and choose compliance and other relationship objectives, rather than attempts at repairing interaction, because these other goals are more easily achieved.

In an important paper on the relations between attachment states of mind and mother–infant interactions, Lyons-Ruth, Yellin, Melnick and Atwood [10] have suggested that along with unresolved trauma, hostile and helpless states of mind may be the representational dispositions that lead to the most dysfunctional mother–infant interactions. In both cases, adaptation to the immediate environment may lead to the elaboration of perceptions of relationships as sources of danger that must be met with hostility or compliance. When such representations are turned toward the infant, when the parent perceives the infant as a source of danger, dysfunctional interactions emerge and problematic relationships that direct future development are formed [9, 10].

Third, in these three aspects of relationship representations (unresolved trauma, hostility, helplessness), young mothers may foster attributions of intent toward their infant that are linked to adaptation in the immediate environment, but lead to problematic maternal behavior. Some examples taken from interviews conducted within our own research program may help illustrate this point:

- 'My baby was quite nasty with me today, moving all over the place even when I told him to stop' (statement made by a pregnant teen).

- 'When my son falls and hurts himself, I really don't want to help him because he has to learn that it is a tough world and that no one is there to help him. He has to make it on his own' (mother of a 12-month-old).

- 'Sometimes she really wants to manipulate me by crying all the time. I have seen her give me the finger when I left her in her chair. She makes me mad and I just won't fall for that' (mother of a 7-month-old).

- 'He is just like his dad. He is very independent and pretty much does what he wants. There is not a whole lot I can do to make him change when he wants something' (mother of a 10-month-old).

Such statements may be reflective of problematic representations that young mothers may have of their infants. They also suggest how adaptation in certain contexts may yield to inaccurate inferences and perceptions regarding infant development and needs in the context of the mother–infant relationship. In fact, it is possible that the many studies that have identified problems in young parents' knowledge of infant development have in part tapped into their representations of relationship organization and attributions of infant intentions [8]. Young parents' understanding of child development may in part be derived from unresolved traumatic experiences or the adaptation imperatives of high-risk environments. In this perspective, one may view the relationship-based representational challenges to young motherhood as involving past experiences, as well as current, ongoing developmental process whose nexus with child development is the mother–infant relationship [7].

7.3 Adolescent mother–infant interaction and the elaboration of attachment

It is perhaps not surprising that in this developmental ecology, and given their representational dispositions towards their social environment and their child, adolescent mothers are at greater risk of interacting in problematic ways with their infant. Several research groups have shown that teen mothers are less sensitive towards infant signals and behaviors, and more often adopt coercive and intrusive interactive behaviors, than low-risk mothers. They less frequently engage in contingent, face-to-face interaction, they vocalize less, less frequently hold their infant and will more often leave infants unattended for long periods of time, being sometimes physically or psychologically withdrawn even when infant signals are clear [7, 8].

Studies have shown that these interactive behaviors are directly linked to the relationship-based representations of young mothers and are important precursors to insecure and disorganized attachments [7, 8, 11]. The hallmark of secure attachment is the infant's ability to benefit from the relationship through proximity-seeking and contact maintenance with their mother, as a secure base for exploration and as a point of reference for emotion regulation challenges. Insecure-avoidant infants have learned to manage distress through exploration, emphasizing their autonomy in their early attachment relationship. Insecure-ambivalent infants will use proximity and contact with parents to manage distress, but will remain upset for long periods of time and remain focused on parental whereabouts and behavior rather than play or exploration. Unlike infants in other forms of insecurity, where relationships seem to be coherent in structure, disorganized infants show a number of problematic behaviors that reveal either breakdowns in strategies to manage distress, an absence of relational strategy or conflicting strategies that prevent infants from interacting effectively with parents in comforting ways. The underlying feature is the fear that the infant experiences, which conflicts with their ability to orient towards the parent in times of distress. Frightened, frightening or highly insensitive parenting has been shown to be linked to disorganized attachment in adolescent mother–infant dyads and other high-risk groups [12]. Insecure and disorganized attachment is considered to place infants at risk for future socioemotional development.

In a meta-analysis, Van IJzendoorn and colleagues [13] have shown that adolescent mother–infant dyads are over-represented in the disorganized (23%) and insecure (60%) attachment categories. Since that study, several researchers have obtained results where over 65% of adolescent mother–infant dyads were insecure, with over 40% being classified as disorganized [11] echoing the findings of other researchers [8].

Problems have also been observed in other spheres of development. Spieker and her colleagues found that children of adolescent mothers are at greater risk for different problems on the level of socio-emotional, language and cognitive development. At six years of age, only 27% of their sample did not show problems in one of these domains [14], underlining the challenges these children face.

Taken together, these results suggest that one of the mediators of infant and early child development – mother–infant interaction and early attachment – shows infants of adolescent mothers to be at high risk, reflected in infant attachment security and organization. As secure attachment is an early indicator of infant ability to organize emotion regulation behaviors around parents in times of distress, to orient themselves with confidence toward parents when alarmed, and to use the parent as a secure base for exploration of the environment, the high levels of insecurity and disorganization that have been found suggest that, by the end of the first year, these infants are already showing signs of the developmental difficulties to come, later reflected in broader indices of socio-emotional health used by public health administrators. In light of this observation, many prevention and intervention efforts have been developed to help foster positive change for adolescent mother–infant dyads.

7.4 Intervention with adolescent mothers and their infants

We and others have argued elsewhere that in structuring intervention with young mothers and other high-risk populations, it is critical that:

1 The targets of intervention be appropriately defined; and that

2 All targets of intervention receive specialized intervention [15].

There are relatively few domino effects in intervention with high-risk populations such as adolescent mother–infant dyads. One type of positive effect does not automatically lead to positive change in other spheres. This is of particular importance in the context of prevention and intervention efforts with young mothers, where the challenges are numerous and on different levels (biological, socio-economic, psychological, interactive and developmental). Strategies that target the biological conditions of pregnancy and neonatal health do not necessarily lead to improvements in maternal adaptation. Likewise, strategies that focus on adaptation often do not change mother–infant interactions and infant developmental processes. Each target of intervention requires intentional efforts aimed at that specific target [15].

We currently focus on two broad categories of strategic action. The first category is intended to improve the psychosocial circumstances of the mother–infant dyad. Among the stated objectives of such strategies are:

- Improved family organization and perceptions of personal competence in different domains, such that maternal stress decreases and general well-being increases during the pre- or postnatal periods;

- Improved networking and the establishment of positive, mentoring relationships with community members and social services to make better use of competent support structures; and

- Improved knowledge of child development and of the factors that favor it.

Many strategies that have favored such objectives have been delivered via community centers, school settings, home visiting professionals, paraprofessionals or volunteers. While much of this work is provided in the context of community health services and remains vastly under-evaluated, especially with respect to young mothers, some strategies have been evaluated in quasi-experimental designs or randomized control trials. For example, Saddler and colleagues [16] were able to show that young mothers who participated in a school-based parenting curriculum, together with school-based help with child-care, showed notable increases in overall adaptation. Mother–infant interactions also appeared to improve but to a lesser degree, as did some aspects of socio-emotional development. Other community-based strategies have been implemented and have shown successful reductions in teen mother adaptation [15].

In the second category, prevention and intervention strategies are specifically focused on improving mother–infant interaction. Such approaches have underlined the importance of mother–infant interaction in different domains of development and have highly structured, manualized programs aimed at increasing maternal sensitivity and responsiveness to infant distress, cues and signals, and the overall contingency of mother–infant interaction. In a randomized control trial of a targeted video-feedback intervention, Moran, Pederson and Krupka [17] showed meaningful improvements in maternal sensitivity between infant ages 6 and 24 months, as well as improvements in infant attachment security. Similar results have been obtained on the level of maternal behavior and infant socio-emotional and cognitive development by several groups of researchers when intervention strategies focused on interactions [15].

Two issues remain to be addressed in the context of a discussion on prevention and intervention strategies with young mothers. First, relatively few evaluations of comprehensive strategies are reported in the literature that address the biological health of mothers during the pre- and postnatal periods, as well as social support and organizational needs and the quality of mother–infant interactions. When they are, the results are not always favorable to such approaches. Perhaps the best-known such approach and the one that has yielded the most convincing results is the nurse–family partnership, developed by David Olds and a number of collaborators [18]. The strength of this approach has been its comprehensiveness, and the consistent finding that exposure to intervention reduces biological risk during the prenatal period and at birth, and increases social support and parental perceptions of competence. One of the advantages of this approach for young mother–infant dyads is the presence of stable, highly trained intervention personnel who establish supportive, mentoring relationships with mothers. Olds and colleagues have underlined how the combination of high levels of competence and the establishment of stable relationships between home-visiting nurses and mothers are critical for the effectiveness of the program. The program has also shown positive impacts on the quality of interactions and markers of infant, child and adolescent development. The methodological rigor of the repeated evaluations, the high level of training given to the home-visiting nurses and the specific concern towards adolescent mothers suggest that a comprehensive model of intervention can be successful.

A second issue concerns some of the variables that moderate the effectiveness of early prevention and intervention, and the limits of this approach for intervening with high-risk dyads. For example, the video-feedback strategy used by Moran and colleagues [17] appeared to be ineffective when working with mothers who reported unresolved trauma during an interview. Likewise, some strategies have been shown to be effective on the level of mother–infant interaction, but less so on the level of maternal indices of adjustment. Other authors have found that maternal adaptation and well-being place certain limits on the effectiveness of prevention and intervention initiatives and that these characteristics of mothers touch on the domain of general maternal representations of their environment and relationships. In response to such findings, Lieberman [19] has strongly argued for targeting the quality of interactions, to address infant developmental issues, but also to move beyond providing support and more positive contexts and to address the more cognitive features linked to the representational domain. A focus on interactions, family support and organization, or on biology, does not preclude therapeutic intervention that addresses representational issues linked to the developmental histories and environments of adolescent mothers. A valuable contribution to future intervention research will be to document the role played by maternal representations of relationships and overall mental health in the effectiveness of early intervention.

7.5 Conclusion

Three different issues and directions for future research are raised in this review of adolescent mother–infant dyads. First, it is important to reiterate that there is no order to the different challenges that adolescent mothers and their infants face. Biology does not necessarily precede representations. Representations of relationships are intimately linked to mental health, in which one finds the problems of substance abuse, nutrition and family organization that are related to how mothers take care of themselves and the fetus during their pregnancy. Interactions can influence biology as well. To the degree that social interactions are involved in the psychological distress that may be at work in fetal programming and, later, in postnatal mother–infant interaction, the social environment is intricately woven into biological development [4]. But biology can precede both representations and interactions – small, underweight infants born to high-risk mothers are more difficult to read and respond in less predictable ways to maternal input, making it difficult to develop harmonious relationships and to engage in positive developmental trajectories. Thus, while we have little information about how the many challenges young mothers face are causally related, we do know that they are important to target in intervention initiatives. Positive change at any level of the processes that have been described appears to modify either maternal or infant development. Relatedly, it is important to reiterate that adolescent motherhood, and being the infant of an adolescent mother, is embedded within this complex ecology. Adolescent pregnancy and childbirth are markers of risk that was already present. The arrival of the infant marks an increase in risk and, in this respect, raises the need for effective clinical initiatives.

Second, there appear to be a number of potentially helpful intervention strategies. These strategies focus on different variables linked to maternal characteristics, mother–infant interaction and infant development. Those that appear most effective in influencing infant development are those that are highly focused on improving mother–infant interaction. Such interventions touch on one of the critical mediators of the link between risk and infant development and seem successful in improving the quality of the most proximal developmental processes. As such, it would seem a priority for intervention strategies that aim to improve infant development to systematically address the factors affecting this critical interaction. The study of such strategies will also be important for scientific reasons. Intervention studies where levels of a given variable are manipulated provide an experimental context for testing causal relations between variables in ways that correlational research (not involving intervention) cannot. Such experimental studies will allow for a clearer understanding of the contributions and potential moderating roles of representational and mental health variables to intervention effectiveness, mother–infant interaction and infant development. Moreover, it will be possible to consider how paternal involvement in the family and the father's characteristics facilitate or hinder intervention effectiveness with the young mother and her child. This information will be critical to establishing the most effective ways of targeting intervention to specific dimensions of the adolescent mother–infant ecology.

Finally, there are several issues regarding adolescent pregnancy and parenting that were not addressed in the current chapter, most notable are those linked to the debilitating effects of chronic poverty on mothers and children, as well as issues related to education, job training and other school or occupational concerns. On a developmental level, such concerns relate to family organization and planning, and to the ability of parents to be empowered to integrate and contribute to the development of their infants and their communities. Such challenges take different forms across cultural and sociopolitical contexts and it will be important for future work to identify both general challenges to young parents as well as those that apply in specific ecologies within and across nations.

7.6 References

1. World Health Organization (2009) *World Health Statistics*. World Health Organization Press, Geneva.
2. Whitman, T.L., Borkowski, J.G., Keogh, D.A. and Weed, K. (2001) *Interwoven Lives: Adolescent Mothers and Their Children*. Society for Research on Adolescence. Mahwah, NJ, USA.
3. Jaffee, S., Caspi, A., Moffitt, T., Belsky, J. and Silva, P. (2001) Why are children born to teen mothers at risk for adverse outcomes in young adulthood. Results from a 20-year longitudinal study. *Development and Psychopathology*, **13**, 377–97.
4. Keenan, K., Sheffield, R. and Boeldt, D. (2007) Are prenatal psychological or physical stressors associated with suboptimal outcomes in neonates born to adolescent mothers? *Early Human Development*, **83**, 623–27.

5. O'Connor, T., Heron, J., Golding, J., Glover, V. & the ALSPAC study team (2003) Maternal antenatal anxiety and behavioral/emotional problems in children: A test of the programming hypothesis. *Journal of Child Psychology and Psychiatry*, **44**, 1025–36.

6. Milan, S., Ickovicks, J.R., Kershaw, T. *et al.* (2004) Prevalence, course and predictors of emotional distress in pregnant and parenting adolescents. *Journal of Consulting and Clinical Psychological*, **72**, 328–40.

7. Spieker, S.J. and Bensley, L. (1994) Roles of living arrangements and grandmother support in adolescent mothering and infant attachment. *Developmental Psychology*, **30**, 102–11.

8. Tarabulsy, G.M., Bernier, A., Provost, M.A. *et al.* (2005) Another look inside the gap: ecological contributions to the transmission of attachment in a sample of adolescent mother-infant dyads. *Developmental Psychology*, **41**, 212–24.

9. Bailey, H.N., Moran, G. and Pederson, D.R. (2007) Childhood maltreatment, complex trauma symptoms, and unresolved attachment in an at-risk sample of adolescent mothers. *Attachment and Human Development*, **9**, 139–61.

10. Lyons-Ruth, K., Yellin, C., Melnick, S. and Atwood, G. (2005) Expanding the concept of unresolved mental states: hostile/helpless states of mind on the attachment interview are associated with disrupted mother-infant communication and infant disorganization. *Development and Psychopathology*, **17**, 1–23.

11. Madigan, S., Moran, G. and Pederson, D.R. (2006) Unresolved states of mind, disorganized attachment relationships, and disrupted interactions of adolescent mothers and their infants. *Developmental Psychology*, **42**, 293–304.

12. Madigan, S., Bakermans-Kranenburg, M., van IJzendoorn, M. *et al.* (2006) Unresolved states of mind, anomalous parental behavior and disorganized attachment: a review and meta-analysis of a transmission gap. *Attachment and Human Development*, **8**, 89–111.

13. Van IJzendoorn, M.H., Schuengel, C. and Bakermans-Kranenburg, M.J. (1999) Disorganized attachment in early childhood: meta-analysis of precursors, concomitants, and sequelae. *Development and Psychopathology*, **11**, 225–49.

14. Spieker, S.J., Larson, N.C., Lewis, S.N. *et al.* (1997) Children of adolescent mothers: cognitive and behavioral status at age 6. *Child and Adolescent Social Work Journal*, **14**, 335–64.

15. Tarabulsy, G.M., Pascuzzo, K., Moss, E. *et al.* (2008) Attachment-based intervention for maltreating families. *American Journal of Orthopsychiatry*, **78**, 322–32.

16. Sadler, L.S., Swartz, M.K., Ryan-Krause, P. *et al.* (2007) Promising outcomes in teen mothers enrolled in a school-based parent support program and child care center. *Journal of School Health*, **77**, 121–30.

17. Moran, G., Pederson, D.R. and Krupka, A. (2005) Maternal unresolved attachment status impedes the effectiveness of interventions with adolescent mothers. *Infant Mental Health Journal*, **26**, 231–49.

18. Olds, D.L. (2007) The nurse-family partnership: an evidence-based preventive intervention. *Infant Mental Health Journal*, **27**, 5–25.

19. Lieberman, A.F. (2007) Ghosts and angels: intergenerational patterns in the transmission and treatment of the traumatic sequelae of domestic violence. *Infant Mental Health Journal*, **28**, 422–39.

8

Psychopathological states in the pregnant mother

Carol Henshaw MD FRCPsych FHEA

Liverpool Women's Hospital, UK

8.1 Introduction

More than a third of pregnant women suffer from a mental disorder [1]. Some will experience a recurrence of a previous illness, while others will suffer from a new onset condition. Conception rates in women with most disorders (with the exception of anorexia nervosa, severe learning disability and possibly schizophrenia) are the same as women in the general population. The advent of atypical antipsychotics, most of which do not impair reproductive function, suggest conception rates in women with psychosis may increase in the future. In addition, pregnancy is a multifactorial stressor and life event which may render women with a history of psychiatric problems, who may be well when they conceive, vulnerable to relapse during pregnancy. There are a number of adverse outcomes associated with pregnancy in women with both psychotic and non-psychotic disorders, not least the women with psychosis or severe depressive illness who commit suicide during pregnancy or post-partum [2]. This chapter will outline the impact of pregnancy on mental disorders, and the issues and outcomes for both mother and child.

Schizophrenia

Women with a history of treatment for schizophrenia have a high risk of difficult reproductive lives. They are more likely than women in the general population to have multiple

Parenthood and Mental Health: A Bridge between Infant and Adult Psychiatry   Sam Tyano, Miri Keren, Helen Herrman and John Cox
© 2010 John Wiley & Sons, Ltd

partners and to be indulging in risky sexual behavior, which confers a higher risk of sexually transmitted infections [3]. Their pregnancies are more liable to be unplanned and they are more likely to have had a termination of pregnancy [4]. Women with psychosis are less likely to have received contraceptive advice from their primary care team and while mental health professionals are usually aware of which of their patients are sexually active, they are much less likely to know if the patient is using contraception and less likely to discuss this with them [5].

Women with schizophrenia have a higher risk of experiencing violence during pregnancy and more likely to have a past history of forced sex [6]. More are socially disadvantaged, single and lacking in social support than women in the general population. Their partners are more likely to be unemployed or disabled. Compared to other delivered women they tend to be either very young ($\leq$ 19) or older ($\geq$ 35) mothers and therefore at increased obstetric risk [7]. Women with psychotic disorders are more likely than controls to use illicit drugs before pregnancy, and to drink alcohol and/or continue to use drugs during pregnancy, which confers additional risks to the fetus.

Even when smoking and other risk factors such as maternal age, education and pregnancy-induced hypertension are controlled for, the odds of poor outcomes such as low birth weight (LBW), small for gestational age (SGA) infants, preterm delivery and stillbirth are higher in women with schizophrenia [8]. Complications such as placental abruption, antepartum hemorrhage, the toxic side effects of alcohol and illicit drugs and infants with cardiovascular congenital anomalies (most commonly patent ductus arteriosus) occur more frequently [7].

Being overweight and folate-deficient when pregnant increases the risk of neural tube defects [9] as does Vitamin B12 deficiency. It is not known whether this relates to poor diet, weight gain on atypical antipsychotics or is a direct metabolic consequence of schizophrenia. Patients with schizophrenia are also at increased risk of impaired glucose tolerance and diabetes, particularly if they are taking certain atypical antipsychotic drugs. When pregnant this renders them at higher risk of gestational diabetes which confers greater morbidity for both mother and fetus. Obesity in pregnancy also increases obstetric risk and is associated with being less likely to have a spontaneous onset of labor, more blood loss in labor, higher-weight babies and longer hospital stays. Many of the examinations and investigations which are part of antenatal care are more difficult in an obese woman. For example, it is harder to palpate the uterus and ultrasound penetrates fat very poorly.

Despite these increased risks, women with severe mental illness are more likely to default from antenatal appointments. This might be because they fear that their baby will be removed after delivery, particularly if this has happened previously or there have been child protection case conferences. Alternatively there may be delusional beliefs about interventions, intimate examinations or health professionals. Negative symptoms and chaotic lives may lead to disregarding appointment letters and lacking the motivation to attend. Even when they do attend, women with schizophrenia receive poorer-quality antenatal care than other women accessing maternity services, with smoking and alcohol consumption less likely to be documented despite the higher prevalence of these risk factors in women with mental illness [10].

There are reports in the literature of schizophrenic women attempting to pull the baby out by themselves, or ask others to do so and one case report of a woman who performed her own Caesarean section. Psychotic denial of pregnancy may lead to refusal of antenatal care or unattended delivery. Some women with schizophrenia are reported to be unaware of the symptoms of labor and have delivered in the toilet believing that they were passing faeces.

If a woman experiences a recurrence or acute exacerbation of positive symptoms during pregnancy this may have an impact on her capacity to consent to any interventions or treatment decisions. Attention, absorption, recall and retention of information may be impaired by symptoms such as hallucinations which distract the woman. Conversation may be difficult if there is formal thought disorder and understanding may be affected by paranoid delusions regarding the treatment, the health-care professionals or the fetus. Command hallucinations may direct an alternative course of action to that advised by the health professional. If capacity is in doubt, an assessment should be undertaken in relation to each proposed treatment decision. If capacity is likely to be impaired during labor when rapid decisions may need to be made, consider the use of advance directives in relation to any likely intrapartum treatment decisions. These directives can made during pregnancy at a time when a woman has capacity and can willingly engage in discussion and decision-making with maternity staff.

Women with tightly defined schizophrenia who remain on medication are less likely to relapse after delivery than women with mood disorders or more broadly defined schizophrenia. However, a fifth of those who have had treatment that includes hospital admissions in the settings studied before they became pregnant will relapse after delivery [11], this relapse being more likely if medication is discontinued. The risk of post-partum relapse and the associated problems must be taken into consideration when making treatment decisions during pregnancy.

Bipolar disorder

Like women with schizophrenia, women with bipolar disorder are more likely to be single and are at increased risk of obstetric complications, specifically placenta previa and antepartum hemorrhage [4].

They have a very high risk of recurrence related to childbirth with up to two-thirds experiencing an episode in the immediate post-partum period and those with a family history of puerperal relapse being particularly vulnerable. The risk remains high even if the woman has been well during pregnancy and for the two years before she became pregnant and even if she is living in good social circumstances with good social support. The risk of recurrence appears to be the same in both bipolar I and II patients but particularly likely if there have been more than four previous episodes. Pregnant women are as likely to relapse as non-pregnant women if mood-stabilizing medication is discontinued and the risk of recurrence is greater with a rapid discontinuation rather than a gradual reduction in dose.

Early studies suggested that bipolar women were less likely to experience an episode of illness during pregnancy. However it now seems clear that this is not the case with between a third and a half of pregnant bipolar women experiencing a worsening of symptoms or a recurrence. Those experiencing symptoms during pregnancy are more likely to have a post-partum episode. Women who are euthymic at conception and stop prophylactic medication are twice as likely to relapse, have a fourfold shorter time to recurrence and a five times greater proportion of weeks during pregnancy spent ill than women who continue with medication (40% of pregnancy vs. 8.8%). Most recurrences were depressive or dysphoric mixed states and almost half occurred during the first trimester [12].

Depression

Depression is as common during pregnancy as it is following delivery although depressive *symptoms* may be more prevalent. A systematic review and meta-analysis of prevalence studies from high-income countries [13] confirmed rates of 7.4%, 12.8% and 12.0% in the first, second and third trimesters respectively.

Risk factors for depressive symptoms in pregnancy include being single, of low educational status, unemployed, having poor partner and/or social support and the presence of stressful life events or chronic stressors. Women with histories of childhood sexual abuse, intimate partner violence or sexual coercion are more likely to report depressive symptoms. Depression in pregnancy is closely associated with smoking during pregnancy, alcohol and drug use. A poor appetite may lead to under-nutrition. Depressed women who smoke find it harder to give up when they become pregnant than women who are not depressed.

Symptoms such as fatigue, lack of energy, excessive sleepiness, food cravings or aversions and weight changes, all of which may be common complaints during pregnancy, mean careful assessment is required in order to distinguish these from the somatic symptoms of depression.

Anxiety disorders

Anxiety disorders may be more common than depression during pregnancy with the following prevalences reported in the literature [14]:

Panic disorder	1.3–2.0%
Obsessive compulsive disorder (OCD)	0.2–3.5%
Post-traumatic stress disorder (PTSD)	0–7.7%
Generalized anxiety disorder (GAD)	8.5%
Agoraphobia	14%
Social phobia	0–4.1%
Specific phobia	2.3%

Common fears are fear of fetal loss or giving birth to a handicapped child, particularly if there is a history of reproductive loss or fertility problems. In addition 7.2% of pregnant women are reported to have a blood or injection phobia which clearly has implications for their care during pregnancy and delivery.

Anxiety disorders may be co-morbid with a depressive disorder; and anxiety during pregnancy, especially if present in the last trimester, is an independent predictor of postnatal depression. PTSD increases the likelihood of a woman also having a substance misuse diagnosis. For a review of anxiety disorders see [14].

Tokophobia is an intense dread of childbirth which can lead to women avoiding pregnancy, terminating the pregnancy of a much-wanted baby, or demanding a Caesarean section in subsequent pregnancies [15]. It may occur in a nulliparous woman (primary tokophobia) or be secondary to previous traumatic deliveries or other traumatic events. It can also occur in the context of a depressive illness or PTSD. The prevalence of severe fear is reported as 5.5% and is associated with subsequent elective Caesarean delivery. In addition to arising from traumatic delivery, tokophobia may occur in response to previous traumatic gynecological examination or a history of sexual abuse or assault.

Women with a history of sexual abuse are less likely to have an uncomplicated vaginal delivery at term.

Obsessive compulsive disorder

OCD may occur for the first time during pregnancy. Up to a third of parous women with OCD reported their first onset as having occurred during pregnancy. Around half of those with pre-existing OCD find their symptoms worsen but about a quarter report improvement. However, those with improvement remain liable to relapse after delivery or following a miscarriage. Obsessions commonly found in pregnancy relate to fears of fetal contamination with associated cleaning and washing compulsions. Obsessions relating to symmetry and ordering are also found, and checking is a common compulsion during pregnancy. Some women experience aggressive intrusive thoughts or images, which may relate to self-harm, harming the fetus or harming the infant after delivery. Such thoughts are less likely to be disclosed to health professionals. Ego dystonic intrusive thoughts require careful assessment in order to distinguish these from thoughts of actually harming the fetus [14].

Panic disorder

There is conflicting evidence regarding the impact pregnancy has on the course of illness in women with pre-existing panic disorder [14]. It may or may not be complicated by agoraphobia. Studies suggest that around a quarter of women notice no change in their level of symptomatology, just under a half experience improvement and a third become worse. There is some suggestion that those with mild symptoms show improvements while women with a more severe disorder are more likely to experience deterioration in their panic symptoms. Even if symptoms improve during pregnancy, they may recur post-partum particularly if prophylactic medication is discontinued and not recommended. Like OCD, panic disorder may also occur for the first time during pregnancy.

Studies have reported contradictory findings when examining whether or not anxiety disorders during pregnancy predict poor outcomes. For example, some have reported lower APGAR scores in the infants, increased risks of pregnancy loss and complications while others have contradicted these findings. A meta-analysis conducted by Littleton *et al* [16] found no significant associations between anxiety symptoms during pregnancy and several perinatal outcomes (length of labor, birth weight, use of analgesia during labor, gestational age and five-minute APGAR score).

Eating disorders

The majority of women with eating disorders (ED) are of childbearing age. Fertility problems have been linked with ED and the fertility rate of women with ED is lower than that of the general population (particularly in women with anorexia nervosa). However, those who have recovered from anorexia, women with bulimia and those with partial syndromes or subsyndromal disrupted eating and extreme concerns about bodyweight do become pregnant. Estimates of the prevalence of disordered eating in pregnant populations range from a probable 2–3% having a clinical disorder and up to 11% with subsyndromal symptoms. Eating disorders have significant implications for the pregnancy and fetus but women with ED may be particularly reluctant to disclose their symptoms to maternity staff perhaps because they fear pressure to put on weight or are ashamed of their behaviour [17].

Several studies report that ED symptoms in women with both bulimia and restrictive anorexia improve during pregnancy although they may return to preconception levels of symptomatology again after delivery. Others find symptoms increase with concerns regarding changes in body shape and weight and there may then be a consequent increase in laxative abuse and/or vomiting. Several studies report an increased prevalence of hyperemesis in women with ED but it is unknown whether this is a true increase or reflects bulimic symptoms [17].

Whether the ED is treated or not may make a difference and it has been reported .that women with bulimia nervosa who had recently received treatment for their ED were less symptomatic in relation to childbirth and in the year after than those women who had not had a child. However, several studies report that women with ED are at increased risk of having a postnatal depressive episode.

Women with anorexia nervosa or bulimia nervosa who are symptomatic during pregnancy are at risk of poorer outcomes including [17]:

- Miscarriage

- Termination of pregnancy

- Hyperemesis

- Poor weight gain

- Gestational diabetes

- Preterm delivery

- LBW infants

- SGA infant

- Infants with microcephaly

- Operative delivery.

Possible mechanisms for these findings include: weight-controlling behavior by restricting intake or excessive exercise, vomiting, using diuretics or laxatives. Such activities may lead to compromised flow of nutrients via the placenta. The use of laxatives and diuretics can lead to metabolic disturbances and may also exert a teratogenic effect. Under-nourishment can impair the immune system which could lead to an increased risk of maternal infection with adverse consequences for the fetus.

As women with ED may not readily disclose their problems, the following should alert clinicians to the possible presence of an ED:

- A body mass index of 19 or less at antenatal booking

- A past history of an ED

- Hyperemesis gravidarum

- Lack of weight gain over two consecutive visits in the second trimester

- The presence of hypotension, bradycardia, cold intolerance, carotinemia, dry skin, lanugo or brittle hair (features which may be present in anorexia)
- Self-induced vomiting can cause:
  - Oral mucosal damage
  - Dental erosions
  - Russell's sign: calluses or abrasions on the knuckles
  - Parotid gland enlargement
  - Laxative or diuretic abuse may cause abdominal pain and diarrhoea.

Questions such as 'Are you satisfied with your eating pattern?' and 'Do you eat in secret?' have been found to distinguish bulimics from normal eaters in primary care settings and may be a useful approach at antenatal booking. With a positive response or if an ED is suspected there should be a sensitive but systematic enquiry about purging, self-induced vomiting, the use and frequency of use of laxatives, diuretics and diet pills. Obstetric review will need to be more frequent and maternity staff need to be aware of the lengths women with ED may go to in order to conceal their true weight when being weighed. Even if there has been improvement in pregnancy, the risk of return to pre-pregnant eating patterns and behavior and the increased risk of depression after delivery must be communicated to the professionals who will be supporting mother and infant post-partum.

Personality disorder

Personality disorder affects 4–12% of the European adult population and yet there is relatively little written in the scientific literature regarding the impact of pregnancy on personality disorder compared with that relating to Axis I disorders. However, the problems that people with personality disorder have lead to reduced ability to function in daily life and subjective distress. They are also more vulnerable to interpersonal and marital problems and more likely to suffer from Axis I psychiatric disorders than the general population so it is very likely that they will have an increased vulnerability to stressful life events such as pregnancy and childbirth.

Pregnancy may be particularly difficult if there have been problems in adapting to previous life changes or if the response to stress is to adopt immature coping strategies and defense mechanisms. There may also be conflicts and problems in relation to motherhood, for example in relation to the woman's own experience of mothering. Women diagnosed with borderline personality disorder are more likely than the general population to have unplanned pregnancies and difficulties in their intimate relationships. These interpersonal difficulties may lead to communication problems and misunderstandings with health-care professionals. However, one recent study from Sweden found no differences in the childbirth experience between women with this diagnosis, women with other psychiatric disorders and healthy pregnant women [18].

Concealed pregnancy

Women who conceal pregnancy are often younger and still living at home with their mothers [19]. Concealment may occur for a variety of reasons including abuse in the home, previous removal of a child and the desire to avoid this again, or pregnancy occurring outside marriage in communities where this may have serious consequences for the woman. Concealment until delivery is estimated to occur in 1 in 2500 pregnancies. The women are more likely to have a personality disorder or psychological difficulties than a formal mental illness although many do not receive a psychiatric assessment. Neonaticide has occurred following concealed pregnancy where delivery happens out of hospital and is assisted. There may be child protection concerns in concealed pregnancy and therefore appropriate referral should be made.

Deliberate self-harm

Deliberate self-harm in pregnancy most often takes the form of an overdose of the most accessible medication: over-the-counter analgesics, iron or vitamins. Problems related to pregnancy and interpersonal difficulties are the most frequently cited reasons for the overdose. Suicidal ideation is more likely to occur in women with a history of physical or sexual abuse [20].

Self-poisoning during pregnancy increases the risk of preterm labor, the need for Caesarean section and blood transfusion and increases the likelihood of respiratory distress syndrome and neonatal death [21]. This large study identified the best predictor of self-harm as substance misuse.

Women with psychosis or severe depressive illnesses during pregnancy who are suicidal tend to use violent methods, most frequently hanging or jumping from a height and are hence more likely to succeed in killing themselves [2].

8.2   General guidelines

Mental health professionals caring for women with serious mental illness, particularly those with bipolar disorder, should discuss with all female patients of childbearing potential the risks associated with childbirth and plans to manage this risk should they become pregnant. Primary care services should ensure that women with serious mental illness receive appropriate contraceptive advice.

All pregnant women should be routinely asked at the antenatal booking interview about current and previous mental health problems. This should include their use of prescribed and non-prescribed medicine, herbal, homeopathic and over-the-counter remedies and legal and illegal substances including tobacco and alcohol. The nature and severity of these problems should be established. The family history of psychiatric disorder should also be enquired about.

If the woman has not been referred to maternity care by the primary care team, maternity services should check with the woman's primary care physician for further information. Midwives should routinely inform the primary care physician that their patient is pregnant and ask for any health or relevant social information.

If primary care physicians are referring to maternity care they should communicate not only with obstetricians, but also with midwives, the details of their patient's previous psychiatric history including that of alcohol and drug misuse.

All pregnant women who have a current serious mental illness or are at identified risk of serious postnatal mental illness should be assessed by a psychiatric team, preferably a specialist perinatal psychiatry service. Each woman should have a clear management plan which is communicated to all involved in her care (maternity and psychiatric services) and is contained in all versions of her records (computerized, paper and hand-held) with details of who to contact if there is a crisis. The plan should include a system of close multi-disciplinary supervision throughout pregnancy, and following birth if she is at risk of postnatal recurrence. Support may be required in ensuring that appointments are attended. If there are child protection concerns, social services must be informed and involved.

Midwives should check on the continuing mental health of all their clients at least twice during pregnancy and following delivery in order to detect new onset disorders which arise after the booking interview. Mental health professionals should liaise with maternity services about any of their patients who become pregnant and ensure that both midwives and obstetricians are aware of the current and planned treatment.

It is also important not to attribute all a pregnant woman's symptoms to her mental disorder if she has a psychiatric diagnosis. Clinicians need to remain alert regarding the possibility of serious physical illness in pregnant women and recognize when tachycardia and breathlessness are not attributable to anxiety and a lack of response may not be due to depression but an acute severe physical illness. Failure to do this and directing the patient to a psychiatric facility rather than a general hospital has led to maternal deaths [2].

8.3 Conclusions

Pregnancy can be a difficult and very risky time for many women with mental disorders and those at risk of onset of a mental disorder. A woman's mental state, associated behaviors or treatment may confer significant risk to her infant. It is therefore crucial that management is proactive and involves all the relevant disciplines with good communication between all parties.

8.4 References

1. Kelly, R.H., Zatick, D. and Anders, T.F. (2001) The detection and treatment of psychiatric disorders and substance use among pregnant women cared for in obstetrics. *American Journal of Psychiatry*, **158**, 213–19.
2. Lewis, G. (2007) *The Confidential Enquiry into Maternal and Child Health (CEMACH). Saving Mothers' Lives: Reviewing Maternal Deaths to Make Motherhood Safer – 2003–2005. The Seventh Report on Confidential Enquiries into Maternal Deaths in the United Kingdom*.CEMACH, London.
3. Dickerson, F.B., Brown, C.H., Kreyenbuhl, J. *et al.* (2004) Sexual and reproductive behaviors among persons with mental illness. *Psychiatric Services*, **55**, 1299–1301.
4. Shah, N. and Howard, L. (2006) Screening for smoking and substance misuse in pregnant women with mental illness. *Psychiatric Bulletin*, **30**, 294–97.
5. McLennan, J.D. and Ganguli, R. (1999) Family planning and parenthood needs of women with severe mental illness: clinicians' perspective. *Community Mental Health Journal*, **35**, 369–80.
6. Coverdale, J., Turbott, S. and Roberts, H. (1997) Family planning needs and STD risk behaviours of female psychiatric out- patients. *British Journal of Psychiatry*, **171**, 69–72.
7. Jablensky, A.V., Morgan, V., Zubrick, S. R. *et al.* (2005) Pregnancy, delivery, and neonatal complications in a population cohort of women with schizophrenia and major affective disorders. *American Journal of Psychiatry*, **162**, 79–91.

8. Nilsson, E., Lichtenstein, P., Cnattingius, S. *et al.* (2002) Women with schizophrenia: pregnancy outcome and infant death among their offspring. *Schizophrenia Research*, **58**, 221–29.

9. Koren, G., Cohn, T., Chitayat, D. *et al.* (2002) Use of atypical antipsychotics during pregnancy and the risk of neural tube defects in infants. *American Journal of Psychiatry*, **159**, 136–37.

10. Howard, L.M. (2005) Fertility and pregnancy in women with psychotic disorders. *European Journal of Obstetrics and Gynecology and Reproductive Biology*, **119**, 3–10.

11. Harlow, B.L., Vitonis, A.F., Sparen, P. *et al.* (2007) Incidence of hospitalization for postpartum psychotic and bipolar episodes in women with and without prior prepregnancy or prenatal psychiatric hospitalizations. *Archives of General Psychiatry*, **64**, 42–48.

12. Viguera, A.C., Whitfield, T., Baldessarini, R.J. *et al.* (2007) Risk of recurrence in women with bipolar disorder during pregnancy: prospective study of mood stabilizer discontinuation. *American Journal of Psychiatry*, **164**, 1817–24.

13. Bennett, H.A., Einarson, A., Taddio, A. *et al.* (2004) Prevalence of depression during pregnancy: systematic review. *Obstetrics and Gynecology*, **103**, 698–709.

14. Ross, L.E. and McLean, L.M. (2006) Anxiety disorders during pregnancy and the postpartum period: a systematic review. *Journal of Clinical Psychiatry*, **67**, 1285–98.

15. Hofberg, K. and Brockington, I. (2000) Tokophobia: an unreasoning dread of childbirth. A series of 26 cases. *British Journal of Psychiatry*, **176**, 83–85.

16. Littleton, H.L., Breitkopf, C.R. and Berenson, A.B. (2007) Correlates of anxiety symptoms during pregnancy and association with perinatal outcomes: a meta-analysis. *American Journal of Obstetrics and Gynecology*, **196**, 424–32.

17. Astrachan-Fletcher, E., Veldhuis, C., Lively, N. *et al.* (2008) The reciprocal effects of eating disorders and the postpartum period: a review of the literature and recommendations for clinical care. *Journal of Women's Health*, **17**, 227–39.

18. Börjesson, K., Ruppert, S., Wager, J. *et al.* (2007) Personality disorder, psychiatric symptoms and experience of childbirth among childbearing women in Sweden. *Midwifery*, **23**, 260–68.

19. Friedman, S.H., Heneghan, A. and Rosenthal, M. (2007) Characteristics of women who deny or conceal pregnancy. *Psychosomatics*, **48**, 117–22.

20. Farber, E.W., Herbert, S.E. and Reviere, S.L. (1996) Childhood abuse and suicidality in obstetrics patients in a hospital-based urban prenatal clinic. *General Hospital Psychiatry*, **18**, 56–60.

21. Gandhi, S.G., Gilbert, W.M., McElvy, S.S. *et al* (2006) Maternal and neonatal outcomes after attempted suicide. *Obstetrics and Gynecology*, **107**, 984–90.

9

When something goes wrong with the fetus: rights, wrongs and consequences

Julio Arboleda-Flórez

Queen's University, Kingston, Canada

9.1 Reproduction and threats to the unborn

The consequences when something goes wrong with the fetus may be immediate, either because of miscarriage and therapeutic abortion or by destruction at birth. If viable and allowed to live, the consequences for the disabled adult are massive in terms of independence, self-determination and personal autonomy. Often, defective fetuses are not viable within the womb and exit the maternal body at an early age in the pregnancy via miscarriages. Genetic abnormalities and organ malformations account for the majority of these cases. External substances ingested by the mother, especially alcohol, cocaine or plain nicotine with or without criminal intent, cause damage in the organs of the fetus and may lead to malformations incompatible with life *in utero*. Blunt trauma, in modern times most commonly caused by traffic accidents, may lead to stillbirths after an indeterminate time following death of the fetus in the womb.

The legalization of abortion on demand before quickening or viability, which occurs about week 23 (see below) has had a salutary effect on the health of the expectant woman, who in the past suffered major infections and risked permanent infertility and death while seeking an illegal abortion. The debate over abortion now is more theoretical in regard to

Parenthood and Mental Health: A Bridge between Infant and Adult Psychiatry   Sam Tyano, Miri Keren, Helen Herrman and John Cox
© 2010 John Wiley & Sons, Ltd

whether the fetus has any rights, or political between those opposed to abortion (pro-lifers) and those who favoured it (pro-choice).

Severely handicapped newborns were usually actively destroyed at the moment of birth or, in modern time with the custom of giving birth in hospital, they are selectively chosen for non-treatment and allowed to die in the neonatal intensive care units [2]. Aristotle asked for a law that no *deformed* child should be allowed to live [3]. Infanticide is an old practice and has been known in any culture and at all times since recorded history. It has also been the subject of famous literary works from Euripides' *Medea* to Chaucer's *The Canterbury Tales*, Goethe's *Faust*, Swift's *A Modest Proposal* and Dickens' *Oliver Twist*. While economic resources in the community or religious ideas would have ended up in the destruction (infanticide) of healthy children, the deformed were mostly the ones targeted for active and openly encouraged destruction, usually with much social approval. This was a rational practice devoid of any feelings or sentiments. As infanticide became a punishable offence, during the Middle Ages 'abandonment' became the common practice to deal with unwanted and deformed babies. Religious superstitions were also a factor in the active killing or abandonment of a defective newborn. Physically deformed or mentally retarded children were considered 'changelings' – supernatural substitutes or 'demon-children' who had substituted the 'real' ones.

The birth of a deformed child may give rise to tort legal actions known as 'wrongful births' if brought up by the parents, and 'wrongful life' cases if originating in the deformed infant. In the former, the parents sue the defendant physicians for negligence in the care of the pregnant mother, or negligent care of the fetus *in utero*. Some claims of this nature are 'wrongful pregnancies' when the woman alleges negligence on the part of the practitioner as contributory to an unwanted pregnancy when she had followed contraceptive advice or undertaken procedures to avoid pregnancies and became pregnant nonetheless. 'Wrongful life' cases are brought in by the infant, alleging that he would have not been born and suffer a life of problems, but for the negligence of the practitioner.

Infanticide and selective non-treatment of defective infants as well as 'wrongful birth' and 'wrongful life' cases should decline with the advent of improved technologies to visualize the fetus and proceed to termination of the pregnancy or to decide for intrauterine surgical interventions. In this respect, technology has eliminated the element of surprise to realize at birth that the baby is deformed. Genetic manipulation and screening may also help in preventing genetically transmissible defects in the fetus [4].

In vitro fertilization and other new reproductive technologies have brought hopes to unfertile couples, but have also opened up a Pandora's box of ethical concerns. For the first time in the history of *Homo sapiens* the three components of parenthood – the genetic, the gestational and the nurturant – can now be separated. Ovum or sperm donation, rent-a-womb schemes or embryo adoptions have become a common occurrence. In the brouhaha of technological success the voices that have not been heard are those of the children, many of whom having been cut off from their genetic heritage.

Furthermore, as humankind becomes more knowledgeable of the mechanics of life, cloning and the use of embryos and of physically deformed fetuses as farms for organs have become a reality [5]. More specifically, the search for anencephalic infants has increased. These fetuses with no hopes of living are purposefully brought to birth solely for purposes of harvesting their organs. Worse, as the present determination of death depends on the activity of the brain stem ceasing, at which time organs may have already started to deteriorate because of hypoxia, claims to change death time are being advanced so as to be able to harvest organs in better conditions for transplantation. Whether the anencephalic baby has a soul, has any legal rights to personhood or is just an integrated living organ farm is not the concern of the clinicians. His low level of neural integration leads to the fiction that he is not alive, but if he is not alive, how could he be declared dead in order to take his organs and parcel them out? Anencephalic babies are nothing else than passive carriers of organs for harvesting; sadly, a 'being' not alive, but not dead, the perfect zombie!

9.2 The rights of the fetus and of the newborn

Whether the unborn have any rights is a debatable proposition. Most philosophies of natural rights would hold that a fetus has rights and legal personhood when it becomes sentient or self-aware, thus defining personhood on a neurophysiological basis requiring substantial neocortical development which is achieved about week 23 (coinciding with 'quickening' – see below). Religious traditions that hold the presence of a non-physical soul as the basis of personhood differ about the time when ensoulment takes place, that is, the moment in which the soul is created or implanted in the fetus. Some hold that this happens at the very moment of conception; others believe at the moment of implantation of the fertilized egg in the uterus; others think it is at quickening; and finally, for others, it happens only at the moment of birth (post-fetal). The presence or absence of a soul permeates the debate about moral justifications of abortion or whether it should be considered murder or infanticide.

The rights of the unborn and of the newborn encompass more than just a right to life; they also include rights to a maximization of possibilities for comfort and security so as to make sure of optimum emotional, intellectual and physical development *in utero* and over the first year of life. A right to personal security consists in a person's legal and uninterrupted enjoyment of his life, his limbs, his body, his health and his reputation. Yet, whether the unborn have any rights clearly spelled out in law may be a moot question because in practice those rights have been upheld on multiple occasions and in many cultures. For example, the murder of a pregnant woman is usually followed by a charge of double homicide, the woman and the fetus that she is carrying. A situation of double homicide charges is contemplated in the *Unborn Victims of Violence Act in the United States* (2004), a law passed after the murder of a pregnant woman (Lacy Peterson) at the hands of her husband. And many women are criminally prosecuted or arrested under child protection statutes for allegedly endangering the life of the fetus especially by the use of alcohol or illicit drugs. Drug addicts have also been accused of supplying drugs to a minor through unintentional transfer of the drugs via the umbilical cord.

Blackstone, while considering life as an immediate gift of God (of nature, for those who may be atheists) explains that it is a right inherent by nature in every individual so that as per contemplation of the laws it begins as an infant is able to stir in the mother's womb (quickening). He further explains that if a woman is quick with child and by potion or otherwise kills it in her womb, or if somebody beats her and the child dies in her body and she is delivered of a dead child, by ancient law it is homicide or manslaughter. However, 'quickening' meaning to reach the stage of pregnancy at which the child shows life ('quick' meaning to be 'alive') when the mother feels its movement inside the womb, which happens about week 20, has not been the only standard for legal purposes about unlawful behaviour against an unborn child. 'Formation', or the point at which the fetus takes on a human shape (much earlier than quickening), has been used for millennia as a rule to consider that the fetus is alive. The Old Testament is specific in stating that killing the fetus is akin to taking a life if it was already perfectly formed. 'Viability' is another standard that has been used to determine that human life has legally begun; it refers to the point when the fetus is potentially able to live outside the womb, even if artificial aid is required. Viability is usually considered to happen at 28 weeks (seven months), but may be as early as 24 weeks.

The concept that life begins at the moment of conception, that is, the very moment the sperm penetrates a mature egg, is enshrined in the *American Convention on Human Rights* that was approved by all Latin American states in 1969. Many other states, however, consider that life begins at the moment of birth when the infant takes in its first breath. Iranian law stipulates that anyone who brings about a miscarriage must pay in compensation a monetary fine commensurate with the stage of development and sex of the fetus. Some other countries have entered fetal rights in their constitutions. The Eighth Amendment of the Constitution of Ireland was passed by popular referendum in 1983 and it recognizes 'the right to life of the unborn'. In 1993 the Federal Constitutional Court of Germany held that the constitution guaranteed the right to life from conception, but allowed some exception to abortion in the first trimester. On the other hand, in Canada, the fetus is a human being only when it has completely proceeded, in a living state, from the body of its mother, whether or not it has completely breathed, it has an independent circulation or the navel string is severed. Fetal rights that also convey on the fetus the power of legal personhood are the major arguments for those who oppose legal abortions (pro-life groups), whereas those who oppose fetal rights (pro-choice groups) do so because they feel it is a slippery slope strategy to restricting abortions. In the Catholic Church it is a matter of dogma that ensoulment happens at conception and emphasizes the dignity and humanity of embryos in its encyclical *Dignitas Personae* [6].

But a fetus does not only have a right to life and security. *In ventre sa mere:* a fetus is supposed in law to be born for many purposes such as having rights to a legacy, or to an estate; it may have assigned guardians, to have estates for their limited use – all as if it had actually been born assigned – *qui in utero sunt, in jure civili intelliguntur in rerum natura esse, cum de eorum commodo agatur* – 'those who are in the womb, are considered by civil law to be in the nature of things, as they are capable of being benefited'.

Thus, although it may not be until quickening or any of the other standards that a fetus acquires rights as a person, the law is clear in that although the fetus may not be considered a person, hence being no better than an object before movements are discernible, tampering with it for criminal purposes at any stage is a crime.

In modern times the human rights of the fetus and the newborn have been recognized in a number of declarations and covenants. In English Common Law the unborn have similar and all the rights of the born, and these rights have been enshrined in constitutions in many countries. In the United States, the unborn have all the rights of the born as stipulated in the Ninth Amendment and all the rights in the Bill of Rights apply equally to both groups. These rights were contemplated in US anti-abortion laws, but were abrogated by the decision on *Roe v. Wade* (410 U.S. 112, 1973) that became constitutional law for the whole country. *Roe v. Wade* was a landmark and very controversial case in regard to both the rights of the unborn and a right to abortion on demand. The unborn were protected after 'viability' – when the mother loses dominion of her body in favor of the protection of the unborn. After viability, abortion could only legally be acceptable if it was required for the protection of the life of the mother. However, before viability, *Roe v. Wade* also legitimized abortion on demand as a fundamental right on the basis that a woman owns her body and has the right to privacy, construed broadly enough as to encompass her decision to terminate her pregnancy.

Whether dominion over her body is absolute at any time including while pregnant, or while pregnant dominion is curbed by a share dominion with the fetus, may be at the basis of the case of a woman addicted to glue-sniffing in Canada. The judge ordered that she be confined to a drug treatment center until the birth of her child. She had been sniffing solvents for over eight years and two of her children had already been born with neurological damage because of her addiction. She herself was very sick with neurological complications from the solvents. The judge's decision, while broadly approved by the Canadian public, unleashed a national controversy between those opining on the rights of the fetus to life and security and those who thought the woman had absolute dominion over her body and liberty to pursue her addiction as she pleased regardless of the needs, and rights, of her unborn child. The poignant question for all was – for a country that permits abortion on demand, how could a judge curtail the freedom of a woman to carry her fetus to term even if she was exposing it to serious harm? Which one of the two should be the social imperative: the rights of the fetus or the freedom of the mother [7]?

9.3 Parental reactions

Parents, especially expectant mothers, are routinely advised to avoid ingesting any substances that may conceivably harm the fetus including alcohol, smoking, street drugs or even medications known to be teratogenic, and to avoid exposure to radiation by X-rays or gamma rays. Some women, especially those suffering from addictions, may not pay attention to these entreaties and play Russian roulette with the wholesomeness of the offspring; they carry on regardless of consequences. However, despite all possible protections and medical care, it does happen that a fetus is deformed for many other reasons than the mother's wantonness. Under these circumstances parental reactions, some of them maladaptive, are to be expected, depending on the emotional investment and even attachment that has already developed with the future child. For those couples who were counting on a happy event, especially when there have been problems in conceiving, the news that something is wrong with the fetus could be devastating. The shock and disbelief and the need to make quick decisions may overwhelm them. To resign herself to proceed to an abortion is always a difficult decision for a woman and therapeutic abortions are not entirely without risks to health. These risks may be physical and immediate such as hemorrhage, infections and perforations, or delayed, such as effects on later pregnancies because of injuries to the cervix, scarring of the fallopian tubes, missed abortions when the fetus was not lodged in the uterus but in the tubes, breast cancer and even deaths especially in late abortions. Risks can also be emotional because even when an abortion is wanted and the procedure provides an immediate feeling of relief, women may experience sadness, guilt, depression and suicidal ideation, which some may try to cope with via drinking and abusing drugs. Such emotional after-effects may also affect relationships as some women may blame the partner, avoid future relationships or may develop sexual dysfunction.

If the couple decides to proceed with the gestation and the newborn child is seriously handicapped, it is possible that the decision to proceed overlooked future encumbrances, deprivations and sacrifices. While some parents may rally to the cause and accept the child and its deformities or handicaps as the will of God, pray for fortitude, praise the joys that they obtain otherwise and obtain a sense of moral fulfillment, others will feel unjustifiably punished and undeserving of their lot, will feel depressed, resenting the constant worry, the medical arrangements and the financial costs that may spell ruin for the family. Many others resort to alcohol and often blame each other for the misfortune or blame the deformed child as the seed of the marital discord. Mutual recriminations not infrequently eventually lead to separation or divorce and, practically inevitably, to the emotional and physical abuse of the child.

9.4 The fate of persons with developmental disabilities

The management of persons with developmental disabilities that often result from genetic defects, from noxious elements internal to the maternal body or from external environmental threats have, for centuries, posed a challenge to social beliefs and political systems. These persons have either being accepted and protected, or rejected and destroyed. The Spartans would throw their defective children down Mt Taygetus rock as, by law in both Sparta and Rome, infants with deformities were not permitted to live. In the Middle Ages, deformed infants were considered to be 'monsters occasioned by the craft and subtlety of the devil' [8] in sexual union with a woman, and put to death. To the contrary, Talmudic law recognized the *shoteh* (those with mental retardation and mental illness) had a limited mental capacity and exonerated them, the deaf and minors from wrongdoing. Zoroaster and Confucius as well as Jewish, Muslim and Christian traditions considered mentally retarded persons as innocent and in need of care and protection. In modern times in less developed economies and rural communities, the defective usually finds a niche in the market structure and contributes to the productivity of the group.

Unfortunately, in more advanced economies, there is no room in the labor market for the defective so the alternative is warehousing in institutions, which while affording some protection from society are usually overcrowded, underfunded and understaffed and where inmates are not uncommonly subjected to abuse. Some of those institutions have become legendary because of their lack of human decency such as Willowbrook State School in New York City Staten Island, which at one time housed up to 5400 inmates and which, along with Vineland Training School, became preferred institutions for unethical research practices. Institutions also became favourite places for involuntary sterilization practices at the order of the superintendent who had legally been permitted to act accordingly on inmates afflicted with hereditary forms of recurrent insanity, idiocy, imbecility, feeble-mindedness and epilepsy (*Buck v. Bell*, 274 U.S. 200, 1927). These practices had been encouraged by the eugenics movement first described by Sir Francis Galton in 1883. Together with social Darwinism, natural selection ideas and survival of the fittest, the eugenic movement strived for the preservation and propagation of only those considered in perfect shape intellectually, physically and emotionally. Those not fitting this selection process were exterminated, warehoused or sterilized.

The practice of sterilization started at the beginning of the 1900s and, by 1913, 12 states had enacted them and similar laws were approved in Denmark, Norway, Sweden, Finland, Canada, etc. At the Michener Centre in Alberta, Canada, sterilizations were still carried out by statute until 1972. These laws were the forerunners of the Nazis *Sterilization Act* or 'Law for the Prevention of Genetically Diseased Descendants' proclaimed on 14 July 1933.

A large list of conditions, including alcoholism and mental illness, were included as 'genetic illnesses' whose sufferers were considered apt for sterilization, 'even against the will of the person' as contemplated in Paragraph 12 of the Act. It is calculated that between 1933 and 1939, 375 000 persons had been sterilized, about 39% involuntarily. The leap from mass sterilization to involuntary euthanasia did not take long afterwards. Already in 1920, Hoche and Binding, a psychiatrist and a lawyer respectively, promoted the idea in their book *Permitting the Destruction of Unworthy Life*, alleging that it could reasonably be applied to terminal patients, idiots, the mentally ill and those rendered unconscious from injuries. The practice was carried out via injections of morphine, asphyxiation or gassing. It was estimated that about 100 000 persons residing in asylums, mostly mentally ill and mentally handicapped and disabled children, suffered this fate. Eugenic beliefs in the first part of the twentieth century led many to fear the deformed as they were deemed dangerous and carriers of poor genetic material. Thus Spartan extermination laws have a modern equivalent in the eugenic movements and in Nazi practices in the twentieth century.

Superintendents and boards of directors used to run their institutions as their own fiefdoms where they were the law and inmates had no rights and no protections. Neither there was any concern from the outside as persons were sent to institutions and forgotten; treatment and rehabilitation were not expected. It was only during the decade of the 1960s that a movement to *normalization* began and the mentally retarded and the mentally ill started leaving the institutions. In the United States, the *Mental Retardation and Developmental Disability Act* of 1964 accomplished this for the mentally retarded in the same way as the deinstitutionalization movement did it for the mentally ill.

Later in life, developmentally disabled persons face limitations in their participation in and understanding of social interactions and functions. After World War II much concern has developed in the Western world about protecting disadvantaged and vulnerable populations. The atrocities committed during the Nazi regime (1933–45) in Germany, with the wholesale destruction of minorities and vulnerable groups of individuals as referred to above, sensitized the public to the need for protection of these populations. The lessons learned at Nuremberg (1945–49), that minorities and vulnerable populations were in need of special protection, have resulted in a myriad of regulations, covenants and declarations purportedly drafted to create special protection for and to ban discrimination against these populations.

Unfortunately, none of these instruments seem enough to counter systemic practices of abuse in institutions, a lack of vigilance of monitoring systems and ignorance of ethical best-practices. Thus, several landmark cases have been used as precedents. In the United States *Wyatt v. Stickney* (325 F. Supp. 781, M.D. Ala 1971 and 344 F. Supp 373, 1972) determined that persons in institutions had a constitutional right to treatment in properly staffed and equipped institutions. In *Jackson v. Indiana* (406 U.S. 715, 1972) the Supreme Court ruled on a lifetime confinement of a mentally retarded person who had been convicted on a minor charge, but was confined to an institution until deemed 'sane'. The court found it an unconstitutional denial of due process which, the court reasoned, requires that the nature and duration of commitment bear some reasonable relation to the purpose for which the person is committed. In *O'Connor v. Donaldson* (422 U.S.563, 1975), the court found that a state cannot constitutionally confine, without motive, a non-dangerous individual who is capable of surviving safely in freedom by himself or with the help of a willing and responsible family member. In *Wyatt v. Stickney* (see above), the court also ruled that a least-restrictive environment should be sought for persons with disabilities, recommending the closure of institutions and residents be placed in the community. Finally, in 1992, the *Americans with Disabilities Act* prohibited any discrimination in employment against persons with disabilities and required reasonable accommodation to their special needs to meet legitimate job criteria.

In Canada, Section 15 of the *Charter of Rights and Freedoms* [9] affirms the equality of every individual under the law and the right to equal protections 'without discrimination based on race, national or ethnic origin, colour religion, sex, age or *mental or physical disability*'. The dispositions of the Charter were applied in *Re Eve* (31 D.L.R. 4th 1 S.C.C. 1986). In this case the parents sought leave to conduct a non-therapeutic sterilization for contraceptive purposes on their disabled daughter on the basis that she could not properly take care of any offspring, given her disabilities. The court, however, ruled that *parens patriae* powers do not extend to competent persons capable of making their own treatment decisions as was the case at hand. *Re Eve* affirmed the rights and entitlements of developmentally disabled persons in Canada.

The European Union, where it is estimated that there are 37 million disabled persons, protects the rights of the disabled as citizens with equal rights entitled to dignity, equal treatment, independent living and full participation in society. The European Community signed the *United Nations Convention on the Rights of Persons with Disabilities* [10] as a legal entity. The UN Convention covers the civil, political, economic, social and cultural rights of people with disabilities. Specifically Article 25 of the Convention states that people with disabilities should enjoy the highest attainable standard of health without discrimination and access to health and health-related rehabilitation should be gender-sensitive.

Many ethical dilemmas arise in the management of disabled persons, most because of dependency needs that should be put together with the need to foster some semblance of independence and self-reliance. Furthermore, the constant demands for supervision for even the most basic aspects of life and activities of daily living may create feelings of despair and futility, anger and resentment among caregivers. Conflicts can also arise when the caregiver assumes the functions of substitute decision-maker. Another set of ethical issues has also developed with the use of genetic counselling that may impinge on reproductive decisions in families affected by ongoing genetic conditions [11].

Implied in the concept of morality and responsibility is the notion that individuals have a basic freedom, or autonomy, to act. Kant expressed the thought that every rational being exists as an end in himself and not merely as a means for arbitrary use by anybody else; a human is an autonomous being. Further, Kant mentioned that persons are not objects and each one has a right to self-determination. There are occasions in medicine, however, when it is not possible to respect these two principles or to respect Mill's injunctions against the use of coercion with the caveat that they apply only for as long as persons are in the maturity of their faculties. Developmental disabilities frequently occur in association with lack of maturity that leads to dependency. The existence of these conditions, then, requires a careful balancing of priorities: protection of the individual for his own good (beneficence) and preservation of his rights and freedoms (autonomy and self-determination). It is proposed that such a balance should flow from a thorough and conscientious assessment of the level of disability so that the less the disability the less the beneficence and the more autonomy and self-determination, and vice versa.

Legal status, obligations and rights are conceded only to humans, not to objects or to animals, although in the case of animals some negative rights prohibiting humans from abusing them are in force in many countries. Legal status and rights enjoyed by persons are related to their being endowed with teleological, moral and legal personhood. The Christian view that all human beings are in possession of an immortal soul – no matter how perverted the person, or for that matter, how intellectually deficient – provides a shield, or natural right, to be cared for, protected and respected. In Judeo-Christian morality, humans are made in *imago Dei*, in the image of God, hence the sanctity of life and an inherent right to life. Many with no religious affiliations may not wish to endorse these points of view; there are other ways, though, in which to recognize the rights of the disabled.

Kant proposes respect for autonomous rational choice, but it has been noted already that intellectually handicapped persons lack capacity to make autonomous and independent choices. Other commentators have proposed a social contract of rights, but social contracts being specific to a moment in history punctuated by socio-political movements would leave the disabled utterly at the mercy of the latest ideologies where they might not fit. Perhaps incompetent persons retain some conditions of personhood even if they cannot retain all the legal rights. The important consideration is that disabled persons are in need of protection, whether they are in an institution or in the community. Incidents of sexual and physical abuse of the disabled in institutions are quite well known and documented, but the community is no better at protections, as is exemplified by the fictional case of Stinking Lizaveta in Dostoevsky's *The Brothers Karamazov*. In this work of the Russian master, a mentally retarded and disabled 'idiot' (Lizaveta) grew and was accepted by her small community with respect for her disabilities and as a member in need of protection. However, the social fabric of the community was rent when a drunkard confessed that he had sexually abused and beaten poor Lizaveta.

Genetic privacy is a basic requisite of genetic counselling and is based on the absolute expectation of confidentiality and a right to privacy for those under counselling. Revelations of genetic limitations may lead to social stigma and discrimination of parents and offspring alike. Alas, massive data banks threaten to invade this privacy so that genetic counselling information may be used to screen for jobs, to determine suitability for a particular task, to be accepted in a marital relationship and many other illegal uses that put the potentially disabled fetus at further risk.

9.5 Conclusions

When something is wrong with the fetus, the problem is not just for the fetus and its parents, but it confronts the whole value structure of society. As it is at present, debate still rages on whether the fetus has any right and legal personhood, whether it can be discarded at the whim of the mother or denied a uterine environment free of traumas of any kind.

New technologies that allow for visualization of the fetus have taken away in most occasions the surprise factor of having a deformed baby; the finding usually leads to abortion, which in many countries is only a decision for the mother to take. Handicapped newborns have been destroyed in many ways and, lately, they may be selectively non-treated in neonatal intensive care units. Worldwide and throughout history there has been a continuum of misfortunes not only for the developmentally disabled, but also for their parents and families. Despite strong religious traditions for their charitable acceptance, most societies still struggle for reasonable accommodations with their disabled populations, even though in many countries they have a right *in se* to their existence and participation in society.

9.6 References

1. Weisstub, D.N. and Arboleda-Flórez, J. (1988) Ethical research with vulnerable populations: the developmentally disabled. In *Research on Human Subjects* (ed. D.N. Weisstub,), Pergamon, Kidlington (Oxford).
2. Weir, R. (1984) Selective Nontreatment of Handicapped Newborns. Oxford University Press, Oxford.
3. Aristotle (1944) *Politics*, in *The Basic Works of Aristotle* (ed. R. McKeon), Random House, New York.
4. Brody, E.B. (1993) *Biomedical Technology and Human Rights*. UNESCO Publishing, Dartmouth.
5. Soupart, P. (1984) *Present and possible future research in the use of human embryos, in Abortion and the Status of the Fetus* (eds W.B. Bondeson, D.T. Engelhardt, S.F. Spicker and D.H. Winship), D. Reidel Publishing Co., Boston, pp. 67–104.
6. Pope Benedict XVI. *Dignitas Personae* (encyclical on the internet). Available from http://www.usccb.org/comm/Dignitaspersonae, downloaded on 15 July 2009.
7. *MacLean's Magazine*. Fetal rights issue raised (article on the internet). Available from http://www.thecanadianencyclopedia.com/index.cfm?PgNM, downloaded 15 July 2009.
8. Paré, A. (1634), quoted by Ferngren, G.B. (1987) The Imago Dei and the sanctity of life: the origins of an idea, in *Euthanasia and the Newborn: Conflicts Regarding Saving Lives* (eds R.C. Mcmillan, H.T. Engelhardt Jr and S.F. Spicker, D. Reidel Publishing Co., Boston, p. 58.
9. Watt, D. and Fuerst, M. (2008) *Tremeear's Criminal Code* – Constitution Act, 1982 (Canadian Charter of Rights and Freedoms), Thomson-Carswell, Toronto, pp. 1739–1818.
10. *The United Nations Convention on the Rights of Persons with Disabilities* (2008).
11. Arboleda-Flórez, J. (2001) Ethical aspects of treatment and research, in *Catalysts for University Education in Developmental Disabilities* (eds B. McCreary, P. Peppin and B. Stanton), Queen's University Press, Kingston, pp. 191–207.

10

Multiple fetuses pregnancy and other medical high-risk pregnancies

Micheline Garel,[1] Elise Charlemaine[2] and Sylvain Missonnier[3]

[1]INSERM, Villejuif, France
[2]Cochin Hospital, Paris, France
[3]Paris Descartes University, France

10.1 Medical high-risk pregnancies: definition

All pregnancies should be evaluated early on in three ways – medically, psychologically and socially – to identify risk factors that are present or conceivable. In fact, medical low-risk pregnancy is now recognized as a period of metamorphosis that simultaneously increases both creativity and biological, psychological and social vulnerability [1]. In this connection, the mother, spouse and the entire family are priority targets for a reasonable primary and secondary prevention policy for problems of parenting, of early parent/fetus/baby relations and of the child's development.

In pregnancies deemed to be medical high-risk, the mother, the fetus or the newborn will be subject to an increased risk of morbidity or mortality before or after the delivery. There are many potential factors (Table 10.1): inadequate prenatal care, past obstetric history, previous illness of the mother, illness caused by the pregnancy, multiple pregnancy, mother too old or too young, and more. All increase the vulnerability inherent in the pregnancy and justify tailored, consistent, multi-disciplinary support.

Parenthood and Mental Health: A Bridge between Infant and Adult Psychiatry   Sam Tyano, Miri Keren, Helen Herrman and John Cox
© 2010 John Wiley & Sons, Ltd

Table 10.1 Antepartum pathologies

Pathologies throughout the pregnancy
Pathologies of the amniotic fluid
Placentary pathologies
Gynecological pathologies
Medical interruption of pregnancy
Fetal pathologies
Twinning (multiple pregnancies)
Pregnancy-induced hypertension
Cardiac pathologies
Diabetes
Hematology
Infectious pathologies that do not affect the fetus
Infectious pathologies that affect the fetus
Neurological pathologies
Muscular pathologies
Respiratory pathologies
Renal pathologies
Digestive, hepatic and vomiting pathologies
Varicose, phlebitis, embolisms
Autoimmune pathologies
Mental problems that complicate pregnancy, delivery and puerperium
Psychological problems
Social problems

In this chapter the psychological aspects of two paradigmatic situations will be developed: multiple pregnancies and pregnancies with HIV infection.

10.2 Psychological aspects of multiple pregnancies

Since the middle of the 1970s the rate of multiple deliveries has risen sharply in France, as in most Western countries. The arrival of multiple children in a family involves a material, social and psychological upheaval for the parents, bringing on what some call 'the stress of multiple births' [2].

The course of a multiple pregnancy

A multiple pregnancy is discovered during a diagnostic ultrasound. The imaginary child is usually dreamt of as a single child, and seeing many on the screen can prove very disturbing for the future mother. Mothers speak of a 'shock', something really staggering. Psychological counseling could be offered at that point [3].

The announcement of a twin pregnancy is not necessarily better accepted when it can be foreseen, as following infertility treatment where it is referred to from the very beginning.

On the other hand, some women who in principle had no reason to have twins can accept the news without anxiety, as being part of the natural order of things.

All pregnancies are accompanied by physiological changes that are generally accentuated in the case of a multiple pregnancy. The future mother must accept the major deformation of her body. Some bear it proudly, but others find it difficult. There are also some mental changes, and the fantasy of intrusion can be especially strong, to the point of giving the woman the feeling she is endangering her own integrity and unity [4]. A woman said,

> Pregnancy with twins was strange. I had the impression with the older one, when he was in my womb, that we were doing things together, and I talked to him all the time. When I was pregnant with the two, I had problems dividing myself up. I had nothing to tell them apart from not to be born too quickly. In fact, I didn't imagine myself with twins. And I didn't feel well in myself. I was too big, too heavy. It wasn't really me any longer.

Sometimes embryo reduction is proposed. The decision to eliminate embryos following a course of fertility treatment is somewhat paradoxical. All the studies emphasize the difficulty of this decision and the key role played by the medical teams in helping the couples that are faced with it [5].

Women who have had recourse to fertility treatment have had to face a painful life of sterility. The pregnancy that eventually ensues may be marked by fear of failure and anxiety of losing the babies [6]. In point of fact, the threat of a premature delivery and the medical risks for the mother are more common among multiple pregnancies. The fear of giving birth prematurely and the worry that one of the children is developing less well are a cause of psychological problems during pregnancy. When bed rest is ordered it is often taken badly and can bring on depression. Frequent hospitalization, causing separation from the husband and the other children, can cause material complications, worries and/or anxiety. It is rare that the future mothers are able to share their experience with other women around them. And if depression occurs, it induces a sense of guilt. The myth that pregnancy is always fulfilling is hard to deny without risking being considered a 'bad mother'.

Women say they need to be better informed and better supported during pregnancy. For all these reasons psychological support could be offered to them as standard during pregnancy.

Delivery

If a vaginal delivery takes place, a strictly medical protocol, allowing for the particular risks related to the delivery, does not always provide for the psychological dimension of giving birth [4]. Some mothers feel they have missed out on something for themselves, as well as in the way in which they welcomed their babies. The delivery also has more chance of happening through Caesarean section. The immediate consequences for the mother of a Caesarean are longer convalescence and contact with the children made more difficult, especially if they are hospitalized in a neonatal department [7].

Post-partum

For the mother of a single birth, the time in maternity hospital is a pause, a moment of transition when the mother–baby relationship starts to develop; the mother of multiple children quickly assesses the importance of the care to be provided and the need very quickly to find a strategy [4]. Sometimes not being able to recognize her children can represent a narcissistic injury for the mother, a violation of her role as mother. Even if they are well and close to their mother, the children generally weigh little and have feeding difficulties, particularly breastfeeding, which some women find very difficult.

Hospitalization of the children

The hospitalization of twins in a neonatal department happens very frequently. Even if the babies' health is not alarming, being separated from them is always difficult for the mother. The separation also complicates already highly complex bonding mechanisms. It can happen that among the same set of babies from a multiple birth that not all of them require the same length of hospitalization, or that one of them remains with the mother. This situation causes organizational and time-management problems and complicates even further the bonding process. It is important that the pediatrician pays attention to possible cathexis differences, which if they persist may impair the development of one of the children.

During the stay in the maternity department everything must be done to encourage mother–baby bonding, all the more so if the mother is separated from her children or from one of them. There are some mothers who are exhausted by the pregnancy and delivery, and who need to get back to themselves prior to having contact with the children. Support by the care team must help each mother discover her own pace and her place as mother.

Death of a child

Pre- and postnatal mortality is much higher in multiple pregnancies. Very often one of the children dies. The death of one of the babies during the pregnancy can lead to serious psychological disturbances in the form of maternal depression and pathological mourning that require psychological treatment to protect the relationship with the surviving child or children.

A mother, one of whose twins died at 27.5 weeks of pregnancy, came for advice when the surviving child was a month and a half old, a few weeks after the live birth. The pregnancy ran till the thirty-third week. She said, 'For a month and a half I had the dead baby in my womb. I did not suffer that she died in my womb because at least she was with me. I was apprehensive of the delivery. It was going to be a wrench. They were going to take her away from me.' She had a Caesarean section under general anesthetic for medical reasons. She said,

> When I woke up, it was the dead baby I saw first. I saw her three times because I had not kept on looking at her. They put a nappy on her. It was only two days later that I saw the other in the mother-and-baby unit. In fact they looked very much like each other. I didn't go there earlier because after the Caesarean I had a great deal of pain and she was in the mother-and-baby unit. In any case, I did not want to see her, I was only thinking of the other one.

When talking of the living twin she said, 'I always see her with her sister next to her. I want her to know that I do not deny the life of her sister. They shared the same uterus. They each take up the same amount of space for me, I love them equally. I am into death and life, in the two simultaneously.'

The death of one of the children after the birth also presents the parents with a very special mourning and the cathexis in the living twin is complicated for the mother because she is caught up in contradictory movements [4]. The relationship with the living child can be difficult, marked by extreme attitudes of rejection or over-protection. Often those around believe that the presence of the living child will remove the sadness for the death of the other. The risk of depression five years after giving birth for mothers who lost a twin after the birth is three times higher than for mothers who gave birth to a single child. In such situations the support offered by health professionals at the time of the death is critical. Its purpose is to help both the loss process and the bonding process.

The role of the father

Few studies have focused on the father during the pregnancy and following a multiple birth. Yet the father plays a key role by his presence, his help and the support that he can provide for the mother at both the physical and psychological levels. He may have difficulties adjusting to the new family context. Fatigue and lack of sleep are important, just as the care to be given to the children. Fathers sometimes feel uneasy in the role of substitute mother [4]. They sometimes keep their distance, putting extra effort into their work. Their partners then object to their lack of involvement in the domestic jobs and those of upbringing. On account of the profound mental changes brought on by childbirth, it happens very frequently that marital relations deteriorate. Dialogue becomes difficult through the lack of availability and the frustrations each one feels towards the other [4].

Key points

Insofar as multiple births are on the increase, it is important to know what problems the families encounter. It is essential to make health professionals aware of the psychological implications of a multiple birth. Psychological assistance can be offered, sometimes from pregnancy. Taking their mental suffering into account is crucial for women's health and might also prevent problems in the relationship with the children and their consequences on bonding development.

10.3   Pregnancy and HIV, a public health problem

From AIDS to HIV under tritherapy

In France about 1500 women infected with HIV give birth each year. Over 60% of them come from sub-Saharan Africa. The AIDS situation has changed greatly since the arrival of tritherapies in 1996. On the one hand the professionals now consider AIDS as a chronic condition, and on the other hand the viral transmission rate from mother to child is today 1%, whereas it was 20% when there was no treatment. With the death sentence of HIV lifted, social and psychological questions followed closely behind the strictly medical issue. It is no longer a question of providing support for the sick until death, but rather to support the life of subjects in relatively good health whose social position has become increasingly precarious.

The specificity of HIV: a traumatic incursion

A woman who has been infected for 15 years said,

> When the doctor told me I had AIDS, it was like the end of the world. Since then I no longer live like others, it's even worse, I am no longer like the others. I always have that exact moment in mind when he told me, the words he used. Since then I take tranquil-lizers and antidepressants to avoid anxiety attacks and to manage to sleep.

In the popular imagination, despite progress in treatment, HIV remains synonymous with death. It embodies the power of death over oneself and others. It also personifies the prohibi-tion and danger of sexuality, so much so that some responsibility is attributed to the carrier, who feels shame and guilt. The origin of this guilt lies in the moment of contamination through sexual relations or taking drugs – two acts of pleasure. The links between HIV and death and sexuality explain why the announcement of being HIV-positive is considered an apocalyptic cataclysm that knocks mental functioning for six, hurling the subject into the abyss of break-down. The diagnosis becomes a traumatic incursion that staggers the person now burdened with a 'parasite', a sort of internal foreign body, which generates a dreadful sense of deperso-nalization. The ego becomes disorganized and can even become split. Denial lets the subject get away from the scary reality of death and protect himself or herself by ejecting a part of their own ego that is deemed a bad object – because sick – to the outside, often the doctor or the treatment, while the other, 'healthy' part is over-invested. This part finds again the mega-lomaniac, carefree existence of its youth, and in this way can continue to believe in its immortality. Beyond the trauma, HIV requires the subject to be in mourning for the ideal of the ego – which Freud [8] conceives as a substitute for the lost narcissism of childhood – and the associated self-esteem. The mental make-up thus tries to put in place a narcissistic protection so that the individual does collapse. The illness, insofar as it represents a narcissistic violation, is comparable to the loss of an object. It is the confrontation of reality with the loss of an object, which will allow the subject to change its libidinous investments.

Pregnancy and diagnosis as HIV-positive

About one third of women infected with HIV discover the infection when serology is offered as standard at the start of the pregnancy. What happens to the mental development in maternity when the trauma of the announcement of being HIV-positive muddies the waters? The woman's psyche is now the seat of contradictory impulses, those of life and death. We believe pregnancy is not an additional trauma, but rather a life force that for the time being protects the future mother from collapse. With the hope of life symbolized by pregnancy, reinforced by an 'invisible virus', while the viral load becomes undetectable, the anxiety about death is anesthetized, suppressed. Thus the traumatized narcissistic stratum and the ideal of the ego see themselves as restored by pregnancy and maternity. Time is no longer suspended or stopped, but turned towards the future, the child to come. This is even stronger among African women for whom having a child is a sign of social recognition and represents a key element in female identity.

Sometimes the future mother gets to announce she is HIV-positive to the father of her child or will ask the doctors to do so. If the partner is HIV-positive, the doubt about who infected who will remain. If he is HIV-negative, will he abandon her? If the patient has children who have remained in the home country, she will live with the anxiety that they too are infected. If in the past the couple had already been tested and found negative, the HIV-positive reveals infidelity on the part of one of them. How will the couple reconstitute itself? Sometimes the woman does not manage to discuss her being HIV-positive with the father of her future child, for fear that he will leave her. Medical confidentiality prevents the carer from letting him know.

HIV, the psychological and social stakes: our experience at Port-Royal

At the Port-Royal maternity department (Cochin Hospital, Paris), HIV-positive, pregnant women are treated by a multidisciplinary team. The team is made up of an obstetrician, several internists, a midwife, a nurse, an orderly, a social worker and a psychologist. The waiting list is about 80–90 women per year; 85% of them come from sub-Saharan Africa.

A number of these patients live in extremely precarious circumstances, with serious social and relational isolation, very far removed from the myth of African communal solidarity and protection. The resulting sense of loneliness is exacerbated by the impossibility of telling those around them of their infection. This secretiveness is motivated by fear of being rejected and stigmatized. One patient said, 'If you open your mouth people move away and abandon you.' These women have officially left their countries, fleeing war, poverty and the absence of a future. However, in truth they are increasingly numerous and one suspects that already in their home countries they were already infected with the AIDS virus and knew that it was only by leaving the country of their birth that they could escape a death sentence. The migration of such women has become in a way a necessary and inevitable exile. The French health system provides them with access to tritherapy, as well as allowing them to obtain identity papers. It also provides them with confidentiality, as against the hospitals in West Africa.

Coming to France is synonymous with a better life and treatment; however, once arrived, living conditions are infinitely harder that what they had imagined [9]. Often the only contact point is the address of someone from their country, a distant cousin whom they have never seen and who can show them the door at any time. One cannot ignore this precarious situation when following treatment during pregnancy is an imperative. For those who refuse or who are not very cooperative, strong denial is usually the order of the day. French law does not permit forcing a pregnant woman to undergo treatment that is intended to protect the fetus against her will. In legal terms the fetus is not a person, so has no civil status or rights. It is only when the child is born that the pediatricians can inform the state prosecutor of the mother's refusal to give him his antiretroviral syrup.

Today every woman who is HIV-positive, if her viral load is undetectable and the obstetric conditions are favorable, can give birth naturally. In fact half of these births take place by Caesarean section, where programming deals mainly with mothers with a bicicatricial uterus (the result of previous deliveries where Caesarean section had been recommended when HIV-positive). D'Yvoire [10] recounts that African women view the Caesarean as an 'indelible mark on the body, evidence of the woman's inability to have children normally'. The counter-indication of breastfeeding is particularly painful for these mothers, who in addition need to explain away to those around them why they are not breastfeeding.

Maternal ambivalence and HIV

HIV-positive pregnant women express a real struggle for life, with the child becoming a motor towards a bleak future. For all that, it does not seem that the cathexis of this baby to come will be easy. In fact, how does one make place for the child when the sickness is monopolizing the entire psyche? How can one invest in it when in mourning for oneself? What does this child represent in the mother's fantasy world? One often meets women who, once certain their child is not HIV-positive, collapse. How does one manage the guilt of risking infecting one's child and at the same time accepting that he will be different from you on account of not being HIV-positive? The future mother is often assailed by both terrible conscious and unconscious feelings of guilt.

Unconscious guilt is based on hate for the child considered as a fantasy figure that exists in every pregnancy and is inextricably tied up with the love the mother also shows for it. This hate can be an unconscious wish to commit infanticide. Infecting the baby would make real this unconscious wish to kill. Paradoxically, if the child becomes infected, which the woman never consciously wanted, she can manifest very powerful maternal feelings; this child who owes her everything, even its sickness, she will be able to keep for herself, never to be separated from it, thereby correcting the wrongdoing she had committed. On the other hand, if it is 'healthy', it is the one who becomes omnipotent and the mother can have it in for it, for not sharing her suffering. She can try to retain her maternal power by contradictory surges of love and rejection, and also by using her power over the knowledge of the child being HIV-positive.

Key points

Handling HIV has developed a great deal. While just a few years ago the lethal prognosis led to a proposal for an interruption or medical termination of pregnancy, today it has become vital to worry about the psychological and social support for future mothers who are HIV-positive. Multidisciplinary handling seeks to let these women distance themselves from HIV in order to be in 'good-enough' physical shape to have their baby.

Clinical vignette

A woman who had been spoken to by the pediatrician went to consult a psychologist because her son was not looking at her. In fact when on the nappy-changing table he was only interested in its edges, actively keeping his look away from his mother. The mother said,

> My baby intimidates me. It's on account of the HIV that I'm intimidated. I learnt I was HIV-positive 15 years ago, and I have never really accepted it. It's a moral thing. That's what intimidates me, as though to be a mother you have to be faultless. The birth reawakened the virus, it's as though the hidden part of the iceberg has appeared. I feel obliged to talk about it one day to my son. One day I want to tell him the truth, so as a result until then I don't want to think about it. I don't want my baby to feel ashamed or upset because of me. I want to tell him because my father hid from me part of his own history. I learnt about it when he died and I suffered from that. He transmitted to me his anxiety and his blocks. Nor could I tell him that I was HIV-positive. I don't want my son to go the

same route. But what should I say about myself to my son? I no longer know what is me and what is the virus. I often ask myself how I would have been without it and basically who am I. For 15 years I have been living handcuffed. Sometimes it acts as a strength and sometimes as an obstacle. It has made me get ahead. I am no longer afraid of much. I feel I am different from the others, I no longer see things like the others. It is a strength, but I also feel very much alone, all the more so since I have had the baby. During the pregnancy my baby was with me and he didn't judge me. His look, for me, is a judgement.

10.4 Conclusion

As clearly indicated by the cases of multiple pregnancies and pregnancies with HIV infection, multidisciplinary support for *all* women faced with a medical high-risk pregnancy, for the spouse and their family is required as a priority for primary and secondary prevention of parenting problems and problems in the early relationship of parents/fetus/baby and in the child's development.

10.5 References

1. Missonnier, S. (2003) *Perinatal Therapeutic Treatment*. Érès, Toulouse.
2. Harvey, D. Bryan, E. (1991) *The Stress of Multiple Births*. Multiple Birth Foundation, London.
3. Bryan, E. (1992) *Twins and Higher Multiple Births: a Guide to Their Nature and Nurture*. Edward Arnold, London.
4. Garel, M., Charlemaine, E. and Blondel, B. (2006) Psychological consequences of multiple births. *Gyn Obst Fertil*, **34**, 1058–63.
5. Garel, M., Missonnier, S. and Blondel, B. (2005) Psychological effects of multifetal pregnancy reduction, in *Multiple Pregnancy* (eds I Blickstein and L.G. Keith), 2nd edition, Taylor & Francis, Paris.
6. Klock, S.C. (2004) Psychological adjustment to twins after infertility. *Best Practice and Research. Clinical Obstetrics and Gynaecology*, **18**, 645–56.
7. Garel, M. and Blondel, B. (1992) Assessment at one year of the psychological consequences of having triplets. *Human Reproduction*, **7**, 729–32.
8. Freud, S. On narcissism (original work published 1914), in Freud, S. (1969) *Sexual Life*. P.U.F., Paris.
9. Jaffre, Y. and Olivier de Sardan, J.P. (eds) (2003) *Inhospitable Medicine*. Karthala, Paris.
10. D'Yvoire, C. (1992) Pregnancy and delivery among West African immigrant women. *Migrants Formation*, **91**.

11

Prenatal self-report questionnaires, scales and interviews

Massimo Ammaniti and Renata Tambelli

University of Rome, Italy

11.1 Introduction

For a woman and for the couple, pregnancy is an extremely important transition phase, during which one prepares to become a parent and to take care of a child who will be immature and dependent for all his first year of life. Research and clinical contributions have lent specific attention to the construction of the maternal identity, defined by Stern [2] maternal constellation, and to the development of maternal capabilities during pregnancy, which are indicative and foretelling of the mother–child relationship after birth, even in at-risk situations.

The psychology and psychopathology of pregnancy have been studied using research tools that have addressed different areas. In this paper we will take into consideration a few of the more relevant research areas for this phase:

1 The psychological dynamics connected to the attainment of the maternal identity, analysed through the mental representations of pregnant women;

Parenthood and Mental Health: A Bridge between Infant and Adult Psychiatry   Sam Tyano, Miri Keren, Helen Herrman and John Cox
© 2010 John Wiley & Sons, Ltd

2 The formation process of the mother's attachment to the fetus during pregnancy, which prepares the stabilization of this attachment after birth;

3 Mental states specific to pregnancy, such as the primary maternal preoccupation [1].

The assessment of prenatal parenting has been done through research instruments with different purposes: semi-structured clinical interviews, self-report-questionnaires and scales. Before describing the instruments more frequently used during pregnancy, here are some brief comments about their use in clinical work and in research.

11.2 Semi-structured interviews

Semi-structured interviews specifically evaluate thematic dimensions of the narration, widely used in the diagnostic and therapeutic context. They require clinical competence and a specific training of the interviewer who has to create a relational context, modulating the different questions in the most appropriate way. These particularly sensitive instruments can capture the complex nuances of the woman's representational world. In research, the training of the interviewers guarantees an adequate concordance between coders.

In the case of self-report questionnaires, the willingness of the participant is most important and for this reason, as well as for the rigidity of questions, they are less suitable for diagnostic purposes.

Semi-structured clinical interviews that investigate the pregnant woman's mental representations, focusing attention on the woman's past experiences, on how she copes with pregnancy and maternity and on how she progressively creates the image of the fetus and of the future child. To study the mental representations the woman has of herself as a mother and of the child in a more systematic way, attention is given to the structure of the narration the woman does during the interview. The interview is very susceptible an instrument for exploring parenting mental representations when they are still not defined and stabilized. Therefore, several researchers have developed interview formats to assess the narrative styles of mothers, such as the 'L'entretien-R' [3], the open-ended descriptions of their mothers – 'Describe your mother' [4] – using the method developed by Blatt et al. [5], and 'The interview on maternal representations' [6].

Among prenatal interviews, the IRMAG-R (Interview for Maternal Representations during Pregnancy, revised version,) [7, 8, 9] must be noted; this is a semi-structured interview consisting of 41 questions which bring women to tell their experience of pregnancy and of becoming mothers: their stories are not evaluated by their content, but on the basis of their narrative structure. The interview is performed between the sixth and the eighth month of pregnancy and is audiotaped and transcribed. The average length of the IRMAG is approximately 45 minutes.

The IRMAG explores the following areas:

1 How the mother organizes and communicates her experience through a narrative structure;

2 The desire of maternity within the personal and marital history;

3 Partner's and family's reactions to the news of the pregnancy;

4 Emotions and changes in personal life, in relationship with the husband/partner and between the two families occurred during pregnancy;

5 Impressions, negative and positive emotions, maternal and paternal representations: space for internal baby;

6 Temporal perspective: expectations for the future;

7 Historical perspective with respect to the mother's past.

The narrative structure of the interview is coded considering the mother's representation of herself as a mother and her representation of the fetus on the basis of seven parameters:

Richness of perception

This refers to the woman's acknowledgement of herself as a mother and of the child: this parameter evaluates the way the episodes, feelings and emotions of the woman herself, of her partner and of the future baby are told.

Openness to change

This dimension evaluates the mother's flexibility towards those physical and psychological transformations which are specific to the experience she is living, referred to herself and to the future baby. It evaluates the capability of recognizing these physical and psychological changes which involve herself, her emotional, sexual and relational life as being part of the process. It evaluates the capability to modify the representation of the baby as the pregnancy goes along.

Intensity of involvement

This dimension is used to measure the breadth of the woman's psychological involvement in confronting experiences connected to the pregnancy, to the child and to her relation with the child; this can be found in the description of the emotional echoes caused by the event as well as in the woman's participation to the interview.

Coherence

The story's coherence is measured, by which the woman, through a well organized and logical narrative flux, gives a comprehensible picture of herself as a mother, of the child and of her relation with the child. Coherence is found in the plausibility of the story told and in the capability to provide evidence and episodes which sustain her considerations and evaluations.

Differentiation

This evaluates the level of the mother's acknowledgement of her personal boundaries, of her stable mental and physical characteristics, of her specific needs and wishes, differentiated from those of her partner and of her parent figures. It evaluates the degree to which the mother is conscious that the child has his own mental and physical characteristics, with specific boundaries and specific needs.

Social dependence

This evaluates the degree of influence and dependence, to the limit of subordination, of the woman's representation of herself as a mother and of the child from the opinions, judgements and messages coming from the partner, the family, friends, the social context, mass media, social and medical institutions. It measures the degree of conformism towards others, which can in extreme cases cause a flatness of representation and a lack of personal elaboration.

Predominance of fantasies

This is used to measure the emerging of fantasies regarding the pregnancy, the future motherhood and the representation of the child, including all those images, metaphors, analogies, open-eye and night dreams, expectations, fears and wishes which characterize the way a woman imagines the pregnancy experience and the representation of herself as a mother and of the child. The fantasies can refer to the pregnancy itself, to the woman's body, to delivery, to rearing, to the integrity and physical health of the baby, his physical and character qualities, to the mother's role; these can all have a more or less realistic quality. It is not only the number of fantasies which must be considered in assigning the score but their relevance and their impact on the representation of the mother and the child.

These seven parameters all refer to the woman's representation of herself as a mother and to her representation of the child and are codified in scales with a five-point range (from 1 to 5). The assignment of the final score individuates three different styles of maternal representation:

Integrated/balanced

The integrated/balanced maternal representations are coherent narrations, in which the description of the experience the woman is living is rich in episodes and moods, and has an intense emotional involvement in an atmosphere of flexibility and openness towards the physical, psychological and emotional transformations the mother is confronting. The relationship with the child is already present during the pregnancy, and the child is considered as a person with his own motives and moods.

Restricted/disinvested

The restricted/disinvested representations emerge from narratives in which a strong emotional control prevails, with mechanisms of rationalization towards the fact of becoming a mother and towards the child. These women talk of their pregnancy, of motherhood and of the child in poor terms, without many references to emotional events and changes. The storytelling has an impersonal quality, is frequently abstract and does not communicate emotions or specific images.

Not integrated/ambivalent

The not integrated/ambivalent maternal representations are those found in confused narrations, characterized by digressions and by the woman's difficulty in answering questions in a clear and articulate way. The coherence of the story is poor, and an ambivalent involvement of the mother towards the experience she is living, towards her partner and towards her family is present. These women often express contrasting attitudes towards their motherhood, or towards the child. The son or daughter is awaited to satisfy the caregiver's needs.

Two independent, trained, certified and reliable judges coded IRMAG interviews according to the above described seven rating scales. Inter-rater reliability for IRMAG scales ranged from 0.89 (coherence) to 0.96 (predominance of *fantasies*), with a mean reliability of 0.92. Inter-rater reliability with respect to the main category was 94% (k = 0.83, p < 0.001). Disagreement was solved by a third rater.

Statistical validity is supported by an exploratory factor analysis using oblimin rotation, performed both for maternal representation of herself as a mother and of her child. The screen plot suggested that two factors should be extracted, in both cases. The two dimensions formulated to define the construct of mother's mental representations of herself as a mother were confirmed by factor analysis and accounted for 70.5% of the post-rotational variance (Table 11.1). Measures of internal consistency (Cronbach's alpha) were conducted

Table 11.1 Factor analysis (oblimin rotation) of the mother's mental representations of herself as a mother (N = 314)

Mother's dimension	Factor 1	Factor 2
A3 Affective engagement	0.87	
A2 Openness to change	0.86	
A1 Richness of perceptions	0.85	
A5 Differentiation	0.80	
A4 Coherence	0.55	
A6 Social dependence		0.83
A7 Fantasies emergence		0.72
Explicated variance	49.67%	20.83%

to examine the reliability of the two dimensions (F1, M = 2.99, SD = 0.40, α = 0.85; F2, M = 2.61, SD = 0.58, α = 0.52).

In the same manner, the two dimensions formulated to define the construct of the mother's mental representations of her unborn infant were confirmed by factor analysis and accounted for 78.95% of the post-rotational variance (Table 11.2). Measures of internal

Table 11.2 Factor analysis (oblimin rotation) of the mother's mental representations of her unborn infant (N = 314)

Child's dimension	Factor 1	Factor 2
B1 Richness of perceptions	0.90	
B5 Differentiation	0.89	
B2 Openness to change	0.89	
B3 Affective engagement	0.89	
B4 Coherence	0.88	
B6 Social dependence		0.86
B7 Fantasies emergence		0.71
Explicated variance	60.94%	18.01%

consistency (Cronbach's alpha) were conducted to examine the reliability of the two dimensions (F1, M = 2 .89, SD = 0.40, α = 0.93; F2, M = 2.63, SD = 0.73, α = 0 .45).

At the end of the interview there are five scales modeled on semantic differentials, each containing 17 pairs of opposite adjectives. The first three scales designate the individual characteristics of the unborn infant, of the woman's self and of the infant's father. Comparing the three lists, it is possible to evaluate if the representation of the baby is more influenced by the woman's self-representation or that of her partner.

The other two scales deal with the maternal characteristics of the pregnant woman and those of her mother. In this case adjectives will refer to affective orientations, personal lay-out, maternal role, maternal sensitivity and competence.

The interview is used to assess how information and emotions concerning the woman herself and her child are organized, whereas the five scales give us a picture of the contents of the representations. The two instruments can be used together[7, 10] and independently [11, 12, 13].

To explore the configuration of paternal representations and their differences from the mother's the IRPAG (Interview for Paternal Representations during Pregnancy) [14] is used.

As indicated in Table 11.3, fathers' representations have a different distribution confronted with mothers' ones.

Table 11.3 Distribution of maternal and paternal representations during pregnancy (IRMAG/IRPAG)

Group	Integrated	Ambivalent	Restricted
Mother (N = 162)	89 (54.9%)	35 (21.6%)	38 (23.5%)
Father (N = 162)	93 (57.4%)	15 (9.2%)	54 (33.4%)

Notes: χ^2 (2, N = 324) = 10.87 g.di l. = 2; p = 0.004.

The results reported in Table 11.3 show that in our sample the integrated/balanced parental representation is equally distributed among women and men, as opposed to the restricted/disinvested one more common among men and the non-integrated/ambivalent one more common among women. These data confirm the differences of psychological orientation of mothers and fathers during pregnancy, even though the mothers' and fathers' attitudes draw closer after birth.

The use of IRMAG-R in at-risk pregnancies allows study of the contents and structure of maternal representations which give significant indication to evaluate parenting capabilities during pregnancy and the postnatal period (Table 11.4).

Table 11.4   Distribution of maternal representations during pregnancy in at-risk and non-risk mothers

Group	Integrated	Ambivalent	Restricted
Normal mothers (N = 239)	60.7% (145)	20.1% (48)	19.2% (46)
At-risk mothers (N = 132)	43.2% (57)	34.1% (45)	22.7% (30)

Notes: χ^2 (2, N = 371) = 11.93 g.di l. = 2; p < 0.003.

In at-risk situations, persistent preoccupations and phobic fears have been found; a specific scale is being created for these. This scale allows us to detect the levels of pervasiveness and intrusiveness of fears in relation to the pregnancy, to delivery and to the rearing of the child. The scale for the evaluation of the risk factors is, like the others, an ordinal scale with a five-point range.

The IRMAG-R can be used for research in the clinical field to study the psychological state of women during pregnancy or for at-risk situations, in medically assisted pregnancies or in projects to support motherhood.

Considering the stability of maternal representation categories between pregnancy and the postnatal period we have: for the integrated representation r = 0.72, the restricted one r = 0.68, the non-integrated one r = 0.64.

Regarding now the predictive value of the interview, women who are more self-conscious and more able to recognize their personal ambivalence during pregnancy are more competent in appreciating the personal features of the baby after birth and the changes during early development [7].

11.3 Self-report questionnaires and scales

Self-report questionnaires and scales have been used to assess attachment processes during pregnancy, when emotional ties start rising between mother and child. The construct of prenatal attachment [15, 16, 17] takes account of the mother's affective investment for the fetus, which is 'the most precocious and basic form of human intimacy' [18, 19]. Condon [16] has suggested a hierarchical model of attachment based on five subjective experiences which derive from maternal love experience and mediate this core experience and overt behaviours. These subjective experiences are expressed in maternal disposition 'to know' the loved fetus, 'to be with' him or her, 'to avoid separation or loss' of the loved object, disposition 'to protect' the fetus and finally 'to gratify' the fetus's needs.

The quality and evolution of the prenatal attachment is influenced by many factors, first of all by the advancing of the pregnancy which entails growing ties between the mother and child, hastened by the appearance of fetal movements. Aside these factors, the personal history of the woman and of the couple have a significant influence on prenatal attachment.

Obviously this attachment is not only present in mothers but in fathers as well, although in 15–20% of the fathers this affective attachment to the fetus seems not to rise [16].

The instruments more frequently used to study prenatal attachment are self-report questionaires.

Maternal Fetal Attachment Scale

The Maternal Fetal Attachment Scale (MFAS) [15] is based on 24 items upon which an agreement score from a range of five points is expressed. The higher the score in the items, the more definite and consistent is the mother's attachment to the fetus. The items refer to five basic components:

- Differentiation of self from fetus

- Interaction with fetus

- Attributing characteristics to the fetus

- Giving of self

- Role-taking.

Measurements of internal consistency (Cronbach's alpha 0.85) are good on the total of the items, while the subscales have lower scores (between 52 and 73). Typical of the MFAS is that the items evaluate the mother's behavior more than her feelings or thoughts. In the validation sample used by Cranley, this instrument was used between weeks 35 and 40. The scale of maternal attachment was later adapted to a specular version which measures the father's attachment to the fetus.

Maternal Antenatal Attachment Scale

In the Maternal Antenatal Attachment Scale (MAAS) [16], based on 19 items, the response is rated on five response options, enquiring as to the frequency and/or intensity of these experiences over the preceding two weeks. The scale was used during the third trimester of pregnancy and has good levels of internal consistency (Cronbach's alpha > 0.80).

It measures, beside a global attachment value, two underlying dimensions: *quality of involvement* and *intensity of preoccupation*. From the characteristics of these two factors, four styles of attachment can be identified:

- Positive-preoccupied

- Positive-disinterested

- Negative-preoccupied

- Negative-disinterested.

The fathers' version is based on 16 items, 14 of which are in common with the mother's, as Condon sustains that prenatal attachment, even though it has a common basis for mothers and fathers, has specific aspects as well.

Besides this, the MAAS has been recognized as having predictive value of the postnatal attachment when the baby is four and eight months old [19].

Prenatal Attachment Inventory

The Prenatal Attachment Inventory (PAI) [17] is based on 21 items. The response to each item is rated on a four-point Likert scale. A higher score indicates greater attachment. In structure it is similar to Cranley's scale but the aspects researched are different. It refers to attachment theory, describing women's thoughts, feelings and relationship towards the fetus. Two constructs, in particular, are extremely relevant in the theoretic model at the basis of the PAI: *attachment relation to the partner* and *adaptation to pregnancy*, because according to Muller [17] these are both positively related to prenatal attachment. The statistical analyses have shown good validity and internal consistency (Cronbach's alpha varies from 81 to 91 in all researches that used it). Muller's instrument does not allow an evaluation of father's prenatal attachment.

Muller's instrument displays a correlation, although not very high ($r = 0.46$), between prenatal attachment and postnatal attachment at the twelfth week of life.

The measurements from the self-evaluation scales described above concern the quality and quantity of the emotional investment of the parents towards the fetus without, however, going into more complex elements (mental representations of the parents, parents' attachment models). Therefore these scales can be used together with other research instruments.

Among the instruments for evaluating prenatal attachment, MAAS is more suitable because it specifically measures the prenatal attachment instead of a positive attitude toward pregnancy. Besides this, MAAS has a high test-retest reliability and an internal consistency and has been translated and standardized in different countries.

11.4 Inventories

Inventories have been used to study the psychic state during pregnancy, such as the primary maternal preoccupation, a mental state Winnicott [1] described as 'almost an illness' that a mother 'must experience and recover in order to create and sustain an environment that can meet the physical and psychobiological needs of her infant'. He hypothesized that this special state begins towards the end of the pregnancy and continues through the first months of the infant's life.

If Winnicott's concept had only a clinical value, it was later explored by means of a semi-structured interview, Yale Inventory of Parental Thoughts and Action (YIPTA) [20] within which an inventory systematically explores the mother's and father's preoccupations and thoughts.

The specific content of the YIPTA covers the thoughts and actions associated with three domains of caregiving (Care), relationship building (Relationship) and anxious intrusive thoughts and harm avoidant behaviours experienced/performed by parents (AITHAB). The YIPTA is designed for the use of experienced clinicians and has been used at the eighth month of gestation, at two weeks after delivery and three months after birth.

The measurements of the early parental preoccupations and behaviours, besides outlining the psychic states typical of mothers, highlight depression and anxiety symptoms that can appear during pregnancy, while the AITHAB measurements highlight intrusive thoughts and harm-avoidant behaviours which are conceptually related to obsessive compulsive disorders (OCD). It can be hypothesized that some forms of OCD that appear in this period are the dysregulative result of this specific psychic state that appears during pregnancy.

Both parents present the highest levels of 'preoccupation' towards their child around birth time (between the eighth month of pregnancy and the second week after delivery). Thoughts about the baby during the period of Winnicott's primary maternal preoccupation occupy the minds of the mothers and fathers for respectively 14 and 7 hours a day.

At the eighth month of pregnancy [20] the following has been found:

- Preoccupations on the baby's health in 95% of the mothers and 80% of the fathers (health, growth, aspect)

- Thoughts of damaging the baby in 37% of the parents (making it cry, shaking or hitting it, dropping it).

These thoughts are a reason of personal distress in 20% of the cases.

The progress of thoughts and preoccupations shows that these tend to appear around the eighth month of pregnancy and reach their climax around the second month after birth to then slowly disappear (Figure 11.1).

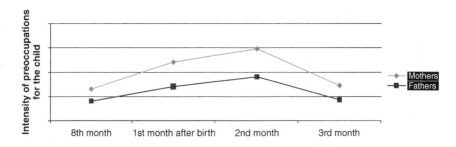

Figure 11.1   Trend of parental preoccupation during pregnancy and postnatal period
Source: Leckman [20], modified.

The YIPTA permits an evaluation of the level of parental preoccupation which is an important psychic state during pregnancy and the postnatal period because it focuses the parents' attention on the baby's health and stimulates better caregiving capabilities. In the mother's depression and in obsessive-compulsive states the level of preoccupations can occupy the mother's mind completely and interfere with her maternal capabilities.

11.5 Conclusion

To conclude, interviews in pregnancy, as we have shown with the presentation of IRMAG-R [9], have at the same time a research and a clinical aim. But what is more specific is the clinical one, because interviews can explore psychological dynamics of the maternal identity and evidence at risk and psychopathological conditions of pregnancy which may interfere with the parental capacity after the birth of the baby. However to use interviews in the proper way, specific training is necessary to lead the interview and to use the coding system to evaluate the text of the interview.

Self-report questionnaires and scales are easier to handle and do not require specific training, but they do not provide a deep exploration of the psychic world of the pregnant woman. They have been used as reliable research and screening instruments which can give evidence of risk situations, as has been shown with attachment [15, 16, 17] and maternal preoccupations [20] questionaires. However after the detection of risk situations, further explorations are required in order to understand better the psychological dynamics of the pregnant woman.

11.6 References

1. Winnicott, D.W. (1956) Primary maternal preoccupation, in his *Through Pediatrics to Psycho-Analysis*. Basic Books, New York.
2. Stern, D.N. (1995) *The Motherhood Constellation: a Unified View of Parent-Infant Psychotherapy*. Basic Books, New York.
3. Robert-Tissot, C., Serpa-Rusconi, S., Bachmann, J., Besson, G., Cramer, B., Knauer, D., de Muralt, M., Palacio-Espasa, F., Stern, D.N. (1989) L'Entretien-R. In: Lebovici, S., Mazet, P., & Visier, J.P. (Eds), *L'évaluation des interactions précoces entre le bébé et ses partenaires*. Eshel, Paris; Médecine et Hygiène, Genève.
4. Priel, B. and Besser, A. (2001) Bridging the gap between attachment and object relations theories: a study of the transition to motherhood. *British Journal of Medical Psychology*, **74**, 85–100.
5. Blatt, S.J., Chevron, S.E., Quinlan, D.M. *et al.* (1992) The assessment of qualitative and structural dimensions of object representations. Yale University, unpublished manuscript.
6. Fava Vizziello G., Antonioli, M.E., Cocci, V. and Invernizzi, R. (1993) From pregnancy to motherhood: the structure of representative and narrative change. *Infant Mental Health Journal*, **14**, 1, 4–16.
7. Ammaniti, M., Baumgartner, E., Candelori, C. *et al.* (1992) Representations and narratives during pregnancy. *Infant Mental Health Journal*, **13**, 167–82.
8. Ammaniti, M., Candelori, C., Pola, M. and Tambelli R. (1999) *Maternite et grossesse*. P.U.F., Paris.
9. Ammaniti, M., Tambelli, R., Odorisio, F. *et al.* (2008) *In the Mother's Mind: Investigations During Pregnancy*. WAIMH, World Congress 2008, 1–5 August, Yokohama, Japan.
10. Ilicali, E.T. and Fisek G.O. (2004) Maternal representations during pregnancy and early motherhood. *Infant Mental Health Journal*, **25**, 16–27.
11. Ammaniti, M., Tambelli, R. and Perucchini P. (2000) De la grossesse à période post-accouchement: stabilité et évolution des représentations maternelles. *Devenir*, **12** (2), 57–74.
12. Pajulo, M., Savonlahti, E., Sourander, A. *et al.* (2001) Prenatal maternal representations: mothers at psychosocial risk. *Infant Mental Health Journal*, **22** (5), 529–44.
13. Pajulo, M., Helenius, H. and Mayes, L. (2006) Prenatal views of baby and parenthood: association with sociodemographic and pregnancy factors. *Infant Mental Health Journal*, **27** (3), 229–50.

14. Ammaniti, M., Tambelli, R. and Odorisio, F. (2006) Intervista clinica per lo studio delle rappresentazioni paterne in gravidanza: IRPAG. *Età Evolutiva*, **85**, 34–44.
15. Cranley, M.C. (1981) Development of a tool for the measurement of maternal attachment during pregnancy. *Nursing Research*, **30**, 281–84.
16. Condon, J.T. (1993) The assessment of antenatal emotional attachment: developments of a questionnaire instrument. *British Journal of Medical Psychology*, **66**, 167–83.
17. Muller, M.E. (1993) Development of the Prenatal Attachment Inventory. *Western Journal of Nursing Research*, **15** (2), 199–215.
18. Condon, J. and Corkindale, C. (1997) The correlates of antenatal attachment in pregnant women. *British Journal of Medical Psychology*, **70**, 359–72.
19. Condon, J. and Corkindale, C. (1998) The assessment of parent-to-infant attachment: development of a self-report questionnaire instrument. *Journal of Reproductive and Infant Psychology*, **16**, 57–76.
20. Leckman, J.F., Myers L.C., Feldman, R. *et al.* (1999) Early parental preoccupations and behaviors and their possible relationship to the symptoms of obsessive-compulsive disorder. *Acta Psychiatrica Scandinavica*, **396**, 1–26.

12

Observational tool: the prenatal Lausanne Trilogue Play[*]

Elisabeth Fivaz-Depeursinge,[1] France Frascarolo[1] and Antoinette Corboz-Warnery[2]

[1]Institut Universitaire de Psychothérapie, Prilly-Lausanne, Switzerland
[2]Lausanne, Switzerland

12.1 Introduction

Adult as well as child clinicians know that the transition to parenthood and co-parenthood begins during pregnancy, and is prepared much earlier, through filiation. Co-parenting designates the manner in which parents cooperate in relation to their child, supporting one another's parenting efforts, undermining or interfering with them [1]. The co-parenting relationship has to be distinguished from the marital relationship which precedes it and continues its separate, though articulated, pathway across the transition to the family triangle. While the marital relationship is a determinant of family-level cooperation and of child socialization, the co-parenting relationship both mediates the influence between the marital relationship and the child development and directly influences it [1]. Thus it is important to have specific instruments for the study and assessment of marital versus co-parenting relationships, and both from an interactional as well as from a representational perspective. The majority of researchers have focused on pregnant mothers'

[*]The research presented in this article has been supported by the Fonds National Suisse de la Recherche Scientifique, grant 32-52508.97.

Parenthood and Mental Health: A Bridge between Infant and Adult Psychiatry   Sam Tyano, Miri Keren, Helen Herrman and John Cox
© 2010 John Wiley & Sons, Ltd

representations of their future parenting. Some have developed individual or couple research interviews to assess the representations of parents-to-be concerning their future co-parenting relationship [2]. In parallel, a very few methods have explored the formation of parenting interactions (see [3]) but none, to our knowledge, the co-parenting interaction in formation during pregnancy. In this chapter, we present such an instrument, the 'Lausanne prenatal Trilogue Play' situation.

A strong argument in favor of studying prenatal relationships between the parents is that researchers studying prenatal maternal stress, in particular Bergman, Sarkar, O'Connor, Modi and Glover [4] have found that prenatal environmental stressors predict child disturbances, such as problems in cognitive development and fearfulness. Interestingly, among the determinant prenatal stressors (unfavorable life events, obstetrical complications, maternal preoccupations, exposure to traumatic events), recurrent couple conflict during pregnancy has been revealed as particularly harmful [5].

What is known at this point shows that a prenatal couple's representations and interactions foreshadow postnatal family interactions. The integrity of the marital relationship is the first predictor which has been identified (see [6]). In particular, several studies of the couple's pre-birth marital relationship have indicated that it may set the stage for greater mutuality in the triadic family process itself (see [1]). Likewise, prenatal marital conflict as well as a weak ego resilience of the father foreshadowed the father's withdrawal in 'who does what' negotiations (how the parents share caretaking tasks) as well as poor co-parenting in family play at three months post-partum [7, 8]. Interviews of the parents during pregnancy about how they anticipated their co-parenting relationship showed that expressions of pessimism regarding the future co-parenting alliance predicted the co-parenting relationship in trilogue play at three months post-partum. The degree of negativity in couple marital conflict, already at the newlywed stage, and then during pregnancy, is predictive of postnatal family interactions as well as of the infant's emotional regulation in family play at three months post-partum [9]. Measuring through a psychodynamic interview the parents' 'triadic capacities' (talk about the future family as a threesome, [2]) showed that triadic capacities were related to the family trilogue capacities at four months. In our view, it was important to add to the above instruments measuring the couples' representations an instrument of observation of their co-parenting interactions. This instrument was developed as one of the versions of the Lausanne Trilogue Play paradigm.

12.2 The Lausanne Trilogue Play paradigm

The Lausanne Trilogue Play (LTP for short) paradigm [10] may be seen as the analogue of the dialogue play situation classically used in parent–infant dyadic assessments, but for three-way rather than two-way play. It was elaborated to systematically observe a family of three – the realistic context in which a first baby is born – from birth to childhood. There are four configurations in which a three-person group may interact:

1 One parent plays with the infant, the other one is the third party;

2 The parents reverse roles;

3 Both parents play together with the infant;

4 The parents talk together and the infant is in the third-party position.

One of the main variables measured through this observation is the family alliance, or how the family and especially the parents work together to scaffold the infant – it ranges from the most cooperative to the most problematic. The system for evaluating family alliances in early infancy is fully described in Frascarolo *et al.* [11]. In families which have the most adaptive alliances, the partners are primed to interact, respect their prescribed roles (active vs. third-party parent) and maintain a joint focus on communal games, while staying in touch emotionally. In families with problematic alliances, partners exclude one another, withdraw or interfere with one another's roles, or fail to establish a joint focus during games or to remain in touch with one another. This conception of family alliances shares a number of similarities with co-parenting conceptualizations.

12.3   The prenatal LTP

As noted above, a prenatal version of the LTP was designed to study the pre- to postnatal transition. It has the same structure in four configurations as the standard version. The goal is to measure the capacity of the parents-to-be to work together as a team in relation to their baby-to-be, in other words, their co-parenting alliance in formation. The point of this observational method is that the parents enact their representations rather than talk about them. For instance, it allows observation of the parents' intuitive parenting behaviors, namely the specific behaviors that humans use with infants, rather than asking them whether they use them; or observation of the actual cooperation between the parents, and their affection towards each other, rather than asking them whether they feel they cooperate or have affection for each other.

Procedure and setting

The prenatal LTP was designed by the third author, A. Corboz-Warnery (for a full description, see [3]). It follows a warm-up interview of the parents on their representations about their baby and their threesome after birth. The facilitator asks the parents to imagine that the delivery has gone well and that it is the first time that they are alone with their baby, asking them to enact this fabulous moment. Then she presents the 'baby', a life-size newborn-looking doll to mother and to father, entraining them in role-playing by addressing the baby in baby talk and expressing her admiration for his/her loveliness. Finally, she asks them to enact this encounter in the four contexts of the LTP and tells them that it usually takes about five minutes. In spite of the surprise that this unusual situation may cause, the vast majority of the parents readily engage in it.

   As an illustration, a brief transcript follows of Lea's father role-playing of his encounter with his baby, while mother is third party. The father has taken the baby in his arms, holding it in a feeding position with much delicacy and tenderness: 'Hello my baby ... Oh but it has tiny hairs ... I am your dad ... You are heavy ...three kilos ... Do you make funny faces? ... You are so cute ... I am proud of you ... You are so beautiful ...' In the meantime, the mother is watching, alternating between laughter and an intense emotion, with tears in her eyes. This is characteristic of the emotions activated in this situation and of the reassuring feeling mothers have when seeing their husbands love their babies.

Coding

The following five-point scales were used, derived from McHale's well-validated coding system of postnatal co-parenting, the CFRS, adding a category for the coding of intuitive parenting behaviors (see [1]). The system is multimodal, in that it takes into account all modalities of interaction, verbal as well as non-verbal. It includes all parts and all interactive levels at once.

1 Playfulness: as this is an unusual situation, it is important that the couple take it playfully, by creating a good-humored space to co-construct their role-playing.

2 Structure of the task: the parents' ability to follow the format in four parts, each lasting for a sufficient duration.

3 The cooperation between the spouses in the face of this unusual context (not only mere absence of antagonism or interference, but active cooperation and support of each other).

4 The expression of warmth between the spouses as well as towards the baby (expressions of affection and tenderness, affective valence as manifested by looks and mutual smiles, shared laughs and affectionate gestures).

5 Each parent's intuitive parenting behaviors (holding, face-to-face orientation, dialogue distance, smiling at infant and baby-talk, rocking, caressing and kissing, exploring the baby's body, caring for the well-being of the baby).

The reliability was found to be good to excellent.

Results

The predictive power of the prenatal LTP was examined in a non-clinical sample (N = 50 families of average to high SES) in relation to the postnatal family alliance measured in the postnatal LTP; it was measured first at 3 months [3], then longitudinally at 9 and 18 months [12].

The results of the pre- to postnatal study showed that the variables which predict postnatal family alliances are cooperation between the parents, warmth and intuitive parenting behaviors. In this regard, it is interesting to note that while intuitive parenting behaviors do distinguish postnatal alliances, they do not distinguish parents' gender, being a father versus being a mother [3].

The results on the trajectories of alliances from pregnancy to 18 months included four measurement points; alliance trajectories were categorized as high (cooperative) versus low (problematic) trajectories [12]. The high-alliance cases, including two-thirds of the sample, maintained a high level of alliance across the study's measurement points. The low-alliance cases maintained a low level of coordination from pregnancy or early infancy on (for details, see [12]). Thus, not only was there continuity between the pre- and postnatal alliances at 3 months, but there was also continuity up to 18 months. It is also of note that our studies examining the triangular capacity of the infant, namely her capacity to interact with both parents simultaneously, showed that this capacity was better developed in families with higher prenatal co-parenting alliances as well as in higher postnatal family alliances [13, 14].

An Italian replication study showed that the pre-natal LTP was applicable to the Italian culture, and had good internal consistency. The results on alliance trajectories were comparable to those of the Lausanne study, with the exception of a decrease of the postnatal alliance at four months and a return to baseline by nine months [16]. This discontinuity might be interpreted as a function of the difference in measurement points (three months in the Lausanne study, versus four months in the Italian study) due to the developmental transition taking place between three and four months. Infants are known to be mainly social at three months, but to develop a more or less exclusive interest for physical objects by four months. By nine months, having integrated their interest for persons and for objects, they return to social cooperation with their parents, including cooperation about objects.

It is also to be noted that a version of the prenatal LTP has been adapted for watching a video of the echography instead of playing with a doll [17, 18].

12.4 Discussion

In sum, the patterns of prenatal co-parenting are already established by the sixth month of pregnancy. They are the central pillar of what will be the family alliance after birth and across the first years. Not only do the results document the continuity between prenatal co-parenting and postnatal family interactions in early infancy, but they also show cross-time coherence of alliances between the prenatal co-parenting alliance and the family alliance up to toddlerhood. It is also well documented that co-parenting and family alliances come to have an imprint on young children's social and emotional development (for a review, see [1]). In particular, our own studies examining the triangular capacity of the infant, namely her capacity to interact with both parents simultaneously, showed that this capacity was better developed in families with higher prenatal co-parenting alliances as well as in higher postnatal family alliances [13, 14].

One may ask: what of the influence of the child on the family alliance? A few studies have attempted to examine the contributions of the infant in moderating linkages between pre- and post-birth family functioning (see [1]). They indicated that the child's temperamental characteristics can amplify or mitigate early co-parenting difficulties, but only in families which are at risk prenatally for developing such problems.

Thus, we have firm grounds to study the co-parenting relationship from its onset during pregnancy, in order to design timely clinical interventions. The earlier the intervention, the more motivated the parents are to work on their parenting, co-parenting and family relationships. From this perspective, it is of note that the LTP paradigm was designed in the systems perspective which considers that assessment is intervention. In fact, going through the prenatal LTP procedure itself is often experienced by parents as a growth-enhancing process. Its association with video feedback allows for brief therapeutic inter-ventions (see [15] for examples).

12.5 Conclusion

In conclusion, knowing, on the one hand, how important the self-esteem of an adult depends on his/her sense of being a good enough parent, and on the other hand, how much good enough parenting depends on the marital and co-parenting relationships and how influential those are for the social development of the child, it is desirable to integrate these perspectives in the treatment of adult patients.

12.6 References

1. McHale, J. (2007) When infants grow up in multiperson relationship systems. *Infant Mental Health Journal*, **28**, 370–92.
2. Buergin, D. and von Klitzing, K. (1995) Prenatal representations and postnatal interactions of a threesome (mother, father and baby), in *Psychosomatic Obstetrics and Gynaecology* (eds. J.Bitzer and M.Stauber), Monduzzi, Bologna, pp. 185–92.
3. Carneiro, C., Corboz Warnery, A. and Fivaz-Depeursinge, E. (2006) Prenatal coparenting and postnatal family alliance. *Infant Mental Health Journal*, **27** (2), 207–28.
4. Bergman, K., Sarkar, P., O'Connor, T. *et al.* (2007). Maternal stress during pregnancy predicts cognitive ability and fearfulness in infancy. *Journal of the American Academy of Child and Adolescent Psychiatry*, **46**, 1454–63.
5. Rusconi-Serpa, S. (2008) Effets du stress prénatal sur le devenir de l'enfant. Conférence dans les journées de prévention dans la petite enfance, Geneva, 13–14 November.
6. Shapiro, A.F., Gottman, J.M. and Carrère, S. (2000) The baby and the marriage: identifying factors that buffer against decline in marital satisfaction after the first baby arrives. *Journal of Family Psychology*, **14**, 59–70.
7. McHale, J., Kazali, C., Rotman, T. *et al.* (2004) The transition to coparenthood: parents' prebirth expectations and early coparental adjustment at 3 months postpartum. *Development and Psychopathology*, **16**, 711–33.
8. Elliston, D., McHale, J, Talbot, J. *et al.* (2008) Withdrawal from co-parenting interactions during early infancy. *Family Process*, **47**, 481–99.
9. Shapiro, A.F. (2004) Examining relationships between the marriage, mother-father-baby interactions and infant emotion regulation. Unpublished doctoral manuscript. University of Washington.
10. Fivaz-Depeursinge, E. and Corboz-Warnery, A. (1999) *The Primary Triangle: a Developmental Systems View of Mothers, Fathers and Infants*. Basic Books, New York.
11. Frascarolo, F., Favez, N., Carneiro, C. and Fivaz-Depeursinge, E. (2004) Hierarchy of interactive functions in father-mother-baby three-way games. *Infant and Child Development*, **13**, 301–22.
12. Favez, N., Frascarolo, F., Carneiro, C. *et al.* (2006) The development of the family alliance from pregnancy to toddlerhood and children outcomes at 18 months. *Infant and Child Development*, **15**, 59–73.
13. Koller, R. (2002) Les affects de l'enfant de trois mois dans l'interaction avec ses deux parents. (The affects of the 3-month old infant in the interaction with both parents). Research report of the Center for Family Studies, University of Lausanne.

14. McHale, J., Fivaz-Depeursinge, E., Dickstein, S. *et al.* (2008) New evidence for the social embeddedness of infant's early triangular capacities. *Family Process*, **47**, 445–63.
15. Fava Vizziello, G.M., Simonelli, A., Bighin, M. and De Palo, F. (in press). Analisi preliminari di validazione del Lausanne Triadic Play pre-natale per lo studio delle competenze genitoriali in gravidanza. *Età Evolutiva*.
16. Fivaz-Depeursinge, E., Corboz-Warnery, A. and Keren, M. (2004) The primary triangle: treating infants in their families, in *Treating Parent-Infant Problems: Strategies for Intervention* (eds A.J. Sameroff, S.C. McDonough and K.L. Rosenblum), Guilford Press, New York.
17. Simonelli, A., Bighin, M., Petech, E. and De Palo, F. (2008) The trilogic competencies in the first year of life: assessment and developmental trajectories.
18. Ammaniti, M., Mazzoni, S. and Menozzi, F. (2009, January) Ecographia in gravidanza ed interazioni genitoriali. Lecture presented at the International conference: La nascita della cogenitorialità in gravidanza. Rome.
19. Ammaniti, M. (1991) Maternal representations during pregnancy and early infant-mother interactions. *Infant Mental Health Journal*, **12**, 246–55.

13

Psychopharmacological treatments during pregnancy: risks and benefits for the mother and her infant

Martin St-André[1,2] and Brigitte Martin[1]

[1]CHU Sainte-Justine, Canada
[2]Université de Montréal, Canada

13.1 Introduction

Pregnancy constitutes a period of dramatic change in the somatic and psychic domains. The future mother experiences profound neurohormonal, intrapsychic and interpersonal challenges that redefine her sense of identity and her capacity for intimacy and nurturing. This enriching period brings multiple moments of joy but is also commonly accompanied by difficult emotional states, particularly among vulnerable women with a fragile personality or a difficult attachment history. These transient experiences and a certain degree of suffering are an integral part of the transition to parenthood and should not be confused with psychopathology.

In many countries, contemporary society and medical culture place great emphasis on autonomy, performance and the preservation of a stable self-image. Developmental tensions are often seen as symptoms to be swiftly eradicated. We are fascinated and seduced by quick technological fixes to various daily and existential problems. Indeed, the utopian promises of neurobiology have raised hopes of somehow being inoculated against moments of distress over the life course. Moreover, the conviction shared by families and clinicians alike that suffering should be prevented at all cost marks a radical departure from traditional

Parenthood and Mental Health: A Bridge between Infant and Adult Psychiatry   Sam Tyano, Miri Keren, Helen Herrman and John Cox
© 2010 John Wiley & Sons, Ltd

cultural values, including Judeo-Christian principles. This shift has allowed the elevation of psychopharmacological intervention to levels unparalleled in the history of medicine.

The real paradox of this situation is that our concern with preventing 'useless suffering' has led a number of clinicians to lose interest in the various layers of meaning that suffering can assume, as is the case during the transition to parenthood. A genuine questioning on the part of parents and clinicians alike about the meaning and context of various symptoms and emotional states during pregnancy is important in order to avoid the unnecessary or harmful medicalization of emotional issues. Any consideration of psychopharmacological treatments should have this line of thinking as its background.

Receiving a psychotropic medication while bearing life is a decision of great significance. Pregnancy often occurs at a time when a woman and her partner feel that joy has finally prevailed over suffering in their lives. A recurrence or an exacerbation of a psychiatric condition is often shamefully experienced as an 'incapacity' to transform oneself. It may also bring the fear of 'turning into' a family member at a life period during which issues of repetition and discontinuity with the family of origin are critical. Taking a psychotropic medication – especially an antipsychotic – also raises issues of stigmatization and fears of being perceived by perinatal teams as unfit or ill-prepared for parenthood. These problems can be circumvented by better educating patients and health workers about common perinatal psychiatric conditions and treatments. Clinicians should validate the patient's ability to identify her emotional needs and to obtain support for herself and her infant at a most vulnerable life period.

Psychopharmacological treatments rightfully emphasize the well-known biological aspects of mental illness. However, clinicians should not minimize the key role of inter-personal factors – notably marital and family of origin issues – in the aetiology and perpetuation of various psychiatric conditions. A systemic and multimodal approach is always necessary in order to optimize treatment and to reduce the sense of guilt and blame experienced by mothers during this sensitive time.

13.2   Depression and anxiety during pregnancy

In contrast with common belief, pregnancy does not protect against depression or anxiety. The prevalence of depression is estimated between 7% and 13% in pregnant women, with 2–6% meeting diagnostic criteria for major depression [1]. Moreover, many women report either an exacerbation of a pre-existing anxiety disorders or clinically high levels of anxiety.

In addition to being a considerable source of suffering for future mothers, a major depression or an anxiety disorder can have various impacts on the course of pregnancy: complicating antenatal care, preventing appropriate preparation for the arrival of the infant, exacerbating interpersonal conflicts, increasing the risk of alcohol or drug use, and raising the risk of postnatal depression and of mother–infant relationship disorders [2]. For the infant, depressive disorders and maternal stress have been associated with an increased risk of spontaneous abortion, pre-eclampsia, prematurity, low birth weight, perinatal complications, low APGAR scores and high cortisol levels [1].

In addition, more than 15 studies have shown a link between high antenatal maternal stress and variations of neurobehavioral development in infants, although the correlations are far from linear and the clinical manifestations in infants are often subclinical. In spite of these data regarding the risk of not treating major depression or severe anxiety disorders during pregnancy or breastfeeding, many mothers decide to stop their treatment when they learn of their pregnancy [3].

Mothers with antenatal depression or anxiety sometimes fear 'becoming crazy' or psychotic in post-partum. In the absence of a personal of familial history of bipolar or psychotic disorders, these fears usually reflect underlying anxiety, such as impulse phobia, and should be treated with reassurance or more specific mood or anxiety treatments. Additionally, clinicians should not confuse culturally sanctioned formulation of anxiety or suffering with psychotic symptoms.

Antidepressants

Structural teratogenesis

Antidepressants are among the most studied medications during pregnancy. A recent large-scale epidemiological survey in Quebec revealed that approximately 3.7% of women were given antidepressants during their first trimester of pregnancy. Table 13.1 summarizes the main published findings regarding the effects of antenatal antidepressant exposure on the fetus and the newborn. Generally speaking, antidepressants do not increase the 3% baseline teratogenic risk for major congenital anomalies, although data will vary from one molecule to another. With more recent or less frequently used medication, current data do not allow to exclude all risks. As studies are still ongoing for many of these agents, the clinician is invited to refer to potential new publications along with the data presented in Table 13.1.

Obstetrical complications

Although two meta-analyses have found an increased risk of spontaneous abortion in women receiving antidepressants, most included studies were not designed to assess this pregnancy

Table 13.1   Safety profile of antidepressive and anxiolytic agents during pregnancy

Medication classes	Teratogenic, neonatal and neurobehavioral developmental effects	Comments and recommendations
Antidepressants		
Selective serotonin reuptake inhibitors (SSRIs) and serotonin-noradrenaline reuptake inhibitors (SNRIs) SSRIs: Citalopram Escitalopram Fluoxetine Fluvoxamine Paroxetine Sertraline	Large epidemiological studies with more than 4000 first-trimester exposures to *citalopram, sertraline* and *fluoxetine* without evidence of an increased risk of congenital birth defects compared to the baseline risk; similar observations but less data available for *escitalopram* and *fluvoxamine* [2, 4]	Despite discrepancy in the quality of the published data, SSRIs are the most studied antidepressants during pregnancy and are considered as first choices for women planning a pregnancy or already pregnant. Experience has been particularly reassuring with *fluoxetine, sertraline* and *citalopram*

Table 13.1   (*Continued*)

Medication classes	Teratogenic, neonatal and neurobehavioral developmental effects	Comments and recommendations
SNRIs: Duloxetine Venlafaxine	More than 5000 first-trimester exposures to *paroxetine*; two studies suggest a small increased risk for cardiac anomalies, although 7 studies did not confirm this association; if present, additional risk for cardiac anomalies is estimated to be less than 1% [4] 1400 first-trimester exposures to *venlafaxine* in prospective and retrospective cohort studies did not reveal an increased birth defects risk compared to the baseline risk [2, 4] No data currently available for *duloxetine* Lower placental transfer for *sertraline* and *paroxetine* compared to *fluoxetine* and *citalopram* Transient and mild neonatal signs affecting central nervous system (CNS), respiratory and digestive systems noted in up to 30% of exposed newborns [5]. Serious effects such as persistent pulmonary hypertension and seizures have been associated with third-trimester use of SSRIs and may affect 1% or less of exposed newborns, although it had not been observed in the latest study Normal neurobehavioral outcomes measured in children up to 6 years old exposed *in utero* to SSRIs in 11 small cohorts; one	*Escitalopram, fluvoxamine, venlafaxine* and *duloxetine* should be reserved as second-line treatments, and *paroxetine* use should be avoided in women planning a pregnancy, although conflicting data suggest only a low absolute risk associated with its use during embryogenesis The great majority of neonatal signs observed at birth are self-remitting and mild; the pathogenesis and the risk factors for these conditions are not known but might possibly include dosage, polytherapy and infant prematurity. The current data do not justify interrupting treatment before birth, since the risk of postnatal depression would be augmented in an unacceptable way. Recent data suggest that a routine follow-up is sufficient for exposed infants. Long-term data, although scarce and limited to preschool follow-up, have not indicated a relationship between SSRIs or SNRIs use and delays in development or other long-term issues

	study found a mild delay in psychomotor development among infants exposed to SSRIs compared to infants exposed to maternal psychotherapy (see text) [7].	
Newer antidepressive agents: Bupropion Mirtazapine	More than 2000 first-trimester exposures to *bupropion* and 350 exposures to *mirtazapine* in epidemiological studies and in the manufacturer's registry without evidence of an increased risk for birth defects compared to the baseline [2, 4] No data on neonatal or long-term effects	Limited data indicate no major risk of birth defects for *bupropion*; *mirtazapine* should be reserved for women in whom other drugs such as SSRIs cannot be considered. Further data, including long-term neurobehavioral assessment, are needed to confirm safety profile. Continuing a newer agent may sometimes be considered, as switching to a better known antidepressant may entail maternal health risks
Tricyclic antidepressants	More than 3500 first-trimester exposures without evidence of an increased risk of congenital birth defects, except for *clomipramine* (twofold increased in cardiac anomalies in one report) [4] Case-reports of neonatal signs possibly related to late-drug exposure (urinary retention, ileus, seizures) Two cohort studies with normal neurodevelopmental outcomes in exposed infants [7]	Although the safety profile of tricyclic antidepressants is well documented, the less desirable side-effect profile of these agents make them second choices for the treatment of anxiodepressive disorders during pregnancy
Other antidepressive agents: Monoamine oxidase inhibitors (MAOIs), Trazodone	400 first-trimester exposures to *trazodone* in small epidemiological studies without evidence of an increased risk of birth defects compared to the baseline risk [2, 4] Limited data for *MAOIs* during pregnancy indicate	The safety profile of *trazodone* is reassuring although data are scarce. *MAOI* prescription should be avoid in women considering pregnancy and reserved to women refractory to other antidepressants

Table 13.1   (*Continued*)

Medication classes	Teratogenic, neonatal and neurobehavioral developmental effects	Comments and recommendations
	a possible teratogenic risk based on 21 exposures No data on long-term effects	
Sedatives – hypnotics and anxiolytic agents		
Benzodiazepines	Most prospective epidemiological studies do not show an increased risk for major congenital birth defects for *benzodiazepines* compared to the baseline risk. However, a meta-analysis of retrospective case-control studies detected a 1.8-fold increase in oral clefts (cleft lip and/or cleft palate). Exposure to *benzodiazepines* during the critical period of palate formation (between the weeks 8 and 11 of gestation) might carry a risk of 2/1000 oral cleft [19] Late pregnancy-exposure to potent *benzodiazepines* with long half-lives such as *clonazepam* or *diazepam* poses a risk of floppy infant syndrome and withdrawal symptoms in newborns. Incidence has not been well defined, but risks are probably low when short-life agents are used, or when these agents are used on an as-needed basis [2] Neurobehavioral sequelaes have been described in children of heavy users who were also abusing substances; these effects have not been shown yet	The current data on this class of anxiolytics do not suggest risks of major anomalies. Use should be ideally restricted during organogenesis, although this period is frequently associated with peaks of anxiety among vulnerable patients. When a *benzodiazepine* is indicated, agents without active metabolites and with a short to intermediate half-life (such as *lorazepam* or *oxazepam*) should be used, especially if prescribed regularly, in order to avoid metabolic accumulation in the infant. Withdrawal symptoms in the infant, rarely observed at usual dosage, are usually helped by non-pharmacological means (swaddling, proper feeding, limited exposure to intense stimuli such as bright lights or heavy noise). Routine postnatal pediatric surveillance is sufficient among exposed infants

	with medical use of *benzodiazepines* [2]	
Zopiclone	More than 600 first-trimester exposures in a small prospective cohort study and a population-based study without evidence of an increased risk for major birth defects compared to the baseline risk [2]	Further studies are needed to confirm the safety profile of *zopiclone*; however, data are reassuring for a woman exposed before knowing of her pregnancy
	No data on late pregnancy exposure or late effects.	

outcome, and the observed rate of 12% was superior to controls but within the normal range for the general population. Selective serotonin reuptake inhibitors' effects (SSRIs) on platelet function have prompted researchers to assess the risk of bleeding at the time of delivery in treated mothers, without evidence of an increased risk of postnatal hemorrhage. An increased rate of prematurity, gestational hypertension, pre-eclampsia and low birth weight were suggested in some studies but not in others [4]. Conclusions from these studies should be interpreted carefully given the frequent lack of control for maternal psychiatric status, multiple confounding factors and the small number of subjects. Overall, the findings are equivocal at best and do not currently suggest stopping or not prescribing SSRIs or serotonin and norepinephrine reuptake inhibitors (SNRIs) when clinically indicated.

Neonatal complications

A neonatal behavioral syndrome has been described following third-trimester exposure to SSRIs and SNRIs (Table 13.1). In the vast majority of cases, these signs are transient, do not delay hospital discharge and do not constitute a life risk [5]. The current data do not justify interrupting treatment before birth, since the risk of postnatal depression would be augmented in an unacceptable way. Recent data suggest that routine follow-up is sufficient for exposed infants [6].

Neurobehavioral development

Research is just beginning to provide information regarding the long-term consequences of antenatal exposure to antidepressants, and several studies are presently ongoing. Eleven of thirteen studies have noted that preschool children who were exposed to SSRIs during pregnancy or breastfeeding had similar psychomotor development compared to unexposed groups [7].

Using the Bayley Scales of Infant Development (BSID-II), one of these studies compared the development of 31 infants exposed *in utero* to SSRIs to infants whose mothers were treated with psychotherapy. Drug-exposed infants had similar cognitive, language and personal-social development but had lower psychomotor development scores and were rated lower on the behavioral motor-quality scale. This slight delay in motor development was suggested to be linked to the regulatory influence of serotonin on muscle tone and other motor output. Another study including SSRI exposure coupled with anticonvulsants and benzodiazepines revealed more abnormal scores in exposed infants.

In a landmark prospective cohort study, researchers showed that IQ, language, behavior and temperament did not differ significantly between children aged 15 to 71 months who were exposed to antidepressants throughout pregnancy and children from non-depressed mothers [8]. However, the authors found that the duration of depression and the number of depressive episodes had a negative impact on children's global IQ and language development. One ongoing research on venlafaxine and SSRIs from the same researchers does not support neurobehavioral sequelaes in children exposed *in utero* to venlafaxine compared to their siblings or to SSRIs-exposed children; however, non-exposed children achieved higher scores on full-scale IQ. Again, maternal psychiatric condition, rather than medication use, was identified as a significant predictor of children's neurocognitive performance.

Selecting an antidepressant during pregnancy

The decision will be guided by the severity of the symptoms, the safety profile of the medication, but also by previous response to a given agent or a class of agents. The clinician will favor a better studied medication, such as the SSRIs sertraline, citalopram and fluoxetine (Table 13.1). As expected, the safety profile of the newer antidepressants is relatively less known; they should be prescribed in more complex clinical situations or when there is non-response or intolerance to a better-studied agent.

Continuing or interrupting antidepressant treatment during pregnancy

The decision to continue or to stop treatment in a woman who just learned of her pregnancy should take into consideration the severity of the maternal condition, the risk of relapse and the accumulated data regarding the medication. Stopping the medication could sometimes be considered, but the risk of relapse is significant and the patient should be offered a close monitoring of her condition. In a single study, two-thirds of women whose depression was controlled and who had stopped taking their medication before conception relapsed, compared to a quarter of women who continued their treatment [9]. The women from this cohort had however a more severe past psychiatric history; the numbers could theoretically be lower for patients without co-morbidity or with a first depressive episode. If treatment is continued, monotherapy should be favored, with the least elevated dose allowing clinical efficacy.

In the case of unplanned pregnancies, which happens near half the time, embryonic exposure has already happened and it is often difficult to wean the patient off the drug before the end of organogenesis: interrupting treatment at this stage hardly reduces the potential risks of structural teratogenesis. Few situations would warrant a change of medication after the onset of pregnancy, since this would expose the mother and the infant to multiple agents instead of one.

Antianxiety agents

The most frequently used class of medication are the benzodiazepines. Agents with a short half-life should be privileged. Occasionally, the use of a longer-acting benzodiazepine could be an alternative among patients who have not responded to a shorter-acting agent and who do not want to receive an antidepressant medication on a continuous basis (see Table 13.1).

Other biological interventions for treating antenatal depression and anxiety

Omega-3 fatty acid supplementation

There is little data thus far on the use of omega-3 supplementation for perinatal depression and results from small studies have tended to be equivocal [10]. However, safety data suggest low risk for obstetrical or neonatal complications with daily supplementation up to 3g beginning after the first trimester. If omega-3 fatty acids are to be prescribed to a pregnant women, careful attention should be given to the choice of a commercial supplement because proper regulation of natural products is lacking in most countries, and mercury and other contaminants may be present in unregulated supplements. Omega-3 supplementation should be avoided among women at risk of bleeding.

St John's wort

As a single study has been conducted on the safety of this herb during pregnancy, the use of agents with a better-known safety profile should be privileged.

Other non-psychotherapeutic treatments for depression and anxiety

Although insufficiently studied, exercise, acupuncture and luminotherapy may all hold promises for preventing perinatal depression and anxiety [10].

13.3 Bipolar disorder

As a chronic condition present in 1–2% of the general population, bipolar disorder can have a very significant impact on pregnancy, both antenatally and postnatally. Recent data has shown that the risk of exacerbation or relapse of bipolar disorder during pregnancy tends to be high. The risk will be clearly increased among women who stop their mood stabilizer before becoming pregnant or during pregnancy [11].

The post-partum period is a particularly vulnerable time for women with bipolar disease, even among women who do not present mood changes during pregnancy. Relapse rates during the first three to six months are as high as 50% and include manic or depressive episodes of various severity [12]. The risk of relapse is higher if the mood stabilizer is stopped abruptly in early pregnancy or if the course of the disorder is marked by four or more mood episodes.

Treatment planning and prophylactic treatment of mothers with bipolar disorder

Personalized recommendations will depend on a proper assessment of the severity of the illness:

- Duration of asymptomatic functioning

- Identified precipitants

- Knowledge about the illness

- Number of prior depressive episodes

- Frequency, type and duration of prior decompensations

- Time elapsed since the last episode

- Presence of various co-morbidities such as substance use or personality disorder.

The clinician will need to document prior response to treatment and the results of past attempts to stop medication. The partner and extended family network will often be solicited as key partners for treatment planning. Importantly, the clinician who is asked questions about pharmacological management should be ready to frankly discuss the patient's readiness for parenthood, especially among very vulnerable patients [13].

If it is decided to stop medication in pre-conception, the interruption should be progressive, during at least two weeks, while monitoring the recurrence of symptoms. According to the assessed risk of recurrence and intensity of symptoms, medication may be restarted during pregnancy, ideally after the period of organogenesis, that is after the first trimester (see Table 13.2).

In more severe conditions, such as in a poorly controlled bipolar I patient, it might be preferable to continue medication throughout pregnancy instead of reintroducing higher doses or multiple medications later during the pregnancy. The general rule will be to use monotherapy with minimal effective doses [14]. The prevention of postnatal depression in bipolar patients is beyond the scope of this chapter, but we should mention that the patient and her family should always be wary of antidepressant-induced manic switches.

Lithium carbonate

Lithium carbonate has been shown to reduces the risk of post-partum psychosis (PPP) two- to fivefold. It is currently considered the first line of prophylactic treatment (Table 13.2). The high relapse rate of bipolar illness justifies in most cases a prophylactic pschopharma- cological intervention, especially postnatally. Indeed, preventing PPP necessitates in the vast majority of cases reintroducing or continuing a mood stabilizer.

Table 13.2 Safety profile of antipsychotic agents and mood stabilizers during pregnancy

Medication classes	Teratogenic, neonatal and neurobehavioral developmental effects	Comments and recommendations
Antipsychotic agents		
Newer antipsychotics: Clozapine Olanzapine Paliperidone Quetiapine Risperidone Ziprasidone	130 first-trimester exposures to *clozapine*, 300 exposures to *olanzapine*, 170 exposures to *risperidone*, less than 40 exposures to *quetiapine* and 50 exposures to *ziprasidone* have been reported in the manufacturers' internal registries, a small prospective cohort study and a population-based study without evidence of an increased risk for birth defects compared to the baseline risk [14, 20]; 300 exposures to *quetiapine* during pregnancy with known outcomes have also been reported to the manufacturer with apparently no pattern of birth defects, but more detailed data are not available [20] Lower placental transfer for *quetiapine* compared to *olanzapine* and *risperidone* [20] Higher rate of large-for-gestational age and higher birth weights among newborn exposed to newer antipsychotic agents in a small cohort [20] Neonatal signs and complications affecting primarily CNS occasionally reported with late pregnancy exposure to *olanzapine*, *risperidone* and *quetiapine*, although a specific syndrome has not been described yet [20]	Manufacturer's internal registries suggest a wide use of atypical antipsychotic drugs during pregnancy, although well-designed epidemiological studies are lacking to support the safety of these medications during pregnancy. Metabolic disturbances, increased body mass index and decreased folate blood levels associated with their use might indirectly lead to increased risks of hyperglycemia, gestational diabetes and possibly birth defects, although the latter has not been shown yet. Until more data is available, the newer antipsychotic agents should be reserved for more difficult clinical situations and should be avoided when better studied medications are available (e.g. benzodiazepines for insomnia)

Table 13.2   (*Continued*)

Medication classes	Teratogenic, neonatal and neurobehavioral developmental effects	Comments and recommendations
	No data currently published for *paliperidone* No published data on neurodevelopment of infants exposed *in utero* [20]	
Conventional antipsychotic agents: Phenothiazines (e.g. chlorpromazine), thioxanthenes (e.g. zuclopenthixol) and butyrophenones (e.g. haloperidol)	*Phenothiazines* use in pregnancy has been associated with a small increase in major birth defects in a meta-analysis [20]; however, a recent population-based study suggests that the psychiatric conditions and related behaviors, rather than the drug itself, can explain this difference; no pattern of birth defects has been described	The safety profile of this class is reassuring, but side effects such as hypotension preclude the use of phenothiazines as first-line agents for psychiatric conditions. For more incisive antipsychotics, close monitoring of extrapyramidal effects is warranted especially postnatally. Although relatively contra-indicated, long-action formulations can be considered when drug compliance is an issue
	More than 400 first-trimester exposures to *haloperidol* recorded in prospective cohort studies without evidence of an increased risk of birth defects above the baseline risk; an increased rate of obstetrical and neonatal complications (prematurity, low birth weight) have been suggested [20]	
	Neonatal signs and CNS complications such as extrapyramidal effects and withdrawal syndromes seldom reported in late pregnancy exposed newborns [20]	
	Few data on long-term developmental effects have been published and do not support a major neurobehavioral teratogenic effect; exposed children appear to be heavier and taller than the general population; the clinical	

significance of these observations is
unknown [14, 20]

Mood stabilizers		
Lithium	Several small epidemiological studies have shown an increased risk for cardiovascular defects, notably Ebstein anomaly, with a frequency estimated to vary between 0.9% up to 6.8% in a small study that probably overestimated the actual risk owing to methodological flaws and a small sample size. The actual additional risk for cardiovascular defects is estimated to be around 1% [14]. The baseline risks for cardiac birth defects and Ebstein anomaly are 1% and 0.005% respectively. Transient neonatal complications (primarily hypotonia and other CNS depression signs, as well as cardiac and renal effects) described in several case reports and clinical studies; these effects tend to be less frequent when lithium treatment is withheld after the onset of labor or 24–48 hours before a planned Caesarean section [14] Few data on long-term effects of prenatal exposure to lithium have been published: mothers of 60 exposed infants reported no adverse effects on their child's development in the Lithium Baby Registry, and 22 infants have been evaluated at one year of age without evidence of impaired development in comparison to a control group [14]	Lithium is a first-choice agent for bipolar disorder in childbearing age women. Depending on the natural course of the disease, lithium treatment can be withheld during the period of cardiac embryogenesis (between weeks 5 and 10 of gestation) to lessen the risks of cardiovascular defects. If exposure occurred during that period, high-resolution fetal cardiac ultrasonography can be offered. Close monitoring of lithium blood levels during pregnancy is warranted because of the pharmacokinetic changes occurring throughout pregnancy. Divided doses should be used. In order to avoid lithium toxicity, good hydration should be maintained. Lithium dosage should be reinstituted at pre-pregnancy doses as soon as possible after delivery. Interactions with NSAIDs should be monitored in post-partum.
Antiepileptic drugs: Carbamazepine Lamotrigine	Increased risk of major birth defects for *valproic acid*, with 10% of exposed newborns	*Valproic acid* should never be considered as a first-line agent for women of childbearing age.

Table 13.2   (*Continued*)

Medication classes	Teratogenic, neonatal and neurobehavioral developmental effects	Comments and recommendations
Topiramate Valproic acid	diagnosed with major structural anomalies, particularly neural tube defects (1–2%). This figure rises when multiple anticonvulsants are used during the first trimester. A possible set of dysmorphic features has been described. A dose-response relationship has been observed, with daily doses exceeding 1000 mg carrying a higher risk [1]. Neurodevelopmental problems such as decreased verbal IQ, learning disorders and impairments in communication associated with autistic spectrum disorder, have been observed in follow-up studies. Nevertheless, numerous confounding factors can bias these observations. Large epidemiological studies for *lamotrigine* have not found an increased risk of birth defects, although a ten-fold increase in isolated oral clefts has been observed in a large registry. The background risk being low for oral clefts, absolute additional risk is less than 1%. Dose-response relationship for birth defects has been proposed in some studies, the risk being slightly higher with daily doses above 200 mg [1]. Assessment of cognitive function at 3 years of age in lamotrigine-exposed children has shown mean IQ values of 101, which were significantly higher than in valproate-exposed children [21]	If indicated, the lowest effective dosage divided in three or four daily doses to minimize serum fluctuations must be given along with preconceptional folic acid. Close antenatal follow-up including detailed ultrasounds is warranted. Exposed children might also need close developmental monitoring Emerging data for *lamotrigine* suggest a very low teratogenic risk. A detailed ultrasound to rule out oral cleft can be offered if first trimester exposure occurs *Carbamazepine* carries a lower teratogenic risk than *valproic acid* and might also be considered an alternative to *valproate*. *Topiramate* should be avoided until further safety studies are available

Carbamazepine has been well studied, and most registries have found birth defects rates similar or slightly higher than the baseline risk, with 2.2–6.8% of children being affected when women are treated with monotherapy [1]. *Carbamazepine* use during first trimester carries a risk of 0.5–1% of neural tube defects. Assessment of cognitive function at 3 years of age in *carbamazepine*-exposed children has shown mean IQ scores of 98, which were significantly higher than in *valproate*-exposed children [21]

Data are still scarce for *topiramate*, and small cohorts from the manufacturer's registry and another pregnancy registry suggest a possible increased risk of oral cleft and hypospadias; incidence can not be estimated from these preliminary data

Antiepileptic drugs

Antiepileptic drugs, notably valproic acid, should be avoided if possible among women with a bipolar disorder, especially during the first trimester (Table 13.2). Lamotrigine could be considered as a second-line agent in women refractory to lithium.

Antipsychotics

The newer antipsychotics are increasingly considered as an alternative or an adjunct for women for whom lithium is an undesirable option. At this time, they should not be considered as first-line treatments (see Table 13.2).

13.4 Schizophrenia

Close to 60% of mothers with schizophrenia report a deterioration of their condition whereas about 30% report some improvement. Cessation of medication during pregnancy has been associated with a relapse risk of 65% [15]. Especially when untreated, this illness is associated with inadequate prenatal care, the use of alcohol, tobacco and substance, spontaneous abortions, low birth weight and stillbirth [15]. When encountered postnatally, delusions or command hallucinations always constitute serious symptoms that interfere with infant care and may lead to severe neglect, infanticide or maternal suicide. The use of pharmacological and non-pharmacological treatments is critical to prevent antenatal or postnatal decompensation among affected mothers.

Treatment planning and prophylactic treatment of mothers with schizophrenia

The principles of treatment planning are similar to bipolar disease. Contingency planning for carefully accompanying mothers and families – and sometimes monitoring parental skills – should be planned with affected parents [16].

Antipsychotics

Independently of exposure to antipsychotics, schizophrenia has been recognized as a risk factor for congenital malformations in some studies [15]. The high relapse rate of schizophrenia justifies in most cases a prophylactic pschopharmacological intervention throughout pregnancy and during the post-partum. Although they have been less studied, the newer antipsychotic agents tend to be increasingly utilized clinically because of their more favorable side-effect profile (see Table 13.2).

Depot antipsychotics

The risks of non-compliance to medical treatment are often high in this population and may require the use of depot antipsychotic medication throughout pregnancy and in post-partum (Table 13.2).

Antiparkinsonians

This class of medication is used in the prevention and treatment of extrapyramidal symptoms sometimes associated with antipsychotics, notably the conventional ones. Although few studies have assessed the use of antiparkinsonians during pregnancy, their safety profile tends to be reassuring overall. Diphenhydramine is the best-studied agent in this class [14].

13.5 Post-partum psychosis

Post-partum psychosis (PPP) is a psychiatric emergency that occurs after 0.1 to 0.2% of all deliveries. This syndrome is associated with a variety of psychiatric disorders, notably bipolar disorder, schizophrenia and schizoaffective disorder [17]. PPP is often the first manifestation of a bipolar disorder. It is observed in 25–50% of non-treated bipolar patients, 75% of bipolar patients with a prior PPP episode and 90% of bipolar patients with a prior PPP and a family history of the disease [18].

Treatment planning and prophylactic treatment of mothers with a history of PPP

In addition to psychoeducation about stress management and sleep hygiene, prophylactic psychopharmacological treatment is a key preventive element of PPP. Since this condition has a very rapid onset, it is critical to educate the patient, her family – and obstetrical teams – about the importance of restarting antipsychotic medication immediately postnatally.

Antipsychotics

Antipsychotics and emergency psychiatric hospitalization are the cornerstones of treatment. Antipsychotics decrease the risks of maternal suicide and infanticide. Dosage optimization should attempt to fully treat maternal psychotic symptoms, while minimizing maternal sedation during supervised visits with her infant. Depending on the underlying psychiatric condition, medical treatment will often lead to a full recovery of maternal functioning.

13.6 Conclusion

The treatments now available to prevent and to treat perinatal psychiatric disorders have the potential to help parents and infants during a most critical period of development. The challenge of balancing a medical–psychiatric view with a more developmentally based approach has become a capital issue for perinatal and infant psychiatrists. Unfortunately, role compartmentalization between adult and infant psychiatrists can lead to a tendency by adult psychiatrists and family physicians to conceptualize and treat antenatal psychiatric disorders primarily or exclusively as an individual psychiatric problem. Insufficient training may be at fault in approaches that include the rest of the family, particularly the infant, in the treatment process. The emerging field of women's psychiatry, for its part, may be facing the same challenges as obstetrics: minimal training is provided in parental role development and the specifics of infant development and psychopathology. Again, more training in infant development, early relationship disorders and infant psychopathology for adult psychiatrists and obstetricians would go a long way to improving the situation.

The growing and cumulative data regarding psychopharmacological treatments during pregnancy helps health professionals make better informed decisions in close collaboration with patients and families. In every situation, psychopharmacological treatment should be integrated within a multimodal treatment plan that will put premium value on emotionally accompanying future mothers and facilitating their transition to parenthood.

13.7 References

1. Pearlstein, T. (2008) Perinatal depression: treatment options and dilemmas. *Rev Psychiatr Neurosci*, **33**, 302–18.
2. Martin, B. and Saint-André, M. (2007) Dépression et troubles anxieux, in *Grossesse et allaitement: guide thérapeutique* (ed. E. Ferreira). Éditions du CHU Sainte-Justine, Montréal, pp. 539–59.
3. Ramos, E., St-André, M., Rey, E. *et al.* (2008) Duration of antidepressant use during pregnancy and risk of major congenital malformations. *British Journal of Psychiatry*, **192**, 344–50.

4. Simoncelli, M., Martin, B.Z. and Bérard A. (2009) Antidepressant use during pregnancy: a critical systematic review of the literature. *Current Drug Safety*, Epub ahead of print.

5. Moses-Kolko, E.L., Bogen, D., Perel, J. *et al.* (2005) Neonatal signs after late in utero exposure to serotonin reuptake inhibitors: literature review and implications for clinical applications. *Journal of the American Medical Association*, **293**, 2372–83.

6. Ferreira, E., Carceller, A.M., Agogue, C. *et al.* (2007) Effects of selective serotonin reuptake inhibitors and venlafaxine during pregnancy in term and preterm neonates. *Pediatrics*, **119**, 52–9.

7. Gentile, S. (2005) SSRIs in pregnancy and lactation: emphasis on neurodevelopmental outcome. *CNS Drugs*, **19**, 623–33.

8. Nulman, I., Rovet, J., Stewart, D.E. *et al.* (2002) Child development following exposure to tricyclic antidepressants or fluoxetine throughout fetal life: a prospective, controlled study. *American Journal of Psychiatry*, **159**, 1889–95.

9. Cohen, L.S., Altshuler, L.L., Harlow, B.L. *et al.* (2006) Relapse of major depression during pregnancy in women who maintain or discontinue antidepressant treatment. *Journal of the American Medical Association*, **295**, 499–507.

10. Raudzus, J. and Misri, S. (2009) Managing unipolar depression in pregnancy. *Current Opinion in Psychiatry*, **22**, 13–18.

11. Viguera, A., Whitfield, T., Baldessarini, R.J. *et al.* (2007) Risk of recurrence in women with bipolar disorder during pregnancy: prospective study of mood stabilizer discontinuation. *American Journal of Psychiatry*, **164**, 1817–24.

12. Cohen, L.S. and Nonacs, R.M. (2005) *Mood and Anxiety Disorders During Pregnancy and the Postpartum*. American Psychiatric Publishing, Washington, DC.

13. Massachussets General Hospital Center for Women's Mental Health. Women's Mental Health.org Internet, cited July 8th, 2009. Available from: http://www.women's mental health.org/.

14. Martin, B. and Saint-André, M. (2007) Maladie bipolaire et troubles psychotiques, in *Grossesse et allaitement: guide thérapeutique* (ed. E. Ferreira), Éitions du CHU Sainte-Justine, Montréal, pp. 561–77.

15. Trixler, M., Gati, A., Fekete, S. *et al.* (2005) Use of antipsychotics in the management of schizophrenia during pregnancy. *Drugs*, **65**, 1193–206.

16. Seeman, M.V. (2008) Prevention inherent in services for women with schizophrenia. *Canadian Journal of Psychiatry*, **53**, 332–41.

17. Spinelli, M.G. (2009) Postpartum psychosis: detection of risk and management. *American Journal of Psychiatry*, **166**, 405–8.

18. Jones, I. and Craddock, N. (2005) Bipolar disorder and childbirth: the importance of recognising risk. *British Journal of Psychiatry*, **186**, 453–54.

19. Dolovich, L.R., Addis, A., Vaillancourt, J.M. *et al.* (1998) Benzodiazepine use in pregnancy and major malformations or oral cleft: meta-analysis of cohort and case-control studies. *British Medical Journal*, **317**, 839–43.

20. Einarson, A. and Boskovic, R. (2009) Use and safety of antipsychotic drugs during pregnancy. *Journal of Psychiatric Practice*, **2009**, 183–92.

21. Meador, K.J., Baker, G.A., Browning, N. *et al.* (2009) Cognitive function at 3 years of age after fetal exposure to antiepileptic drugs. *New England Journal of Medicine*, **360**, 1597–605.

14

Psychotherapeutic, psychosocial, individual and family interventions for abnormal states during pregnancy

Prabha S. Chandra,[1] Geetha Desai[1] and Veena A. Satyanarayana[2]

[1] National Institute of Mental Health and Neurosciences, Bangalore, India
[2] Washington University School of Medicine, St. Louis, USA.

Clinical vignette

Ms B is a 21-year-old woman from India who is pregnant for the second time. Now in her second trimester, she is anxious about the health of her fetus, having had complications in her first pregnancy. She lives with her parents because her husband is a migrant worker and has to stay away from home. He visits her once a month for a few days and during this time consumes alcohol and occasionally is violent towards her. Her firstborn is a female child and, due to the pressure of her in-laws, she is anxious about the sex of this fetus. She has of late become listless, is unable to sleep and is irritable towards her older child who is now two years old. She has also been found to be anemic owing to her poor nutritional status. She

Parenthood and Mental Health: A Bridge between Infant and Adult Psychiatry   Sam Tyano, Miri Keren, Helen Herrman and John Cox
© 2010 John Wiley & Sons, Ltd

had wanted to wait for a few more years before her second baby but had an unplanned pregnancy.

14.1 Introduction

Mental health problems in pregnancy present an enormous challenge to clinicians. Once considered a time of emotional well-being, and 'protecting' women against psychiatric disorders, it is now well established that several psychiatric disorders are common during pregnancy, with depression being most common. The case vignette above depicts a common scenario among women from deprived backgrounds who have unplanned pregnancies, face violence and in certain countries face problems related to the gender of the children they bear. Depression and anxiety are common correlates of such psychosocial situations. A recent meta-analysis of 21 studies [1] found that the mean prevalence rate for depression across the antenatal period was 10.7%, ranging from 7.4% in the first trimester to 12.8% in the second trimester.

Despite the fairly high prevalence of mental health problems and the serious consequences of untreated psychiatric disorders in pregnant women, most mothers and families hesitate to take treatment for fear of being prescribed psychotropic drugs that might cause harm to the fetus. It is hence important to offer psychological and social forms of treatment to pregnant women with mental health problems that can be managed without medications.

This chapter focuses on psychological and psychosocial treatments for common mental health problems during pregnancy. Most mothers with severe mental illness need pharmacological treatment, as psychosocial treatments, though supportive, are not very effective as primary forms of treatment. The focus hence in this chapter will be on the non-psychotic forms of mental illnesses namely, depression, anxiety disorders, eating disorders, substance abuse and suicide.

The literature on interventions in pregnancy is sparse compared to that on post-partum psychiatric problems. This is despite the fact that depression and anxiety during pregnancy have been associated with poor obstetric outcomes and higher rates of post-partum psychiatric morbidity. Most of the literature focuses on depression and to some extent on anxiety. Interventions studies on other disorders are few.

14.2 Maternal–fetal attachment disorders

Maternal–fetal attachment (MFA) and bonding begins fairly early in pregnancy. While some women instinctually bond with their fetus, other women have difficulty engaging in behaviors and interactions that increase their affiliation with the fetus. In a recent meta analysis [2], 72 studies published between 1981 and 2006 were reviewed to examine predictors of MFA. Findings indicated that MFA increased with gestational age, when mothers perceived good availability of social support and (where applicable) with every ultrasound used for prenatal testing, when mothers could see the fetus growing.

Maternal mental health significantly influences MFA. While individual therapy with mothers at risk for MFA-related problems is important, involving family members in treatment and care is crucial. Adequate family support is almost always what the pregnant woman yearns for and therefore activating this informal support network is likely to enhance maternal well-being. Further, social and cultural stereotypes and expectations glorify pregnancy and motherhood and place immense pressure on the woman to enjoy this life event. This creates conflict and dissonance in women who are experiencing negative emotions. Normalizing these emotional states when transitory is important to alleviate this anxiety.

Women and couples are often encouraged to participate in parenting workshops to be better prepared for the adjustments they have to make before and after the arrival of their newborn. Couples are motivated to spend quality time together to enhance maternal mental health and MFA. A recent review included 26 studies to examine the effectiveness of group-based parenting programs in improving maternal mental health [3]. The findings indicated that parenting programs have the potential of improving maternal mental health in the short term. Due to a lack of longitudinal follow-up studies, there is no evidence as yet to support supporting maintenance of these benefits in the long term.

14.3 Anxiety disorders

Pregnancy is a major life event for all women and it is normal to experience some anxiety during pregnancy, either related to the well-being of the fetus, or to the process of childbirth. Though they are quite prevalent, anxiety disorders are not as widely researched in pregnancy as mood disorders. Contrary to the popular belief that pregnancy is a state of well-being with low rates of mental health issues, studies have indicated that anxiety disorders are common during pregnancy. Anxiety symptoms are as common as depression after delivery and possibly more prevalent during pregnancy [4]. Anxiety during pregnancy has been identified as an independent predictor of childhood behavioral and emotional problems and also a predictor of post-partum depression. Common themes of severe anxiety during pregnancy include fear of fetal loss or fetal abnormality. Interventions in anxiety disorders during pregnancy are important because of the association of these disorders with a variety of poor outcomes. These include:

- Pre-eclampsia
- Increased nausea and vomiting
- Longer sick leave during pregnancy
- Increased number of visits to obstetrician
- Spontaneous preterm labor
- Preterm delivery
- Low birth weight
- Admission of infant to neonatal care and elective cesarean section [5].

The effect of anxiety disorders on low birth weight is however, still a subject of scrutiny with a meta-analysis on this relationship failing to demonstrate a significant link.

The psychosocial interventions discussed below pertain to following anxiety disorders: generalized anxiety disorders, panic disorders, phobias, obsessive compulsive disorders and post-traumatic stress disorders.

Panic disorder

Due to the physiological changes that occur during pregnancy a woman may be at increased risk of onset or recurrence of panic disorder. Physiological symptoms such as fear and autonomic arousal symptoms like shortness of breath, pounding heart and dizziness may be misinterpreted in catastrophic ways in relation to the pregnancy. Anticipatory anxiety about future attacks and consequences of the attacks on the fetus can be significantly disabling.

Generalized anxiety disorder

Pregnant women with generalized anxiety disorder (GAD) experience excessive worry about a number of life domains along with various physical symptoms such as tension headaches, muscle aches, irritability and poor concentration. Pregnancy itself is associated with role changes, health concerns for the fetus and bodily changes and may form the content of these worries.

Psychological treatments have been used successfully in treating anxiety disorders. Cognitive behavior therapy (CBT) has found wide acceptance in the treatment of anxiety disorders. The basic tenet of CBT is that emotional responses are caused not by situations per se but by the person's belief and interpretations of these situations. Understanding the cognitive and behavioral factors that underlie anxiety disorders is important in formulating a treatment strategy. Before venturing into treatment it is important for a proper assessment of any co-existing medical disorder that may explain the current anxiety, or another psychiatric disorder that can hamper treatment. There is limited research evidence in the use of CBT in pregnant women with anxiety disorders. However, if the anxiety is mild to moderate it is best to consider psychological management as a first line of treatment.

Phobias

A phobia is an irrational fear of an object or a situation leading to avoidance. There is no literature on the exact prevalence and impact of specific phobias such as social phobia or agoraphobia during pregnancy. A specific type of phobia that has been discussed in relation to pregnancy and child birth is tokophobia, which is defined as an intense fear of childbirth. This can lead to women avoiding pregnancy, terminating pregnancy of a very much wanted baby or demanding Caesarean section in subsequent pregnancies. It has been classified as:

- Primary, in a nulliparous woman

- Secondary, if she has had previous traumatic deliveries

- Secondary to depressive illness or post-traumatic stress disorder (PTSD) during pregnancy [6].

The reported prevalence of serious fear of childbirth was 5.5 % in women. It is also important to consider factors influencing this fear, namely, history of sexual or physical abuse, a traumatic gynecological examination, previous experience of childbirth and related anxiety and also myths about labor and childbirth. Fear of childbirth may also be a symptom of PTSD associated with childbirth.

Interventions for anxiety disorders

Tokophobia

Specific interventions have been developed for tokophobia. Sjogren and Thomassen [7] reported encouraging outcomes in a study that compared 100 pregnant women with fear of childbirth with a matched reference group of women with the same condition. The study group received individualized psychological and obstetric support from psychosomatic gynecologists during pregnancy. Results showed that in the study group the request for Caesarean sections reduced from 68% to 30%. Obstetric outcomes in those who had vaginal deliveries were overall similar in the study and control groups, but women in the study group were more likely to have induced labor, epidural anesthesia or a pudendal nerve block. A randomized controlled trial of an intervention comparing intensive and conventional therapy for 176 pregnant women with fear of childbirth was conducted in week 26 of their gestation. Intervention in the intensive therapy group produced a reduction in unnecessary Caesarean sections, pregnancy and birth-related concerns and shorter labor when compared with the control group who received conventional therapy only [8].

The ultrasound examination also has been used for reducing childbirth-related anxiety: 40 women randomized to video and verbal feedback during three ultrasound examinations were compared with a group which received no feedback. Women in the feedback group were found to have lower scores on the Spielberg State Trait Anxiety Inventory and fewer delivery complications [9].

Bastani *et al.* [10] studied the role of applied relaxation therapy in reducing stress and anxiety among 110 primigravida women in their second trimester. Seven sessions of applied relaxation therapy were compared with usual antenatal care in pregnant women. The intervention group was found to have significant reductions in anxiety symptoms and perceived stress, indicating the benefits of applied relaxation therapy on anxiety.

The role of counseling by midwives in reducing anxiety has however shown mixed results. Midwives trained in counseling talked to the women and invited them to express their fears and devised individual birth plans. Although women were very satisfied with their care, those in the intervention group had more frightening experiences of delivery and higher rates of PTSD symptoms than those in the control group. The authors concluded that the counseling received by the women in this study did not accord them the same positive experience of childbirth as the average parturient at the unit, and that more effective forms of treatment may be necessary [11].

Post-traumatic stress disorder

There has been a recent surge of interest in PTSD among pregnant women. PTSD is seen in women who have experienced a traumatic event. It is characterized by re-experiencing of a traumatic event with hyperarousal symptoms and avoidance of stimuli relating to the traumatic event. Most reports on PTSD are related to a traumatic childbirth in previous deliveries. Rates of PTSD have been reported around 7.7% in disadvantaged pregnant women [12].

Predictors of PTSD symptoms include:

- Perception of low levels of support from staff and partner
- Pain in the first stage
- Low perceived control and feelings of powerlessness in labor
- Medical interventions in pregnancy and labor
- Trait anxiety
- Past history of mental health problems and
- A history of sexual trauma and poor social support.

No treatment trials have been conducted for PTSD during pregnancy. Various psychological treatments that are used in treating PTSD have been recommended in pregnant women, with CBT showing most promising results.

Obsessive compulsive disorder

OCD may have its first onset during pregnancy or post-partum [13]. There are reports of OCD occurring during pregnancy and resolving spontaneously after delivery. The obsessional content may involve the fetus. The psychological treatment that may be used in pregnant women is exposure and response prevention that has evidence of being effective in non-pregnant women with OCD, though no treatment trials are available in the literature.

14.4 Eating disorders

Most women with eating disorders are of childbearing age. Despite fertility rates of women with eating disorders being lower than those in the general population, a study screening women for eating disorders in an antenatal clinic found that 5% scored above threshold on the Eating Attitudes Test.

The consequences of eating disorders in pregnancy are poorly understood, as existing studies have differing sample sizes and varying study designs. Several studies report improvement of symptoms during pregnancy but return of symptoms in the post-partum period. Other studies have found an increased rate of relapse.

The impact of eating disorders on pregnancy [14] includes an apparently increased chance of hyperemesis and increased risk of:

- Postnatal depressive episode
- Pregnancy termination
- Preterm delivery and perinatal mortality
- Gestational diabetes

- Low birth weight in infants, small for gestational age baby

- Caesarean section

- Miscarriage

Eating disorders are associated with nutritional problems, weight loss and concerns about body image.

Management

There are no controlled studies for treatment of eating disorders during pregnancy. A case report of a pregnant woman with anorexia nervosa highlights the need for a multidisciplinary approach [15]. For effective management of pregnant women with eating disorders, a multidisciplinary approach is highly desirable. The team should include where possible physicians, gynecologists, a mental health professional and nutritional experts. The mental health professional should coordinate with other team members regarding the progress of the treatment. Women with eating disorders may mask their weight by using certain strategies; it is hence important to be careful and at the same time to avoid being critical of the behaviors.

A thorough medical evaluation is necessary to rule out the metabolic complications associated with eating disorders. Nutritional assessment is vital to advice regarding the diet. Serial monitoring of weight during the pregnancy is important. Inability to gain weight during pregnancy may be an indicator of underlying eating disorders.

14.5 Depression

Interventions studied for depression are of three types: education, interpersonal therapy (IPT) and Brief Interpersonal therapy (IPT-B). Spinelli [16] piloted IPT among a small group of depressed antepartum women and found it to be a feasible, acceptable and useful intervention. Subsequently the author studied the efficacy of IPT among 50 low-income, recently depressed migrant women from the Dominican Republic [17]. The participants met for 45-minute weekly sessions with therapists. IPT was administered over 16 weeks in a manualized form. This was compared with parenting education programs in reducing depression. During parenting education program sessions, the therapist emphasized the developmental stages of pregnancy, delivery, parenting and early childhood. The therapist also facilitated attaining concrete services (housing, etc.) but did not provide specific emotional support. Twenty-five depressed women were randomly assigned to the experimental treatment IPT group and 25 to the parenting education. Thirty-eight women remained in the study and were included in the data analysis. Depressed mood was measured with the Edinburgh Postnatal Depression Scale (EPDS), the Beck Depression Inventory (BDI) and the Hamilton Depression Rating Scale (HDRS). The Clinical Global Impression (CGI) and the HDRS measured recovery. The authors found that IPT had a significant advantage over parenting education in reducing depression scores measured by the EPDS. Both groups showed marked improvement over the course of treatment. The mood of the women in the IPT group however, improved significantly more than the parenting education program control group on scores on the EPDS.

Grote *et al.* [18, 19] in two separate studies have shown the efficacy of IPT-B in the treatment of depression among antepartum mothers. The first was a pilot study with a small convenience sample of disadvantaged women in a public obstetrics hospital in the USA. The second, more recent study was a randomized controlled trial which used enhanced IPT-B and compared it with routine care. IPT-B, similar to IPT, is designed to treat depression by helping patients resolve one of four interpersonal problem areas (that is, role transition, role dispute, grief and interpersonal deficits). For example, to reduce treatment burden and activate change in the participant, the format of IPT-B treatment is restructured into 8 rather than 16 sessions and a focus on the long-term problem area of interpersonal deficits is avoided. Enhanced IPT-B has been described by the authors as a multi-component model of care consisting of an engagement session, followed by eight acute IPT-B sessions before the birth and maintenance IPT up to six months post-partum. This was augmented with modifications to make it culturally relevant to women who were socio-economically disadvantaged.

The IPT-B study demonstrated that among pregnant women with low incomes who scored >12 on the EPDS in a public care obstetrics and gynecology clinic, those who were randomly assigned to receive enhanced IPT-B and maintenance IPT, compared with those assigned to usual care, obtained significantly greater reductions in depression diagnoses and depressive symptoms before childbirth (three months after baseline) and at six months post-partum. They also showed significant improvements in social functioning at six months post-partum. Patients in the IPT-B group showed significantly higher rates of treatment engagement and retention than patients in the usual care group, with 68% (N = 17) of the IPT-B group compared with 7% (N = 2) in usual care completing a full course of treatment, defined as seven to eight sessions.

The above studies are the only well-tested reported interventions for depression in antepartum women. Dennis *et al.* [20] in a Cochrane review on the subject has discussed the lack of well-designed randomized clinical trials on the topic and the need for further investigation.

One of the important learnings from the limited research described above is that effective interventions in antepartum women are desirably brief, delivered either in the community or in the obstetrics setting and culturally relevant. Grote *et al.* [18, 19] and Spinelli and Endicott [17] studied low-income women in different parts of the USA, who were culturally disadvantaged. They emphasize that despite the intervention being manualized, an ethnographically defined motivational engagement session is an important part of the intervention. Also, the intervention should be cost-effective and accompanied by provision of support for real life needs such as social services, housing and developing wider social networks.

The psychosocial risk approach to intervention

Several clinicians and researchers have advocated the risk approach to intervention in pregnant women with mental health problems. This includes screening of women for possible risk factors (enumerated below) and subsequently offering targeted interventions depending on the nature of the stress.

The psychosocial risk factors that need to be assessed include:

- Past history of depression and anxiety disorder

- Past history of abuse or poor parental care

- Lack of current emotional or practical supports

- Poor quality of relationship with, or absence of, a partner

- Domestic violence (past or current)

- Current major stressors or losses

- Low self-esteem

- Drug and alcohol abuse and

- Dysfunctional personality or coping style.

The greater the number of risk factors, the more likely it is that the mother requires added supports or more specific interventions, irrespective of the presence of current symptoms. Whether there is an advantage to the combined use of a structured risk questionaire or interview with the EPDS in identifying vulnerable women remains to be formally assessed through adequate trials. Once 'at risk' or symptomatic women are identified, there need to be mechanisms in place for the formulation of clear management guidelines. Austin [21] emphasizes the importance of the particular risk factors and clinical symptomatology identified at antenatal psychosocial assessment for each woman leading to specific referral pathways. Examples include referral to antenatal groups for mothers needing stress management skills; those with a history of abuse or suboptimal parenting needing specific psychological or social interventions; those needing medication, to see a psychiatrist; and referral to a social worker for those with experience of domestic violence or relationship problems. The interventions offered will obviously be determined by the availability of local resources.

Other therapies

Some of the other treatment modalities which do not strictly fall under the banner of psychosocial therapies but are targeted at common mental health problems include acupuncture, massage, yoga and mindfulness meditation and relaxation. In a pilot feasibility study, the authors tested the hypotheses that a seven-week mindfulness yoga intervention would reduce salivary cortisol levels as well as self-reports of distress operationalized as perceived stress, anxiety and pain. There were significant improvements in perceived stress and trait anxiety. For women beginning the intervention in third trimester, anxiety and perceived stress had greater attenuation. For women beginning the intervention in second trimester, the physical pain that normally increases over time was minimized. Second-trimester women also appeared to develop increased physical well-being over the seven weeks of sessions while third-trimester women did not experience increased physical well-being but had less psychological distress [22]. A randomized trial evaluated self reported anxiety, maternal heart rate, and serum cortisol concentrations before and after 45-minute periods of active and passive relaxation in 58 pregnant women, and outcomes in both groups significantly improved from pre- to post-treatment [23].

14.6 Suicide

Women experience a gamut of intense emotions during pregnancy, the most damaging being severe depression leading to suicide. A recent report from Australia highlighted the finding that psychiatric illness including suicide is a leading cause of maternal death during the perinatal period in the UK and Australia [21]. A review of the prevalence of suicide during pregnancy and post-partum from the USA indicated that 20% of post-partum deaths were due to suicide. Further, the prevalence of suicidal ideation was estimated as between 5 and 14% [24].

Some women are likely to be at a higher risk for suicide during pregnancy. This includes women who are victims of sexual abuse/rape, intimate partner violence and those who have an unplanned and/or unwanted pregnancy. While depression, hopelessness and suicidal ideation can result in the mother not taking adequate care of herself or her fetus, suicide attempts can lead to a range of adverse consequences on the mother and her developing fetus. Therefore early identification, prevention and psychosocial interventions with women at risk for antenatal and post partum psychiatric disorders are important for two reasons:

1 Intervention during pregnancy can prevent the occurrence of a post-partum psychiatric disorder, and

2 The woman, her family and the treating team are better prepared to deal with exacerbations of symptoms during the postpartum period.

Several types of psychological interventions have been conducted with pregnant women: supportive, interpersonal and CBT. Decision regarding the type of therapy to be conducted depends largely on the client's presenting complaints, their severity and the clinician's speculations about the possible causes for client's distress. For instance, a pregnant woman presenting with severe depression and suicidal ideation stemming from marital problems and a lack of support from spouse is likely to benefit from couples therapy. Crisis intervention has been found useful for women who have attempted suicide. Home visits are also recommended but there is insufficient evidence for their effectiveness.

Depending on the severity of distress, women may also benefit from intensive in-patient treatment and care. Psychological distress may intensify around delivery and women may report suicidal or homicidal tendencies. Women are usually admitted to in-patient intensive care units where round the clock supervision and monitoring of the mother and her child is possible. Clinicians may also recommend physically separating the mother from the child, although the child is brought to the mother for feeding and this occurs in the presence of a nurse. After the first few weeks, there is likely to be attenuation in distress and the woman may start bonding with her child. Women often report feelings of guilt associated with suicidal and homicidal tendencies at this stage.

Mental health professionals often face a sense of time urgency in working with pregnant women. This sometimes seems like an insurmountable challenge because on the one hand, decisions have to be taken quickly and on the other hand, the woman is so distressed that she cannot think rationally, weigh pros and cons and take an informed decision. Whether it is to facilitate decision-making about continuing pregnancy or alleviating distress during pregnancy, there is often a pressure to restore maternal health as early as possible, before it can impact the mother and/or her child adversely. Although psychosocial intervention for pregnant women at risk for suicide is recommended, empirical studies are yet to demonstrate its effectiveness. Nonetheless, routine screening for suicidal ideation and early intervention among pregnant women is underscored.

14.7 Substance use

Literature on psychosocial treatment of substance use during pregnancy has focused primarily on women who drink alcohol and/or smoke tobacco prior to conception, and during pregnancy. Relatively few studies have reported the effectiveness of psychosocial interventions on women using other illicit drugs during pregnancy. Studies from several developed countries have reported high prevalence rates of problem drinking among women of childbearing age. While research has consistently documented a broad range of adverse effects of excessive maternal alcohol use on her fetus, there is inconclusive evidence on the association of moderate alcohol use with obstetric and neonatal outcomes.

Preventive interventions are necessary to create awareness and educate women and couples who plan to conceive. This may be disseminated through media and school-based programs and by gynecologists during routine well woman examinations. While some women choose to cut down or quit substances before planning to conceive, others voluntarily cut down or quit using substances when their pregnancy test is positive. Among the latter, depending on the severity of substance use, some damage may already have been caused to the fetus during the time lag between conception and receiving its confirmation through a pregnancy test.

Substance use during pregnancy is associated with stigma as many societies have criminalized substance-using pregnant women rather than encouraging them to seek treatment. Negative attitudes of treatment providers have also been documented as a potential barrier. Women therefore do not volunteer this information or may try to conceal or deny the same on self-report assessments. Although urine toxicology reports have been used as an objective report of substance use, women may be unwilling to get tested if they perceive the clinician to be judgemental. Therefore, either the treating clinician or a mental health professional will have to verbally and non-verbally communicate acceptance and a non-judgemental stance which will facilitate disclosure and provide an opportunity to instill positive attitudes about seeking psychological help.

Pregnancy offers a 'window of opportunity' for intervention; women are highly motivated to cut down or quit using substances in order to protect the fetus. While increasing awareness and providing information about harmful effects of the substance on both maternal and neonatal health outcomes is important in any individual-, couple- or group-based intervention, specific cognitive behavioral techniques are often used to enhance and sustain women's motivation to maintain abstinence and prevent relapses. Among the CBT techniques, motivational interviewing and contingency management are commonly used. Motivational interviewing (MI) or motivational enhancement therapy is a directive, client centered therapy that promotes readiness for cognitive and behavioral change. Contingency management (CM) is based on the principle of operant conditioning, which uses positive reinforcement as a means to facilitate and sustain behavioral change. However, two recent reviews concluded that there was insufficient empirical evidence for the effectiveness of MI. Comparative outcomes between MI and CM found that people treated with CM had better retention in treatment and achieved drug abstinence compared to those treated with MI [25, 26].

Another recent review examining the effectiveness of educational or psychological interventions to reduce alcohol consumption during pregnancy included four studies (N = 715) [27]. The findings indicated that while these interventions improved abstinence and reduced alcohol consumption, they did not provide sufficient evidence for the effectiveness of any one type of intervention.

Conclusive inferences from the above three reviews could not be made due to the availability of very few controlled studies, small sample size, poorly representative samples and inadequate study of obstetric and neonatal outcomes.

Although empirical evidence is limited, cognitive behavioral strategies found to be clinically effective are also recommended for use where relevant. These include: relaxation training, assertiveness training, cognitive restructuring and discussing alternative methods of dealing with high-risk situations for relapse, problem-solving and conflict resolution skills [28]. Intensive therapeutic efforts in the first few months are essential to prevent further fetotoxic and teratologic effects on the fetus. Frequent follow-up contacts are also necessary to ensure abstinence and to prevent relapses until the baby is weaned.

While intensive therapeutic work is focused on the individual, conjoint sessions are often conducted if a significant other is available. The significant other is often the spouse, partner, a close family member or friend who also functions as a co-therapist and helps the woman maintain sobriety. In addition, pregnant women, spouses and family members may be involved in skills training programs focused on enhancing parental childrearing abilities, strengthening parent–child attachment and encouraging family support systems [28]. Although multidisciplinary, community-based family-centered interventions may be recommended to improve maternal and child health outcomes [29], some women may benefit from residential treatment and care.

Mental health professionals desirably work in liaison with the clinicians or workers in a childbirth (or obstetrics) team to plan prevention, early identification and intervention efforts. Maternal substance use in pregnancy is a public health concern and, more importantly, it is one of the known and most easily preventable causes of developmental abnormalities in the newborn child. While integrated perinatal addiction services are essential, prevention of substance use prior to conception remains a priority.

14.8 Conclusions

It is clear from the above discussion that interventions for mental health problems in pregnancy are important for the well-being of the mother and the unborn fetus, and for the health of the mother–infant unit after birth. There is however a large gap between interventions developed and described for antepartum compared with post-partum mental health problems. Interventions are needed that are friendly to women, can be delivered easily and are accessible to them. Cultural considerations are important during pregnancy and any intervention should take into account the social and cultural context. A risk approach may be the best start as a model for providing targeted interventions. Unfortunately, the involvement of fathers has been minimal in intervention studies and attention needs to be paid to fathers and families acting as a resource.

14.9 Acknowledgements

Time on this chapter was supported by the Fogarty International Center ICOHRTA Training Program in Behavioral Disorders (Grant No. TW05811-08; VA Satyanarayana, Fellow).

14.10 References

1. Bennett, H.A., Einarson, A., Taddio, A. *et al.* (2004) Prevalence of depression during pregnancy: systematic review. *Obstetrics and Gynecology*, **103** (4), 698–709.
2. Yarcheski, A., Mahon, N.E., Yarcheski, T.J. *et al.* (2009) A meta-analytic study of predictors of maternal-fetal attachment. *International Journal of Nursing Studies*, **46**, 708–15.
3. Barlow, J. and Coren, E. (2009) Parent-training programmes for improving maternal psychosocial health. *Cochrane Database Systematic Review*, 1:CD002020.
4. Ross, L.E. and McLean, L.M. (2006) Anxiety disorders during pregnancy and post partum period: a systematic review. *Journal of Clinical Psychiatry*, **67**, 1285–98.
5. Alder, J., Fink, N. and Bitzer, J. (2007) Depression and anxiety during pregnancy: a risk factor for obstetric, fetal and neonatal outcomes? A critical review of the literature. *Journal of Maternal-Fetal and Neonatal Medicine*, **20**, 189–209.
6. Hofberg, K. and Brockington, I.F. (2000) Tokophobia: an unreasoning dread of childbirth. A series of 26 cases. *British Journal of Psychiatry*, **176**, 83–85.
7. Sjogren, B. and Thomasspon, P. (1997) Obsteric outcome in 100 women with severe anxiety over child birth. *Acta Obstetricia et Gynecologica Scandinacvica*, **76**, 948–52.
8. Saisto, T., Salmela Aro, K. and Nurmi, J.-E. (2001) A randomized controlled trial of intervention for fear of child birth. *Obstetrics and Gynecology*, **98**, 820–26.
9. Field, T., Diego, M. and Hernanadez-Reif, M. (2006) Prenatal depression effects on the fetus and newborn: a review. *Infant Behaviour and Development*, **29**, 445–55.
10. Bastani, F., Hidarnia, A., Kazemnejad, A. *et al.* (2005) A randomized controlled trial of the effects of applied relaxation training on reducing anxiety and perceived stress in pregnant women. *Journal of Midwifery and Women's Health*, **50**, 36–40.
11. Ryding, E.L., Persson, A., Onell, C. *et al.* (2003) An evaluation of midwives counseling of pregnancy women in fear of child birth. *Acta Obstetricia et Gynecologica Scandinavica*, **82**, 10–17.
12. Loveland Cook, C.A., Flick, L.H., Homan, S.M. *et al.* (2004) Post traumatic stress disorder in pregnancy: prevalence, risk factors and treatment. *Obstetrics and Gynecology*, **103**, 710–17.
13. Abramowitz, J.S., Schwartz, S.A., Moore, K.M. *et al.* (2003) Obsessive compulsive symptoms in pregnancy and the puerperium: a review of the literature. *Anxiety Disorders*, **17**, 461–78.
14. Franko, D.L. and Spurrell, E.B. Detection and management of eating disorders during pregnancy. *Obstetrics and Gynecology*, **95**, 942–46.
15. Dinas, K., Daniilidis, A., Sikou, S.H.O.K. *et al.* (2008) Anorexia nervosa in pregnancy: a case report and review of the literature. *Obstetric Medicine*, **1**, 97–98.
16. Spinelli, M.G. (1997) Interpersonal psychotherapy for depressed antepartum women: a pilot study. *American Journal of Psychiatry*, **154**, 1028–30.
17. Spinelli, M.G. and Endicott, J. (2003) Controlled clinical trial of interpersonal psychotherapy versus parenting education program for depressed pregnant women. *American Journal of Psychiatry*, **160** (3), March, 555–62.
18. Grote, N.K., Bledsoe, S.E., Swartz, H.A. *et al.* (2004) Feasibility of providing culturally relevant, brief interpersonal psychotherapy for antenatal depression in an obstetrics clinic: a pilot study. *Research on Social Work Practice*, **14**, 397–407.
19. Grote, N.K, Swartz, H.A., Geibel, S.L., *et al.* (2009) A randomized controlled trial of culturally relevant, brief interpersonal psychotherapy for perinatal depression. *Psychiatric Services*, **60** (3), March, 313–21.

20. Dennis, C.L., Ross, L.E. and Grigoriadis, S. (2007) Psychosocial and psychological interventions for treating antenatal depression. *Cochrane Database Systematic Review*, **18** (3). July, CD006309.
21. Austin, M.P., Kildea, S. and Sullivan, E. (2007) Maternal mortality and psychiatric morbidity in the perinatal period: challenges and opportunities for prevention in the Australian setting. *Medical Journal Australia*, **186**, 364–67.
22. Beddoe, A.E., Paul Yang, C.-P., Kennedy, H.P. *et al.* (2009) The effects of mindfulness-based yoga during pregnancy on maternal psychological and physical distress. *Journal of Obstetric, Gynecologic, and Neonatal Nursing*, **38**, 310–19.
23. Teixeira, J., Martin, D., Prendiville, O. and Glover, V. (2005) The effects of acute relaxation on indices of anxiety during pregnancy. *Journal of Psychosomatic Obstetrics and Gynaecology*, **26** (4), 271–76.
24. Lindahl, V., Pearson, J.L. and Colpe, L. (2005) Prevalence of suicidality during pregnancy and the postpartum. *Archives of Women's Mental Health*, **8**, 77–87.
25. Terplan, M. and Lui, S. (2007) Psychosocial interventions for pregnant women in outpatient illicit drug treatment programs compared to other interventions. *Cochrane Database Systematic Review*, **4**, CD006037.
26. Lui, S., Terplan, M. and Smith, E.J. (2008) Psychosocial interventions for women enrolled in alcohol treatment during pregnancy. *Cochrane Database Systematic Review*, **3**, CD006753.
27. Stade, B.C., Bailey, C., Dzendoletas, D. *et al.* (2009) Psychological and/or educational interventions for reducing alcohol consumption in pregnant women and women planning pregnancy. *Cochrane Database Systematic Review*, **2**, CD004228.
28. Kumpfer, K.L. and Fowler, M.A. (2007) Parenting skills and family support programs for drug-abusing mothers. *Seminars in Fetal and Neonatal Medicine*, **12**, 134–42.
29. Lester, B.M., Andreozzi, L. and Appiah, L. (2004) Substance use during pregnancy: time for policy to catch up with research. *Harm Reduction Journal*, **1**, 5.

15

Perinatal loss: its immediate and long-term impact on parenting

Miri Keren

Tel Aviv University Sackler Medical School, Israel

Case vignette 1

A 25-week-pregnant woman was referred for psychiatric consultation by the well-baby care nurse because she claimed not to be feeling fetal movements, in spite of normal monitor and ultrasound. As opposed to the worried nurse, the mother looked stern and detached, and was reluctant to talk about herself in general and her pregnancy specifically. She had immigrated from the former USSR a few years before, her family had stayed there and she had no social support in Israel, except for her husband. Being pressed to tell her obstetrical history, it turned out that this pregnancy was subsequent to a stillbirth. Mother was at first completely disconnected from her unresolved grief, as well as from her current pregnancy, and refuted the link between her lack of feeling the fetal movements and her psychological condition. Still, she agreed to come for a few sessions, mainly because she felt alone in the country and missed her own mother. An intense, unresolved grief was unveiled. She eventually gave birth to a healthy baby, and did not develop any post-partum disorder.

Case vignette 2

A 25-year-old mother is referred to the Infant Mental Health Unit by the well-baby care nurse with her 4 month-old baby girl because of suspected post-partum depression. The primipara pregnancy was described as uneventful by the nurse, and no special antecedents were noted in the chart. A significant mother–infant relationship disorder was diagnosed and dyadic psychotherapy was initiated. After two sessions, the therapist discovered this child was literally a replacement child: the mother had dreamed of her late sister, who died in a car accident at the age of nine years, and told her in the dream, 'I can't wait anymore.' This dream was interpreted by the mother as an order to get pregnant so her late sister could 'relive'. The sister did not come back to life … but the ambivalence and turmoil that characterized their relationship were transmitted to the baby girl …

15.1 Introduction

The uniqueness of perinatal grief

For parents, the simultaneous event of looking forward to life that turns into death puts them into a bewildering, unthinkable state. 'I am a mother, without being a real one. I feel amputated from what I was with that child' said a 27-week-pregnant woman [1, p. 669]. Losing a child is obviously very traumatic for parents, but grieving over somebody who did not or hardly lived is especially complex. This complexity is not only on the psychosocial level, but also on the societal level: in many countries, there is no death certificate for stillborns, nor premature infants who were born at less than 18 weeks of gestational age, and did not survive. The absence of birth and death certificates means that only the live and viable newborn has civil rights; from the juridical perspective, it is a dead child who was never born … Contingently, their parents have no parental social rights, such as coverage of hospital and funeral or incineration expenses, maternal leave, protection of employment and so on. This lack of recognition from society makes the parents even more isolated in their grief, as one parent wrote: 'We would like our late baby be registered as a civilian. We need the official recognition of our little boy … Our life has been so changed that we do not want, we cannot do as if nothing happened' [1, p. 671].

Definitions

Perinatal loss is a broad term that encompasses several different situations: early pregnancy miscarriage, induced abortion following the ultrasound diagnosis of a lethal fetal anomaly after 24 weeks of gestational age, stillbirths, and death shortly after birth. Each of these differ in their circumstances, but all of them are unexpected and traumatic. In a study [2] that compared long-term psychological responses of women following a pregnancy termination due to ultrasound-detected fetal anomalies with those of women following a late spontaneous abortion or a perinatal death, no differences were found between the groups.

15.2 Historical and cultural perspectives

Before the end of the nineteenth century, infant deaths in Europe in the first year of life were around 150 to 200 per thousand live births. Public health measures led to a significant improvement at the beginning of the twentieth century, but only the introduction of safe blood transfusion, sulphonamides and penicillin in the 1930s and 1940s made the real difference: by 1945, perinatal deaths had fallen to 45, and by 1981 to 12 per 1000 births [3]. Since that time, there has been only a marginal change [4].

Attitudes to the loss of a newborn, and recognition of perinatal loss as a significant bereavement, differ in function of normal expectancies. Nowadays Western parents anticipate their pregnancies being successful, and therefore are deeply shocked by the loss of their infant, in contrast with parents from developing countries, where infant mortality is still very high, and where people protect themselves by postponing their attachment to the child [4].

An additional change, linked with advances in medical technology is that, in the past, perinatal losses were always spontaneous and unexpected. Today, the use of ultrasound in pregnancy has made prenatal diagnosis of fetal lethal malformations possible and, contingently, many couples find themselves in the position of choosing to terminate planned and wanted pregnancies. Issues such as how to announce the lethal anomaly, and how to prepare the induced abortion, have been new issues that had to be dealt with, by nursing and medical staff [1].

Most research about psychological impact of perinatal loss have been conducted in the United States, in western Europe and in Australia, with under-representation of minorities [4]. An exception is a qualitative study [5] on low-income African–American couples, where socio-economic hardship was a risk factor, and the use of spirituality a protective factor, in coping with perinatal loss. In a small study of middle-class Indian women after perinatal loss [6], substantial grieving and common family blame for not producing a healthy child were reported. Among Taiwanese women, the theme of strong social expectancy of producing continuity of the family was found as a significant determinant of their psychological reactions [7].

15.3 Psychological effects of perinatal death on *mothers*

In the weeks following perinatal loss, regardless of timing and type, mothers experience grief, i.e. the normative affective response to loss of a significant person, including sadness, irritability, guilt and somatic symptoms [8]. The severity of the symptoms gradually decreases, but are normal for up to one to two years [9]. Besides depression and anxiety symptoms, mothers' self-criticism alone explained 36% of the variance of their coping difficulty [10]. The woman's sense of being causal in the loss has been linked with the increased frequency of unresolved classification of the Adult Attachment Interview found in women with history of stillbirth [11].

Risk factors for prolonged grief include poor social support, pre-pregnancy mental health problems and more 'neurotic' pre-loss personality. Factors such as difficulty in conceiving, greater maternal age, sex of the baby, socio-economic status and religious observance were not significantly associated [12].

Puerperal psychosis following perinatal death is slightly higher than post-partum psychosis, but still is a rare reaction [13].

15.4 Psychological effects of perinatal death on *fathers*

In contrast with the vast array of studies on the psychological impact of perinatal loss on mothers, it is only recently that fathers' reactions have been reported systematically.

Qualitative studies have shown that, in addition to grief, fathers perceive the need to provide emotional support to the mother, at the cost of denying their own grief and remaining strong in the face of the mother's distress [14, 15]. Quantitative studies converge on the finding that fathers have a lower level of grief [16, 17], anxiety and depression [18], but higher than in a control group [19]. Vulnerability factors were the same for fathers and mothers [16]. Low levels of marital adjustment are predictive of increased grief, for men more than for women [10]. It is notable that these reactions were the same for any kind of perinatal loss, including sudden infant death syndrome [19] (still, we do not deal in this chapter with sudden infant death syndrome, because it is a different phenomenon with its own biological and psychological characteristics).

15.5 Impact of perinatal loss on the *couple*

Like any serious adverse life event, perinatal loss puts the couple relationship at strain, especially if parents do not experience grief reactions at the same pace and intensity [20]. For instance, Franche's findings [10], that perinatal loss is mostly relevant to women's self concept and to men's perceived marital adjustment, strengthen the notion of gender difference in stress coping, and may explain, at least partly, the increase in relationship break-up reported in longitudinal studies [20, 21].

15.6 Impact of perinatal loss on the *subsequent pregnancy*

From the *parents'* perspective

Taking on a new pregnancy after previous loss is fraught with apprehension, fear of additional loss and a sense of failure that remains across pregnancy [22]. Pregnant women with a history of perinatal loss, compared with those without loss, have less strong prenatal attachment [23], have altered self-concepts and may experience post-traumatic stress [21]. Post-traumatic stress reactions during the subsequent pregnancy have been reported among mothers as well as among fathers [24], lasting *at the most* for one year post-partum.

From the *child's* perspective

Even after a successful birth, mothers with loss histories are more concerned about their new baby's health and about differentiating this baby from the baby that dies [25]. Although the two psychodynamic concepts of 'vulnerable child syndrome' [26] and 'replacement child syndrome' [27] were introduced a long time ago to describe the ways in which perinatal losses may impact upon the child born subsequent to loss, the existing literature is mainly descriptive. In the replacement child syndrome, the infant grows under the impact of parental projections of an idealized lost child. The infant is perceived as failing to fulfil this idealization, and may grow into an 'as if' personality [28]; some of these children are at risk for scapegoating, neglect and abuse. The vulnerable child syndrome is explained as the result of the infant's internalization of the parental anxiety, growing into an anxious individual, excessively concerned with his or her own health and survival.

Recent quantitative controlled studies have brought findings that may support these two theoretical psychodynamic constructs. Disorganized attachment behavior was found in 53 infants next-born after a stillbirth [29] at a significantly higher frequency than among 53 control infants of primigravid infants. It was strongly associated with maternal own unresolved status of the loss, as measured by the Adult Attachment Interview, a finding that may suggest a causal link between the mother's state of mind with respect to her perinatal loss, and her next child's subsequent attachment behavior.

This same cohort of infants were followed and examined again at seven years of age [30] and an association was found between the attachment disorganization scores they had as infants, and teacher-rated symptoms of attention deficit hyperactivity disorder (ADHD), but not ADHD cases. In parallel, the mother–child interaction was assessed in both study and control groups [31]. There were no significant group differences in child cognitive or health status, nor in teacher-rated child difficulties.

The interesting finding was that mothers with a past of perinatal loss tended to report increased child difficulties and peer problems, and exhibited significantly more negative interactions with their child, than mothers with no history of perinatal loss. More specifically, they exhibited higher levels of criticism and controlling behavior, less positive affect and less engagement with their child. As the authors suggest, these maternal behaviors may be the expression of unconscious rejection and/or fear of loss. Still, the clinical significance for the child of these modest stillbirth-related effects is not clear. *No clinical cases* were detected among these post-stillbirth children.

Following up these children into adolescence may confirm whether or not there is any long-term developmental impingement of a less-than-optimal mother–child relationship. One study has looked at mental health, self-esteem and parent bonding of 77 young university students whose parents had experienced early child loss [32], as compared with 223 controls. The loss group recalled their mothers as more protective/controlling than non-bereaved participants, but no differences were found in their mental health status nor their self-esteem (as measured with self-report questionaires). None of these studies has looked at father's nor family functioning as risk and/or protective factors in the development of these children, in spite of the association found between the experience of stillbirth with a threefold increase in subsequent family breakdown [31].

It is of interest to note that four famous artists were 'replacement children': Chateaubriand, Van Gogh, Ludwig van Beethoven, Salvador Dali . . . each with his own strengths and vulnerabilities . . . One may wonder the role of their familial perinatal loss in their talented but tumultuous lives . . .

15.7 Clinical implications

The vast majority of bereaved parents go through mourning, i.e. the process of recovery, with gradual lessening of distress and return to routine life [4].

Our aim therefore should be to detect the small but significant minority of parents who will develop abnormal grief. Still, we do have a preventive role in managing the loss in a way that facilitates recovery, in identifying the factors that impinge on it, and in planning for specific interventions for those parents at risk for pathological grief. The definition of normal mourning is quite loose, and pathological grief is usually defined as either prolonged (above six months) with impaired functioning, or absent. Surprisingly, a small minority of parents shows a low level of distress after loss, and perceive themselves as coping quite well [16].

Announcement and preparation of induced abortion

At the moment of the announcement of the death *in utero*, parents are in shock, because of the suddenness and unpredictability of the event. The same goes for the announcement of a severe malformation, that is perceived as the immediate disappearance of the baby. 'We don't have a child anymore', announced a mother to her husband after the ultrasound [1, p. 677]. The moment of shock is often followed by intense negative feelings towards the fetus: 'I would look at my belly with horror, I had the feeling I had a monster in my insides ...' [1, p. 677]. Then comes the phase of preparing the parents to take the dead baby out. Most parents value receiving structured information as well as support in helping them make sense of the event [34].

When the baby was born alive, but doomed to die shortly after birth, the benefit of giving parents a role in decision-making for their dying infant has been shown as lessening their experience of helplessness and angry feelings. Still, for some parents, this principle of autonomy may not be adequate at a time when they are in shock.

Holding the dead infant

The suggestion to the parents to hold their dead infant has been a common clinical impression-based recommendation for years. There is recent evidence that physical contact with the dead baby may actually induce depression, and even more significant parental post-traumatic stress disorder and post-loss infant's disorganized attachment [29]. This recent knowledge has led to a change in the guidelines [1]. Acts aimed at forming memories – such as seeing photographs of the infant (taken by the staff at the delivery), giving a name, bringing clothes that had been brought in advance for the newborn, doing some funeral ritual – are suggested to the parents in a non-patronizing manner. Each of the parents decides for her- or himself. When parents do wish to see their dead infant, a 'humanized presentation' is recommended: it should be cleaned, properly enveloped in clothes, and held in the midwife's arms. The positive, reparatory impact of such an event has been well put in words by a mother:

> I expected to see a something of a nothing, and in fact it was a well-done baby, with black hair, looking very much like his older brother, it was a boy. We gave him a name. I remember vividly the midwife's tender look, she had put clothes on him ... I felt proud of my baby, he was beautiful, and he was not a monster ... I did not give birth to a monster. [1, p. 682]

Follow-up of the parents after the loss

In the light of the high frequency of couple breakdowns after a perinatal loss [31], and the link found between future adjustment to the loss, levels of self-criticism in mothers and of marital satisfaction in fathers [10], couple counseling should be routinely recommended, with a focus of increased mutual dependency. Still, in most places, follow-up consultations are offered mainly to women, and the extent of their beneficial impact is not clear. On one hand, more than 90% of a sample of 204 post-perinatal loss women [35] felt a follow-up clinic would have been beneficial, but preferred to be seen by a doctor rather than a midwife or a counselor; on the other hand, routine follow-up was not associated with reduced psychological morbidity. These seemingly contradictory findings became clear when the content of the follow-up sessions was analyzed: Post-perinatal loss women wished to learn more about the possible reasons for the infant's death and the recurrence risks in subsequent pregnancies, but they also wished to be given the opportunity to discuss feelings, and felt the staff was somehow 'blocking' expression of feelings.

A referral for psychiatric assessment is indicated in the presence of psychosis, suicidal ideas, or if the severe depression continues beyond six months. Post-traumatic stress disorder should be detected and treated. Psychiatric management may include antidepressant medication, short-term use of hypnotic medications for sleep problems and psychological treatments. It is notable that to this day, to our best knowledge, there is no systematic study on the efficacy of these different treatment modalities for perinatal bereavement.

About the timing of the next pregnancy

As we have shown above, stillbirth is indeed a risk factor for depression and anxiety in the subsequent pregnancy; these in turn may have a significant impact on the pregnancy outcome (for further details, see Chapter 5, 'The impact of stress in pregnancy on the fetus, the infant, and the child'). Therefore, the clinical recommendation for bereaved parents to postpone pregnancy for six or twelve months makes a lot of sense, and is indeed a common clinical practice, including in our own. Still, parents often do not welcome this 'paternalistic' advice, nor clinicians [36], and they find support in the empirical studies that have shown that subsequent pregnancy predicts less grief and psychopathology [37]. These disparate findings and conclusions may owe much to their methodology. It seems today that individual choice regarding a subsequent pregnancy may be more relevant to parental grief than pregnancy per se: the decrease in active grief occurred particularly in women who were pregnant, but also in women who were *volitionally* deferring pregnancy [38].

Accompaniment of the parents along the new pregnancy

In the light of the data reviewed above in the section on subsequent pregnancies to perinatal loss, it seems justified to recommend that any pregnant woman who has experienced a previous perinatal loss should be screened by the community nurse for feelings of depression and anxiety during the new pregnancy and, even more important, to detect early signs of poor mother–infant interaction during the first year after delivery (that may lead to the development of the vulnerable child syndrome or of the replacement child syndrome). Fathers' vulnerability to anxiety and post-traumatic stress disorder during a pregnancy subsequent to perinatal loss should be recognized [24]. Fathers need support in their own right, rather than simply as an adjunct to their partner.

15.8 Conclusion

Perinatal death, early as well as late in the course of pregnancy, represents a significant bereavement for both parents. Defined guidelines of the way to approach and support the parents at the time of the infant's death have been evidence-based determined, including not to automatically encourage contact with the dead baby. Parents value receiving information about the nature of the problem, and should be given the possibility to be involved in decisions on care of their critically ill newborn. Parents, as well as heath professionals, should expect that, by six months after the loss, they will start resuming their usual train of life, though significant depressive and anxious feelings may take much longer to subside. Professionals need to intervene when the severity of the depression and/or post-traumatic stress disorder is such that the parent's functioning is impaired for longer than six months, and/or when symptoms of psychosis are present. Pregnancy subsequent to perinatal loss should be screened for depression and anxiety, and mothers with high levels of these should be accompanied during the first year of life, with the aim of preventing the syndromes of replacement/vulnerable child.

Research is still needed in order to identify the most vulnerable parents to lasting psychological/psychiatric morbidity, though previous psychiatric disorder and poor social support have already been identified as risk factors. Empirical trials are needed to determine the effectiveness of psychological and pharmacological therapies for psychiatric morbidity triggered by perinatal loss.

15.9 References

1. Dumoulin, M. (2004) Le deuil de l'enfant de la grossesse (Grief over pregnancy), in *La grossesse, l'enfant virtuel, et la parentalité (Pregnancy, the Virtual Child, and Parenthood)* (eds S. Missonnier, B. Golse and M. Soule), Presses Universitaires de France, Paris, pp. 669–94.
2. Salvesen, K.A., Oyen, L., Schmidt, N. *et al.* (1997) Comparison of long-term psychological responses of women after pregnacy termination due to fetal anomalies and after perinatal loss. *Ultrasound Obstetrical Gynecology*, **9**, 80–85.
3. Williams, S. (1997) *Women and Childbirth in the Twentieth Century.* Sutton Publishing, Cornwall.
4. Badenhorst, W. and Hughes, P. (2007) Psychological aspects of perinatal loss. *Best Practice and Research Clinical Obstetrics and Gynaecology*, **21**, 249–59.
5. Kavanaugh, K. and Hershberger, P. (2005) Perinatal loss in low income African American parents. *Journal of Obstetrical, Gynecological, and Neonatal Nursing*, **34**, 595–605.
6. Mammen, O.K. (1995) Women's reaction to perinatal loss in India: an exploratory, descriptive study. *Infant Mental Health Journal*, **16**, 94–101.
7. Hsu, M.T., Tseng, Y.F. and Kuo, L.L. (2002) Transforming loss: Taiwanese women's adaptation to stillbirth. *Journal of Advanced Nursing*, **40**, 387–95.
8. Kennell, J.H., Slyter, H. and Laus, M.H. (1970) The mourning response of parents to the death of the newborn infant. *New England Journal of Medicine*, **283**, 344–49.
9. Janssen, H.J.E.M., Cuisinierm M.C.J. and Hoogduin, K.A.L. (1996) A critical review of the concept of pathological grief following pregnancy loss. *Omega (Westport)*, **33**, 21–42.

10. Franche, R.L. (2001) Psychologic and obstetric predictors of couples' grief during pregnancy after miscarriage or perinatal death. *Obstetrics and Gynaecology*, **97**, 597–602.
11. Hughes, P., Turton, P., Hopper, E. *et al.* (2004) Factors associated with the unresolved classification of the Adult Attachment Interview in women who have suffered stillbirth. *Development and Psychopathology*, **16**, 215–30.
12. Janssen, H.J.E.M., Cuisinier, M.C.J., De Graauw, K.P.H.M. *et al.* (1997) A prospective study of risk factors grief intensity following perinatal loss. *Archives of General Psychiatry*, **54**, 56–61.
13. Kendell, R.E., Chalmers, J.C., Platz, C. *et al.* (1987) Epidemiology of puerperal psychoses. *British Journal of Psychiatry*, **150**, 662–73.
14. Samuelson, M., Radestad, I., Segesten, K. *et al.* (2001) A waste of life: fathers' experience of losing a child before birth. *Birth*, **28**, 124–30.
15. O'Leary, J., Thorwick, C. *et al.* (2006) Fathers' perspectives during pregnancy, postperinatal loss. *Journal of Obstetrical, Gynecological and Neonatal Nursing*, **35**, 78–86.
16. Zeanah, C.H., Danis, B., Hirshberg, L. *et al.* (1995) Initial adaptation in mothers and fathers following perinatal loss. *Infant Mental Health Journal*, **16**, 80–93.
17. Theut, S.K., Zaslow, M.J., Rabinovich, B.A. *et al.* (1990) Resolution of parental bereavement after a perinatal loss. *Journal of American Academy of Child and Adolescent Psychiatry*, **29**, 521–25.
18. Wilson, A.L., Witzle, D., Fenton, L.J. *et al.* (1985) Parental response to perinatal death. Mother-father differences. *American Journal of Diseases in Children*, **139**, 1235–38.
19. Vance, J.C., Najman, J.M., Thearle, M.J. *et al.* (1995) Psychological changes in parents eight months after the loss of an infant from stillbirth, neonatal death, or sudden infant death syndrome – a longitudinal study. *Pediatrics*, **96**, 933–38.
20. Najman, J.M., Vance, J.C., Boyle, F. *et al.* (1993). The impact of a child death on marital adjustment. *Social Science and Medicine*, **37**, 1005–10.
21. Turton, P., Hughes, P., Fonagy, P. *et al.* (2004) An investigation into the possible overlap between PTSD and unresolved responses following stillbirth. *Attachment in Human Development*, **6**, 241–53.
22. Cote-Arsenault, D. (2007) Threat appraisal, coping, and emotions across pregnancy subsequent to perinatal loss. *Nursing Research*, **56**, 108–16.
23. Armstrong, D. and Hutti, M.A. (1998) Pregnancy after perinatal loss: the relationship between anxiety and prenatal attachment. *Journal of Obstetric, Gynecologic, and Neonatal Nursing*, **27**, 183–89.
24. Turton, P., Badenhorst, W., Hugues, P. *et al.* (2006) Psychological impact of stillbirth on fathers in the subsequent pregnancy and puerperium. *British Journal of Psychiatry*, **188**, 165–72.
25. Theut, S.K., Moss, S.A., Zaslow, M.J. *et al.* (1992) Perinatal loss and maternal attitudes toward the subsequent child. *Infant Mental Health Journal*, **13**, 157–66.
26. Green, M. and Solnit, A.J. (1964) Reactions to the threatened loss of a child. *Pediatrics*, **34**, 58–66.
27. Cain, A.C. and Cain, B.S. (1964) On replacing a child. *Journal of American Academy of Child and Adolescent Psychiatry*, **3**, 443–55.
28. Sabbadini, A. (1988) The replacement child. *Contemporary Psychoanalysis*, **24**, 528–47.
29. Hughes, P., Turton, P., Hopper, E. *et al.* (2001) Disorganised attachment behaviour among infants born subsequent to childbirth. *Journal of Child Psychology and Psychiatry*, **42**, 791–801.

30. Pinto, C., Turton, P., Hughes, P. *et al.* (2006) ADHD and infant disorganized attachment: a prospective study of children next-born after stillbirth. *Journal of Attention Disorders*, **10**, 83–91.

31. Turton, P., Badenhorst, W., Pawlby, S. *et al.* (2009) Psychological vulnerability in children next-born after stillbirth: a case control follow-up study. *Journal of Child Psychology and Psychiatry*, 9 July (Epub ahead of print).

32. Pantke, R. and Slade, P. (2006) Remembered parenting style and psychological well-being in young adults whose parents had experienced early child loss. *Psychology and Psychotherapy: Theory, Research, and Practice*, **79**, 69–81.

33. Turton, P., Evans, C. and Hughes, P. (2009) Long-term psychosocial sequelae of stillbirth: Phase II of a nested case-control cohort study. *Archives of Women's Mental Health*, **12**, 35–41.

34. Saflund, K., Sjogren, B. and Wredling, R. (2004) The role of caregivers after stillbirths: views and experiences of parents. *Birth*, **31**, 132–37.

35. Nikcevic, A.V., Tunkel, S.A. and Nicolaides, K.H. (1998) Psychological outcomes following missed abortions and provision of follow-up care. *Ultrasound Obstetrical Gynecology*, **11**, 123–28.

36. Davis, D.L., Stewart, M. and Harmon, R.J. (1989) Postponing pregnancy after perinatal death: perspectives on doctor advice. *Journal of American Academy of Child and Adolescent Psychiatry*, **28**, 481–487.

37. Franche, R.L. and Bulow, C. (1999) The impact of a subsequent pregnancy on grief and emotional adjustment following a perinatal loss. *Infant Mental Health Journal*, **20**, 175–87.

38. Barr, P. (2006) Relation between grief and subsequent pregnancy status 13 months after perinatal bereavement. *Journal of Perinatal Medicine*, **34**, 207–11.

16

Transition to parenthood

Antoine Guedeney[1,2] and Susana Tereno[1*]

[1] Hôpital Claude Bernard, APHP, Paris, France
[2] University Denis Diderot Paris VII

16.1 Introduction

Becoming a parent is an upheaval, usually more for mothers than for fathers. There is no such thing as a good-enough mother alone, could we say after Winnicott's famous sentence [1]. We could add that it takes a village to raise a child, following a famous African saying. Not until the last half of the twentieth century, however, did the transition to parenthood become the subject of intensive analysis by sociologists, psychologists and health and mental health professionals. Major life changes and transitions can create conditions of risk; new challenges can outstrip existing resources, trigger new problems, or amplify pre-existing vulnerabilities and inadequacies. Nevertheless, challenges of

Acknowledgements: The CAPEDP adventure would not have been possible without Tim Greacen's expertise, friendliness and enthusiasm and without support from the strong executive group: T. Greacen, F. Tubach, R. Dugravier, T. Saias, along with the support of Richard Tremblay. We would like to thank the CMP Binet staff and the Bichat hospital maternity ward staff (Pr. D. Mahieu- Caputo), along with the nine other APHP maternity wards who took part in the recruitment (Beaujon, Robert Debré, Jean Rostand, Louis Mourier, St Antoine, Pitié-Salpêtrière, Tenon, Lariboisère, Trousseau) and the administration of Bichat Claude Bernard hospital APHP for their help in our CAPDEP project. Thanks to the A Capedp attachment lab staff, led by Susana Tereno, PhD, and inspired by Nicole Guedeney, MD, PhD. This project was supported by the PHRC 2005 and 2009 (Département à Recherche Clinique et au Développement, Assistance Publique–Hôpitaux de Paris (PHRC AOM05056, Clinical Trials.gov Identifier: NCT00392847) and by INPES (2005 and 2009). This work was supported by a research grant from the French Ministry of Health and the French Institute for Prevention and Health Education.

Parenthood and Mental Health: A Bridge between Infant and Adult Psychiatry Sam Tyano, Miri Keren, Helen Herrman and John Cox transitions can also stimulate the development of new coping skills and higher levels of adaptation. The transition to parenthood is an interesting test case for lifespan development theories because, unlike most expected and unexpected traumatic transitions, becoming a parent is widely regarded as a positive change in the life of a couple. Taken as a group, studies of the transition to parenthood show that new parents experience shifts in five domains:

1 The quality of relationships in the new parents' families of origin;

2 The quality of the new parents' relationship as a couple;

3 The quality of relationship that each parent develops with the baby;

4 The balance between life stress and social support in the new family;

5 The well-being or distress of each parent and child as individuals [2].

This work will describe some of the main theories built to understand the psychological transition to parenthood and its challenges. There is a large literature on the topic, but mainly made of hypothesis, with limited evidence of what is really at stake in the different stages of pregnancy and parenthood, and with little explanation for the great variability in the way young parents go through the transitions of parenthood. We will then address the issue of the increased psychopathology in this period. Denial of pregnancy could be considered as the prototype of a failure of transition to parenthood. In the third part of this work, the central issue of prevention will be considered.

16.2 Pregnancy and emotional upheaval: risks and resiliency

Pregnancy may be considered as no easy time; the idealized version of the pregnancy as a cruise on a calm river is definitely not the most frequent. While emotional upheaval is normative, and may be even leading to a better outcome, it gives way to a great amount of vulnerability, which is the major characteristic of the period. Young parents are in need of a lot of social support to achieve the transition goals, which are mainly to be ready to become a 'good-enough' caregiver. Especially when parents have been through early experiences of disorganized attachment, or early or later experiences of abuse or neglect, they will need their secure base needs to be filled, even though they may not be conscious of the need and may have not learned to call for help or have lost hope to get it, as Fraiberg's pioneer work has taught us [3].

Pregnancy is a time of a demanding transition, giving hope of transformation, achievement and reorganization on one hand, but is also intrinsically one of disruption, of crisis and of potential disorganization on the other, even when pregnancy is planned and wanted. The problem is, to which extent this emotional upheaval, this developmental crisis and reorganization crisis will lead to good-enough parenting and caregiving, or will be the basis for early and potentially long-lasting disordered patterns of relationships between parents and child.

Pregnancy is a time of enormous changes, physically, with hormonal, neurochemical shifts, and changes in self-identity, strong reactivation of attachment and caregiving systems, and changes in internal representations. It is the prototype of an

'In Between' situation, in which the sense of identity allows for some major transformations. Within this situation, variations are huge, depending whether the woman wished to
be pregnant or not, had a stable and pleasurable relationship with the father or not, is
isolated or may use a large network of social support and has or not achieved most of the
preconditions to become a parent.

16.3 The psychological unfolding of pregnancy

A lot of women feel they are pregnant before they realize they miss their period. Even if the
fetus has no real existence in her mind yet, the newly pregnant women often may be making
changes in her diet and activity level, and quitting smoking and alcohol drinking. Early
routine ultrasonography does help make the baby feel more real and deepen the mother's
and father's feeling of bonding to the fetus. Caregiving is biologically based: Feldman [4]
has shown that higher plasma oxytocin levels during the first trimester of pregnancy are
associated with more positive mother–child attachment at four months. Bibring [5] was
about the first to describe the inward stance taken by the pregnant women, turning her
psychological orientation inward as she imagines the baby more realistically and feels him
moving and kicking, at four to five months of pregnancy.

Quite a lot of authors, mainly psychoanalysts, have tried to retrace the psychological
journey of the pregnant women. Bibring [5] has described it in terms of developmental
phase; however, this transition phase fits better with the definition of a reactive transitional
crisis, with an increase of mental symptomatology, and a lot of affective instability. In fact,
maternity is no more considered as the 'final developmental phase' for all women; a lot of
women do develop fully without becoming a mother. However, that a crisis may take place
in pregnancy is more than understandable, when one thinks of all the psychological tasks to
achieve in a matter of months. The major task is probably to come to terms with the
woman's internal representation of a mother, mostly based on her past childhood experience. As Slade [6] puts it, one of the ways that a mother comes to feel like a mother is by
identifying with her own mother. For some mothers, pregnancy will stir up very conflicting
and very ambivalent memories; for some, early relationships with their mothers were so
painful and traumatic that reworking will be difficult, if not impossible.

A mother-to-be has several other psychological tasks, as she already has several roles:
daughter, wife/partner, citizen, member of a culture and of a community and very often
now a working woman. She may be already a mother, and has then to make room for the
new child. Becoming a mother may conflict with some of these roles, and in fact it will
conflict with most, to a more or lesser extent. Regression, anxiety, transient depression,
emotional upheaval and ambivalence are natural consequences of these shifts. Trad [7] has
suggested that these shifts cannot help but trigger ambivalence. This healthy ambivalence
has to be acknowledged to be accepted by the woman and worked through, as it is key to a
successful adaptation to pregnancy. Winnicott [1] has beautifully termed the reasons a
woman may have to hate her baby, and he could add to hate her fetus. Some psychoanalysts
have insisted on the Oedipal value of the pregnancy in the relationship with the parents of
the pregnant women, but this looks like more like fantasy than real psychic life, at least for
women in the normal range of mental life.

A problem we face in studying the psychological transition in pregnancy is that most
descriptions are based on the psychodynamics of childhood infantile sexuality theory,

which was itself mostly based on retrospective observations made with disordered adults, and very little on normal development of infants and toddlers. We lack longitudinal studies on mental health in pregnancy and in the perinatal period, which could consider the wide array of individual variations. That the wish to have a baby is based on the wish the little girl had to have one from her father may be a secondary sexualization of troubled relationships in childhood. Initial descriptions of motherhood and pregnancy by psychoanalysts were mostly retrospective and based on few cases. Studies bases on larger, non-clinical samples longitudinally studied should help us know better what is at stake in pregnancy from a psychological point of view. The psychic life of pregnant women is no more transparent than that of others, but the priorities shift in pregnancy, as Stern [8] as shown in his Motherhood Constellation model.

Finally, one key point is the idea that there is no such thing as a dyad, but a triad from the very onset of pregnancy. This will become more evident as the pregnancy unfolds; even if at times, the mothers to be seem mainly preoccupied with herself and with the unborn baby. The fact is very few women effectively want to have a child alone, just for themselves. The desire to have a child most of the times comes in the context of a couple relationship, be it between heterosexual or homosexual couples, or for adopting couples. The breaking of the relationship with the father during pregnancy or right after delivery is linked with an increase of symptomatology in the infants and later in childhood, and with a higher rate of postnatal depression in the mother.

During the last trimester, women gain the most weight, with restricted mobility. In the last weeks, preparation begins for childbirth, likely related to oxytocin release immediately prior to delivery. Winnicott [1] termed this the beginning of 'Primary Maternal Preoccupation'; influenced by the negative effects of maternal depression he had observed in his own mother, he thought that this almost psychotic like state of mind was necessary for the mother to adjust to the demands of the child without impinging on his developing self. This may not be true. Tronick [9] has brilliantly shown that usual good-enough mother–infant interaction is off the base 50% of the time, but what is important for development is the repair process within the interaction. But what about the evolution of representations of self and of the fetus during pregnancy? By the third trimester, differences among women in their capacity to imagine the baby and to imagine themselves as mothers can be quite striking [6]. These are also fairly consolidated and stable: representations tend to be stable from pregnancy to one year of after birth, and women with balanced representations in pregnancy are more likely to have secure infants at one year. Factors that may lead to a change in representations are income level, single parenthood, history of abuse and depressive symptomatology. A woman's attachment security predicts maternal fetal bonding as well as the quality of prenatal representations of the baby and of the self as a mother [6].

Attachment and caregiving-related representations are the core of changes specific to motherhood. Attachment relationships are defined by reactions of the child to situations of stress, separation, fear, pain or distress; caregiving is the ability of the caregiver to answer these cues adequately. Pregnancy and early parenthood are times of high stress, which stirs up the attachment system. Becoming a mother – or a father – stirs up 'memories in feelings', about attachment relationships in the past. In the balanced, secure mothers, there is confidence and ability to seek help and establish a working alliance, when needed. The pregnant mother becomes more and more dependent, and her ability to tolerate this situation, particularly feelings of helplessness, and to seek and use help will be very useful.

Attachment and caregiving are two behavioral systems that help the survival of the child, but are even more important to the humanization of the child. These are behavioral systems that help develop emotional regulation, and social abilities, among which mentalization seems the most important. The capacity to reflect on one's emotions, feelings and thoughts, the ability to figure out what the other can feel and think is specific to humans, and seems to be a byproduct of secure attachment, provided by a sensitive caregiver with good-enough ability to think about the baby's mind and to keep the individual mind of the baby in mind. The point is to keep that ability even in stressing situations, without disorganizing behavior from the caretaker. Disorganizing behavior , such as frightening the child when he or she need to be comforted, leads to the collapse of the attachment secure base behavior. Parents who have had disorganized parents tend to be disorganized themselves, and to reproduce the disorganizing behaviors they have suffered from. Disorganization may arise from stress, from mental disorders, or from unresolved trauma. Disorganization of attachment, i.e., the collapse of attachment strategies within the child, appears to be the highest mental health risk factor in pregnancy, and therefore the main target for intervention and prevention.

Attachment is a strategy to cope with stress, and not a feature of pathology, as several strategies may be developed by children, i.e. secure, resistant or avoidant, depending on the different styles of caregiving the child has been exposed to.

16.4 Psychopathology in pregnancy

Pregnancy and the year after giving birth are a time when a woman is most at risk of increased mental symptomatology, increased vulnerability of triggering of a latent susceptibility to mental disorders (above all affective disorders), or reactivation of an existing psychopathology (above all borderline personality disorders). Several factors may play a role in this diathesis process: relationships above all, with the key role of past relationships, particularly with mother; the role of the partner as support and the key role of intimate relationships within the couple; and social support in general. But also the role of past traumatic events, particularly if there was some physical/sexual abuse in the past, which may lead to a very difficult feeling of helplessness about labor and giving birth. The presence of trauma symptoms – such as dissociation, numbing and re-experiencing – has a negative effect on prenatal attachment; those symptoms have direct negative effects on the mother's reflective functioning, hampering the capacity of the mother to imagine the child and to imagine herself as a parent in a coherent way.

Finally, any event that has impact on the fetus or on the child has great impact on the mother's and father's mental balance: any structural anomaly seen on ultrasonography, or premature birth, particularly when a fetus was lost in a previous pregnancy or in stillbirth. The role of social and cultural support cannot be overstated: giving birth away from homeland, and away from the help of a mother, of women from the extended family or from the community who can help you after delivery, and give support and advice on how to take care of yourself and of the child may be a traumatic experience in itself, but it is a situation that has become more and more frequent. This situation is even more difficult when migration was decided for economic reasons, with low or no legal and financial support, and lesser access to care and help.

Depression has a large lifelong prevalence in women, and is no specific disease in pregnancy. However, prenatal depression and anxiety have been shown to have impact on the development of the child. Depression in pregnancy may be more intense and frequent than in post-partum. Two peaks of onset of postnatal depression (PND) are evident, at eight weeks and six months post-partum. Its prevalence makes it the most frequent medical complication of pregnancy and delivery (10–15%); it is therefore of utmost importance that PND be screened for during pregnancy and postnatally, in an adequate interview, using adequate screening tools (Edinburgh Postnatal Depression Scale). Post-partum blues (PPB, maternity blues) is sometimes classified into post-partum disorders, since severe post-partum blues overlap with PND. However, PPB appears to be quite different from an affective disorder: it is much more frequent (40–60%); frequency does not increase with pregnancies; it is transient and it has more variability than depression. One hypothesis could be that PPB could play a role in helping establishing the bond between the infant and mother. Post-partum psychosis has become much less frequent, probably because of early recognition and prevention, and is now much more linked with an onset of affective disorder than with the reactivation of an earlier psychotic state. Anxiety disorders generally increase during early pregnancy and decrease towards the end of it. But individual variations are large and the rule of thumb is that no general prognosis can be made, on caregiving abilities for mother's or on the effects of parental psychopathology on parent–infant relationships, only on the basis of mother's psychiatric diagnosis.

Denial of pregnancy appears to be much more frequent than thought before, its recognition being limited by the denial of partner, family and maternity staff. It is not linked with a single psychopathological or social profile, but is often seen in teen pregnancy. For adolescent mothers, pregnancy gets easily in conflict with the adolescent's personal agenda, which explains why the outcome of such pregnancies in terms of parental abilities of the young mother and fair development of the baby are highly dependent on family support.

16.5 Prevention and early intervention

Since pregnancy is such a time of increased psychic vulnerability, and such a time of acute and rapid changes, prevention becomes a key issue. Culture has provided women with a sort of cradle of care beliefs, habits and information, with the idea that the pregnant woman should be specially taken care of, with her urges and wishes met immediately ('I feel like eating cherries now, please go and get some'), with presence and help during labor (midwives, *Doulas*), with a period of presence of the grandmother in the house during a whole month to help start things with the baby. Culture has wisdom, since this In Between situation is a demanding one, when new parents have to make room for the child and to find the cues of its functioning and identity. But this mobilization of support and competences around the new mother is seldom found nowadays, with more and more young parents finding themselves alone. Reaching hard to reach people for a home-based preventive intervention becomes the goal.

A home-based experience of a secure relationship and working alliance may help new parents work through hard memories and increase their mentalizing abilities, allowing them to become sensible and resilient caregivers [10]. In that sense, we may help them fulfill their most important wishes, i.e. to give more to their children than they have received themselves [3]. CAPEDP is such a preventive intervention. It was designed following Slade's Minding the Baby program, with the goal of enhancing reflective functioning in high-risk mothers [6].

16.6 CAPEDP-Attachment: a French project to promote parental skills and decrease disorganized attachment

Developmental theories recognize that social and family environment have long-term effects on the psychological functioning of individuals. The development of good-quality early relationships allows infants to explore their environment safely and contribute to the establishment of a broader range of social skills. Moreover, infants are particularly sensitive to precarious contexts that generate significant stress in their families. The psychological suffering of parents (especially depression), and difficult social context can have a deleterious impact on their development.

Attachment is considered a vital component of social and emotional development in the early years, and individual differences in the quality of attachment relationships are believed to be important early indicators of infant mental health. The way a child learns to develop relationships is vital for her subsequent psychosocial relations, since the use of an attachment figure as a secure base allows her optimal development and her ability to explore the world. Many studies have shown that attachment quality influences the ability to manage situations of alarm or distress and the infant's subsequent mental health. Literature also suggests that the mother's attachment organization may be transmitted to the infant, specifically through the mean of her auto-reflexive skills and by sensitive or disrupting behaviour.

Intervention programs targeted on high-risk populations have been developed in North America and in other different contexts over the years 1960–70. The project CAPEDP (Compétences Parentales et Attachement dans la Petite Enfance: Diminution des risques liés aux troubles de santé mentale et promotion de la résilience –i.e. Parenting Skills and Attachment in Infants: Reducing Mental Health Risks and Promoting Resiliency) started in Paris in 2006. CAPEDP is a randomized research and action program to promote mental health of young infants, conducted by the infant department of the Hospital Bichat, and the Research Laboratory of the Hospital Maison-Blanche. The goal of the research project is to assess the effect of a preventive intervention in a group of young parents with psychosocial vulnerability, defined as being a first-time mother, being young, having a low level of education, living in poverty and feeling isolated.

The general project is CAPEDP. CAPEDP-A (for Attachment) is the ancillary study in a subsample of CAPEDP, with closer and specific measures of child disorganization and attachment quality and of parental disorganizing behaviour and mentalizing abilities. For this, we compare the effect of the preventive intervention at home in an intervention and a control group.

To achieve this aim a subsample of 120 mother–infant dyads was selected from the intervention and control randomized groups of CAPEDP general (60 of 220 of each CAPEDP group). When they are 12 months old, infants' attachment is assessed with the Strange Situation Paradigm [11] (ABCD) in our laboratory and later, at infants' 18 months, the Waters' Attachment Q sort [12] is used to assess attachment quality at home. The maternal disrupting behaviors are assessed by the AMBIANCE scale [13]. Finally, the parental reflexive capacity is assessed by the Insightfulness Assessment Interview [14].

Regarding the intervention program, we provide specific training and supervision to the intervention psychologists on the use of home video feedback for the promotion of maternal sensitivity, promotion of maternal mentalizing skills, prevention, detection and reduction of maternal atypical behaviour and infants' disorganized attachment. This type of approach is relatively recent in this kind of program. By using the video the parent is his own model of intervention. This is an opportunity to focus on the baby's signals and expressions, while stimulating the mother's observation skills and her empathy with her child. It also enables positive reinforcement moments of sensitive behaviour that the parent evidences on the video. The success of the videoscopy strategy is based on it occurring within a supportive relationship that continually recognizes the individuals' and the family's strengths, and recognizing the broader context to which they belong.

A pamphlet entitled 'Infants' Emotional Development' is also used by the intervention psychologists, aiming to give knowledge to the parents on babies' and infants' emotional life. The French pamphlet was developed as part of this research and is based on the results of recent attachment longitudinal studies. Our aim is that the mothers work through it with the psychologists and then read it and reread it when a problem in this area arises or when they are in doubt, as a tool to help them to face the challenge of raising their first child.

In conclusion, even though our data collection is still in progress, CAPEDP hopes to offer new perspectives on preventive mental health, as well as the opportunity to develop specific training on the work involving projects of early mental health promotion. CAPEDP-Attachment, by clarifying our understanding of the mechanisms implied in the secure attachment strategies and in the disorganization of attachment and caregiving, intends to contribute in a significant way to refine parent–infant's early preventive intervention in contexts of psychosocial vulnerability.

Of course other approaches are possible. Becoming a parent is never simple, requiring that a lot of childhood issues be solved. A lot of information and support are also needed. Nowadays, in developed countries, young parents are less and less helped into this transition by an extended family network and by effective social and cultural support. Prevention of maladaptive transition to parenthood therefore has become a major goal. However, the key issue seems to be able to detect who is in need in this period of great changes, even though some of the women may not ask openly for help, because of their prior experience of deception, trauma and sometimes abuse. The general goal of enhancing mentalization is difficult to reach because of these frequent antecedents, and this population has a high level of drop-outs, particularly in great cities. More work is needed to assess the effectiveness and the efficiency of prevention in mental health within the high-risk groups.

16.7 References

1. Winnicott, D.W. (1956) Primary maternal preoccupation, In *Through Pediatrics to Psychoanalysis*. Basic Books, New York, pp. 300–5.
2. Cowan, C. and Cowan, P. (1995) Interventions to ease the transition to parenthood. *Family Relations*, **44** (4), October, 412.
3. Fraiberg, S (1980) *Clinical Studies in Infant Mental Health: the First Year of Life*. Tavistock Publications, London.
4. Feldman, R., Weller, A., Sharon-Zagoory, O. and Levine, A. (2007) Evidence for a neuroendocrinological foundation of human affiliation. *Psychological Science*, **18** (11), 965–970.

5. Bibring, G., Dwyer, T.F., Huntington, D.C. and Valenstein, A.F. (1961) A study of the psychological processes in pregnancy and the earliest mother-child relationship. *Psychoanalytic Study of the Child*, **16**, 9–44.

6. Slade, A., Sadler, L.S. and Mayes, L. (2005) Minding the baby: enhancing parental reflective functioning in a nursing/mental home visiting program. In *Enhancing Early Attachments* (eds. L. Berlin, Y. Ziv, L. Amaya-Jackson and M. Greeberg), Guilford Publications, New York.

7. Trad, P.V. (1990) On becoming a mother: in the throes of developmental transformations. *Psychoanalytic Psychology*, **7**, 341–61.

8. Stern, D.N. (1995) *The Motherhood Constellation*. HarperCollins, New York.

9. Tronick, E. (2007) *The Neurobehavioral and Social-Emotional Development of Infants and Children*. WW Norton & Co., New York.

10. Olds, D., Sadler, L.S. and Kitzman, H. (2007) Programs for parents of infants and toddlers: recent evidence from randomized trials. *Journal of Child Psychology and Psychiatry*, **48**, 355–91.

11. Ainsworth, M., Blehar, M., Waters, E. and Wall, S. (1978) *Patterns of Attachment: A Psychological Study of the Strange Situation*. Lawrence Erlbaum, Hillsdale.

12. Waters, E. (1987) Attachment Q-set (Version 3). Retrieved (2008) from http://www.johnbowlby.com.

13. Lyons Ruth, K., Bronfman, E. and Atwood, G. (1999) A relational diathesis model of hostile-helpless states of mind. In *Attachment Disorganisation* (eds. J. Solomon and C. George), Guildford Press, New York, 33–69.

14. Koren-Karie, N. and Oppenheim, D. (2004) The Insightfulness Assessment Coding Manual (1.1). Unpublished manuscript. University of Haifa, Israel.

17

Role of parenting in the development of the infant's interpersonal abilities

Deborah Weatherston[1] and Hiram E. Fitzgerald[2]

[1]Michigan Association for Infant Mental Health, USA
[2]Michigan State University, USA

A child learns to love through his first human partners, his parents. We can look upon this miraculous occurrence as a gift of love to the baby. We should also regard it as a right, a birthright for every child. S. Fraiberg [1]

17.1 Introduction

The promotion of healthy development requires attention to relationships between mothers and infants, fathers and infants, within families and with practitioners. Development occurs within the context of early caregiving relationships. These relationships, most optimally with parents who provide primary care, shape who the baby is and will become, and provide a sense of emotional security and trust that promotes self-confidence and self-worth. These relationships mediate a young child's capacity to enter into warm and positive social relationships with others from infancy through adulthood.

Although the importance of parenting has been common knowledge for thousands of years, modern developmental sciences have drilled down to determine exactly how parenting practices affect child behavior in an effort to determine how best to maximize positive developmental outcomes for all children. Parental advice such as 'Spare the rod and spoil

Parenthood and Mental Health: A Bridge between Infant and Adult Psychiatry   Sam Tyano, Miri Keren, Helen Herrman and John Cox
© 2010 John Wiley & Sons, Ltd

the child', with its origins in antiquity, speaks to the importance of discipline, although modern knowledge of disciplinary practices replace the rod with more nurturing and constructive approaches.

How a parent responds to the infant, beginning in the first postnatal months, shapes the nature of the parent–child relationship and affects the infant's social and emotional development. This relationship provides a context for the infant's development and change, awareness of self and other, and capacity for empathy, all skills that are crucial for social and emotional health. Moreover, the parent–infant relationship evolves within the context of a family system (Figure 17.1) which regulates the dynamics of a set of complex relationships that influence family organization and cohesion. The system's complexity and organizational structure is also affected by a wide range of factors external to the family.

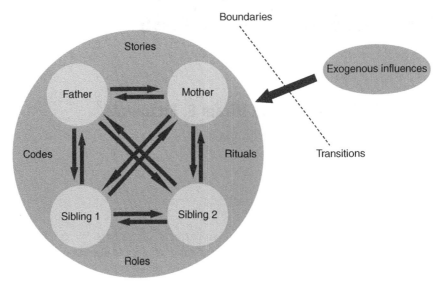

Figure 17.1   Transactions within a family system and influences from external systems
Source: Adapted from Loukas, A., Twitchell, G.R., Piejak, L.A. *et al.* (1998) The family as a unity of interacting personalities, in *Family Psychopathology: The Relational Roots of Dysfunctional Behavior* (ed. L. L'Abate), Guilford, New York, pp. 35–59. With permission

Our understanding of the parent–infant relationship and the relationships inherent in complex family systems has emerged from a variety of transformative theoretical contributions and research findings primarily from the twentieth century. Prior to the twentieth century there was no common concept of childhood or sense that the prenatal to postnatal periods of infancy and toddlerhood were particularly important in human development beyond survival. The transformative changes in knowledge about human development in general, and the earliest years in particular, occurred when the study of early development shifted to systematic and interdisciplinary inquiry and when knowledge of organizing competencies of the human infant were demonstrated.

The contemporary aspect of this work highlights the importance of parenting practices for the development of relational skills, self-regulation, and mental representations of the world as they emerge from the co-constructive processes that influence the organization of internal models of self and others. Of specific interest is the quality of parent–child relationships that contribute to individual differences in early development, particularly as such differences help to shape positive and negative developmental pathways across the life span.

A key tenet advanced in this chapter is that the quality of parent–child interaction is critical to the organization of children's relationship skills and their overall mental health. We focus on contemporary understanding of the importance of the parent (mother)–infant relationship for structuring the infant's capacity to relate to others as informed by:

1 The theoretical transformations of the twentieth century that gave definition to the concept of development [2];

2 The empirical verifications of the infant's active role in constructing the meaning of experience; and

3 The deeper understandings of the mental structures that shape what the infant learns to expect from others and how to regulate dynamic interactions and interpersonal relationships.

17.2 Transformative theoretical concepts of human relationships

Many contemporary theorists, researchers and clinical practitioners draw attention to the importance of infancy and early relationship experiences to health and growth throughout the life span. Their perspectives have been shaped by changes in our understanding of the importance of early human development in five core domains:

1 The centrality of the mother–infant relationship;

2 The cognitive context of early experience;

3 The socio-emotional context of early experience;

4 The organization of behavior from a systems perspective; and

5 The co-constructive nature of the infant's working models of social relationships.

What follows is a discussion of these as they relate to social and emotional development in the first years of life.

Centrality of the mother–infant relationship

Psychoanalytic theory was the first systematic attempt to frame the centrality of the mother–child relationship and to link it to interpersonal dynamics across the life span [3]. Freud described that relationship as: 'unique, without parallel, established unalterably for a whole lifetime, as the first and strongest love object and as the prototype of all later love relationships' (p. 188).

Freud's thoughtfulness about mothers and early relationship experiences led to other fundamental and influential ideas:

1 An emotional attachment, established in infancy, influences a person throughout the life span;

2 Inadequate early care may lead to emotional and relational conflicts at each stage of life; and

3 To the extent that the first relationship in the baby's first year is satisfying and need-fulfilling, the baby will be more likely to establish a healthy sense of self.

Anna Freud played a vital role in extending classical psychoanalytic thinking to include normality and pathology in early childhood [4]. Her elegant descriptions of developmental lines and defensive structures provided a way to understand achievements and failures from infancy through adolescence. From her perspective, early development is fueled by the quality of the mother's attention, responsiveness and the ability to provide appropriate care. Individual profiles of risk and normality are influenced by the mother's provision of care.

Erik Erikson provided a framework that evolved from an emphasis on psychological structures, early experiences, relationships and drives. Erikson took into account the infant and young child's development within a broad, social context, linking a young child's feelings and experiences with external realities [5]. Erikson proposed that the child's identify is established within the context of the developing parent–child relationship, the relationship to the family, and the relationship to the larger social world. Adaptive and interactive, the infant matures within these relationships. Trust, autonomy and initiative emerge within the context of relationship experiences in the early years.

The cognitive context of early experience

In the early part of the twentieth century, Jean Piaget published the first of numerous books that offered a structural alternative to the then dominant positivist view of human developmental [6, 7]. When working with Alfred Binet in Paris, Piaget became fascinated with children's reasoning, rather than their actual answers to questions on the Binet intelligence test. His book on the child's conception of experience [6], though relatively unknown to US developmental and cognitive psychologists until the 1960s, helped to transform Western theoretical perspectives on the role that the infants and young children play in constructing knowledge from experience. Piaget believed that cognitive development was organized in major developmental periods. He proposed that two functional invariant processes, assimilation and accommodation, guided the transformation of cognitive schemas (mental representations of events) through various organizing stages within major re-organized periods of development (sensori-motor, pre-operational, concrete operations) during infancy and childhood. Events consistent with existing schemas were assimilated into that schema, adding depth, but not provoking systemic change. Events inconsistent with existing schemas forced an accommodation, a systemic change in the organizational structure transforming it into something not reducible to its prior level of organization.

Piaget understood cognitive growth as increasingly organized, complex and differentiated. The infant was viewed as an active and interactive being who learns about the world by engaging it and internalizing knowledge models that would move from simple expectancies in infancy to logical propositional thought in adolescence. The very young child learns through continuous interaction and experience, gradually constructing an understanding of the world and establishing a sense of self as separate from objects. The infant's knowledge of others transforms from 'out of sight, out of mind' to understanding that others exist even when they are not immediately present. This transformational event reflects internalized knowledge, or a mental representation, that the others exist and are (or are not) available when needed or desired. It is as if the toddler knows that 'if I cry, she will come because I *know* that she is there'. Thus, Piaget's significant contribution to understanding the importance of the parent–child relationship is his demonstration that representational models of experience are constructed during the earliest years of life, including models of socio-emotional relationships. Somewhat simultaneously, developmental psychoanalytic researchers were discovering similar processes within the socio-emotional domain.

The socio-emotional context of experience

Perhaps inspired by the Freudian hypothesis that inadequate care may lead to developmental challenges for infants and young children, psychoanalytic researchers began to examine the impact of non-home rearing environments on early development [8, 9]. These classic studies demonstrated the negative impact of poor-quality, institutional care on infant development and led to systematic studies contrasting infants reared in institutional settings and infants reared at home [10]. Sally Provence and Rose Lipton concentrated on a broad range of outcomes related to institutional care, assessing infants' capacities to move about, communicate, interact with others, and establish close and affectionate ties. Infants who were well held and cared for by their mothers in their own homes learned that their needs would be met and developed trusting relationships that grew more complex as each month passed. They were playful and showed pleasure in people and toys. On the other hand, infants who were raised in institutions and deprived of adequate nurturing in the first year appeared delayed in motor development, were less able to communicate their wants and needs, had a diminished interest in people or playthings and were unable to seek out the attention of adults for comfort when distressed. Clearly, infants in these two contexts developed qualitatively different mental representations or internal working models of socio-emotional relationships.

Donald Winnicott was among the earliest investigators to note the importance of tactile comfort for promoting the infant's emotional health and growth [11, 12]. Winnicott focused on the role of the parent, the nurturing other, who holds and feeds the baby, responds sensitively and contingently to the infant's wants and needs, soothes the baby's distress, and interacts with warmth and affection. It is this care that assures the baby's underlying sense of security within the first year of life. In the process of providing and receiving care, the infant and parent awaken emotionally to the other and develop a healthy relationship over the course of the first year of life. It is this relationship that provides a foundation for the baby's sense of self and worth. Winnicott's commitment to the importance of holding provides a window into the attachment process and informs us about the important transactions between parent and infant that contribute to the infant's emergent security of attachment [13].

Systems and the organization of behavior

While psychoanalysts, child psychiatrists and child developmentalists were advancing new understandings of the infant's competencies and of the importance of the parent–infant relationship, other scientists were challenging the prevailing paradigms about the nature of human nature. Ludvig von Bertalanffy's [14] general systems theory challenged the dominant positivist philosophy of science of his day. Von Bertalanffy's view of systems was motivated by the paradox between order, organization and maintenance, within the context of continuous change, goal-seeking, and the apparent purposefulness of behavior [15].

General systems theory paved the way for understanding developmental processes as hierarchically organized, self-maintaining, dynamic, emergent and open. The infant who knows that 'out of sight is not out of mind' reacts emotionally to maternal separations and introduces new regulatory aspects to the emerging mother–infant relationship. Parent and infant now have to negotiate or accommodate to a changing relationship, one that has as much impact on the infant's socio-emotional development as it does on the parent's socio-emotional reactions to an infant who is no longer perceived to be passive. Each member of the dyad (or triad) has been transformed and it is the quality of that transformation that now shapes new expectancies about the nature of the relationship.

Within the framework of general systems theory, Sameroff and Chandler [16] developed a transactional model that anchored early infant development in a relational framework. From their perspective, the baby's development is intimately linked to experiences within the caregiving environment. Interactions with parents and other caregivers shape the infant's emerging identity, but simultaneously shape the parent's caregiving behaviors, thoughts and feelings about the baby and early parenthood. Sameroff's transactional model is dynamic and underscores the importance of working with the infant and parent(s) together as they co-construct their relationship and their separate but synergistically organizing identities of self and other.

Sameroff and Emde [17] framed the importance of relationships within the transactional model, beginning with the infant's first relationship experiences, and the devastating consequences of disturbed or disordered relationship patterns. Developmental and clinical practitioners were advised to keep the relationship at the center of their work to promote social or emotional well-being and reduce the risk of relationship failure for parent and child. The transactional model takes into account the social and cultural context in which infant and parent interact. The developing parent–infant relationship has an impact on and is affected by experiences within the larger family and community (see Figure 17.1).

The co-construction of the infant's working model of socio-emotional relationships

Perhaps the seminal theoretical contribution to contemporary study of early socio-emotional development was John Bowlby's theory of attachment [18]. Bowlby integrated concepts from psychoanalyic theory, control systems theory, cognitive developmental theory and ethological theory and launched a broad-based interdisciplinary scientific investigation of the factors that influence the organization of the infant's relationship skills embodied within the attachment framework. Survival of the human infant depended on being in close proximity to a nurturing and responsive caregiver. Bowlby examined specific care-seeking and caregiving behaviors that assured the baby's proximity to the caregiving adult when the baby was frightened or under certain stress. These behaviors led him to acknowledge the significance of early relationships to development, as well as the importance of separation and loss to security of attachment across the life span [18, 19, 20]. Attachment theory anchors us in understanding the significance of caregiving behaviors as they promote a young child's social and emotional health.

Bowlby took a careful look at the infant within a relational context. He emphasized the importance of the infant's signals as well as the importance of the caregiver's response. The baby, an active participant in the developing relationship, elicits attention from his caregiver by looking, smiling, crying, cooing and clinging. In turn, the caregiver responds to the baby's signals. She (his early observations were of the mother) looks, smiles, talks, moves a little closer and picks the baby up. The baby learns to trust that his needs will be responded to reliably and predictably. The baby grows increasingly safe within that relationship. Later infant behaviors, for example, crawling, walking, talking and following, assure that the baby is able to keep the caregiver in view when he needs her and as he seeks out interesting playthings and activities. Each is a partner in the creation of a safe and secure relationship that the baby can use and return to when frightened, sick or under stress. It is an attachment that is specific and fuels the baby's sense of trust in the caregiving environment as well as his self-confidence and security. Bowlby called this a working model of relationship that shapes the individual's expectancies about relationships throughout the life span [21]. Mental models or schemas incorporate expectancies about events, trigger decision processes, and affect the way that we process information, accommodate to novel events, and reconstruct (change) familiar events (see Figure 17.2).

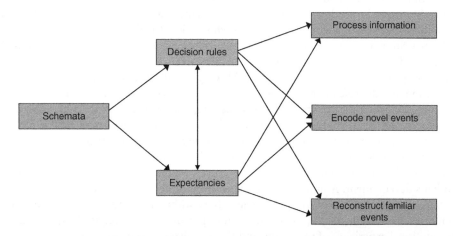

Figure 17.2 The relationship between mental representations (schemas, working models) and the formation of expectancies and decision processes that impact how we perceive information, process it, and reconstruct memory of events. These processes are thought to contribute to the organization of autobiographical memory, intersubjectivity, identity, a sense of self, and are hypothesized to have impacts on the organization of behavior over the life span

The nature of the attachment relationship has powerful implications for the infant's development and developing interest in the larger social world. Secure in the emotional relationship with his primary caregiver, his safe base, the infant reaches away with curiosity and returns to the caregiver for comfort and support as needed. By contrast, the infant who is insecure is less certain about his safe haven. Hesitant or fearful, he appears less able to explore his environment or to seek out new experiences with people or playthings.

Whereas Bowlby articulated an integrated, powerful species-level theory about the importance of the mother–infant relationship for the development of interpersonal competencies, Mary Ainsworth examined individual differences in the nature of the young child's tie to his or her mother [22]. Her research method, the Strange Situation, is regarded by some as the gold standard for measuring the quality of the infant's attachment relationship. The procedure involves a sequence of parent present, parent absent, and stranger present, stranger absent, with observers rating the infant's reactions to the sequenced separations and reunions with mother (or father).

Ainsworth and her colleagues identified two major classifications of attachment in infancy: secure and anxious, the latter category subdivided as avoidant or resistant. Infants identified as secure are curious, responsive, able to seek, and to use comfort when distressed. Infants described as resistant were identified as uncertain in the parent's presence, very distressed during parent absence, and unable to be comforted upon the parent's return to the room after a brief separation. Infants described as avoidant were described as somewhat playful, unsmiling, ignoring of the parent when the parent returned, and unable to seek comfort or use the relationship when the parent returned.

Studies of the antecedents of the attachment classification focused on maternal sensitivity and responsivity to the infant's signals and were related to the infant's attachment classification at 12 months of age [23]. Mothers who are described as sensitive, accepting, cooperative, consistent, available and skillful in providing infant care tend to have babies who are rated as secure. Mothers who are described as less sensitive to the infant's cries and cues, inconsistent, unavailable and rejecting tend to have babies who are identified as insecure [24].

Daniel Stern has provided significant contributions to the understanding of both infancy and early motherhood. Throughout his career, Stern has focused on the early relationship between parent and infant [25], emphasizing the importance of reciprocal interaction and the role of emotion in organizing early experiences, affective monitoring, the core self and interpersonal relationships [26]. Stern-Bruschweiler and Stern [27] introduced the term 'motherhood constellation' to describe challenges that a mother faces in adapting to the care of her new baby. It is within the new caregiving context that a woman begins to alter her identity as a mother. Like Winnicott, Stern-Bruschweiler and Stern consider holding and handling to be crucial aspects of both the infant's and the mother's development. A mother recalls experiences of her own early care while holding, feeding, diapering or comforting her baby. It is within this present context that old memories are stirred [28, 29]. This offers an opportunity for thoughtful exploration of the emotional experience of caregiving and the meaning of the infant's care.

The new parent's internal working model of relationship, developed from her own experiences of early care, affects the ways in which she is now able to care for her own child [30]. The parent's adjustment will be influenced by her own relationship history. Who took care of her? How available, consistent and responsive was her caregiver? What was the nature of that relationship and how enduring is the tie? What happened to the new parent in her early years now influences the care she gives to her baby. We see in this newly developing relationship remains of the old parent–child relationship [31]. It is this internal model of relationship or template that shapes the new parent's care of the baby and adjustment to her new mothering role. Recent evidence from five major longitudinal studies affirms that parents tend to rear their children in much the same way that they were reared, particularly when the parent's own rearing was harsh [32]. Clearly, working models or schemas can be powerful regulators of parenting behavior.

Early mothering memories are particularly vivid and accessible to the new mother in the first months of her baby's life [33]. They may be made more concrete through a clinical interview or therapy experience, enabling a new mother to recall experiences in which she was well cared for, as well as experiences which she remembers as painful or difficult. Given the opportunity to have thoughts and feelings about her own early care in the presence of her infant, a new mother may deepen her understanding of the daughter she was and the mother who took care of her, to become the mother she wants to be. Daniel Stern's expansion of the concept of this present remembering context is a powerful catalyst for transformation and change in the early developing relationship between parent and child [29, 34]. His work helps to integrate what we understand about attachment in infancy and the importance of maternal sensitivity and responsivity [35] with the adult's representations of attachment [36], caregiving history [31] and parenting role.

Consider for a moment the qualities of the caregiving relationship that are so critical for an infant's development. Attachment theorists and researchers believe that consistency of care, parental sensitivity, responsiveness and emotional availability are fundamental for healthy relationship development and for optimal developmental outcomes. It is the quality of interaction between parent and infant that leads to relationship-building. Parent and infant jointly determine the quality of their relationship which as early as 12 months can be characterized as secure, insecure or disorganized.

For many parents, good-enough caregiving qualities are intuitive [37]. They bring the baby home from the hospital and establish a routine fairly easily. They notice when their babies are hungry or uncomfortable, tired or upset. They quickly learn their baby's cues and respond appropriately to their baby's needs. They are predictable in the care they provide. All of these behaviors reinforce the infant's trust in the caregiving environment as well as the parent's feelings of competence and self-worth. What about the baby? What do infants contribute to the interaction and the relationship? Infants, small and dependent on the parent for protection and basic care, especially in the first months, are powerful contributors. They arrive with the capacity to look and listen, follow faces and respond to sounds. They cry out when hungry or wet or uncomfortable; they quiet when picked up or spoken to; they settle when held, wrapped securely and fed. In later months, they laugh and vocalize, respond with enthusiasm, imitate, initiate, protest, creep and follow. They engage parents and primary caregivers in a loving relationship that is described most optimally as safe and secure. Or, when these elements are not present, the relationship organizes in insecurity, doubt and distress, characteristics that negatively impact the expectancy matrix (Figure 17.2).

From this perspective, the infant is a partner in the relationship, a partner who reinforces his mother's caretaking and response. The baby quiets when she looks and holds and rocks him. The baby smiles when she talks to him. The baby molds against her when she picks him up to comfort him. She slowly learns what he wants or needs and understands her importance to him. Microanalytic studies and the use of videotaped sequences of interaction have reinforced understanding of the many ways in which babies influence the parent's ability to provide affectionate and sensitive responses [38]. Within the context of relationship, mother and baby learn to regulate their interactions with one another and discover their new and separate roles. This reciprocity and adaptive regulation is particularly important for infants with difficult temperaments or other challenges, for parents with presenting state characteristics such as depression or antisocial personality disorder, or for families struggling with poverty, disease or exposure to violence [39, 40, 41].

Clearly, parents and infants are partners in the construction of enduring relationships [42]. What they establish in the first year promotes confidence and competence in following years. What they set in motion promotes capacity for emotion regulation, positive interactions and healthy relationships with others when the child enters school.

Equally important, the parent–infant relationship is the foundation for constructing the very young children's autobiographical memory of the events of early experience [39, 43]. Mother and infant co-construct and rehearse event memories that give depth to the infant's representational models of others and of self–other relationships. As infants come to understand that their intentions, feelings and thoughts can be understood by others, they too come to understand that they can embrace the intentions, feelings and thoughts of their caregivers. Moreover, mothers who elaborate their stories and challenge their toddlers with high rates of memory questions tend to have toddlers who have richer autobiographical memories [44]. Toddlers who were developmentally more advanced in self-recognition also tended to have richer autobiographical memories of shared events.

Self-representation is related to autobiographical memory, representational models of attachment, and other internalizations that require a sense that 'I know that I know'. It is directly connected to parent–child interactions evoking construction of shared meaning, both in the sense of who I am ('What a smart, cute little boy you are', versus, 'You dumb, mean boy, you are just like your stupid father!'), and how I relate to the world ('You had a really fun time at the zoo today, didn't you?'). This intersubjectivity [26, 45, 46] is a co-constructed process, aided early on by the quality of the mother's mind-mindedness, or the extent to which she vocalizes and/or physically expresses what she perceives to be the infant's internal emotional state. It is also aided by the extent to which the mother rehearses the infant's memory store of events and constructs a sense of shared meaning of those events.

17.3 Infant mental health service structure

What might account for a parent's inability to provide a warm and nurturing relationship in which the infant can grow? The reasons vary. The parent might be alone, isolated from family and friends, without resources to provide for a baby. The parent might be unprepared and inexperienced, adolescent by age or behavior. The parent might have a significant history of trauma or loss, making it difficult to enter into a loving relationship with an infant. The pregnancy might have been problematic. The labor and delivery might have been complicated. The baby might be difficult or unrewarding to care for. These are risks that we take seriously in the service community, offering early developmental support and clinical treatment for the parent and infant together with the relationship as the focus of the therapeutic work and the therapeutic relationship as the instrument for change [47].

What do infant mental health services offer? They assure a commitment to the emotional health of infants and parents as they develop in relationship to one another in the first years of life. Primary therapeutic tasks include:

- The careful observation of an infant or toddler in interaction with a parent;

- The exploration of feelings that threaten appropriate and affectionate parental response;

- Questioning that offers a parent the opportunity to wonder, reflect, recall and understand reactions;

- Supportive listening;

- The clarification of thoughts and feelings a parent has about the infant; and

- Empathic response.

The underlying therapeutic goal is to create a context in which a parent is able to explore the emotional connections between past and present experiences or relationships and to build a relationship with their infant or toddler that is free from chronic ambivalence, pain, sorrow, anger or distress. Crucial to the approach is the presence of both the infant and the parent. Of equal importance is the therapist's attention and response to emotion as expressed either non-verbally in the interaction between parent and infant or in words. Believing that the developing relationship between parent and child is affected and shaped by both present realities and past experiences, the infant mental health therapist is a careful observer in the moment and a thoughtful listener to the parent's dialogue. The infant–parent therapist uses what is seen and heard to assist parents in recovering and understanding thoughts about caregiving as well as feelings for the infant or toddler in their care. It is an intervention that keeps the infant and parent in mind, offering opportunity for the parent to explore what is going well and what is making the care of the baby difficult. It is an effort to reduce the risk of early relationship failure, better assuring the promotion of healthy social and emotional development between parent and child [31, 48]. To the extent that an infant mental health practitioner is able to understand, support and sustain parents in interacting and responding sensitively to their infants' or toddlers' emotional needs, a significant goal will have been reached.

17.4 Summary

In summary, one cannot overlook the importance of early parental care to nurture and support a baby's social and emotional well-being. Attention to the dynamics of parent–child interaction is crucial. Support for the relationship needs of parents and infants in the first year of life better assures the parent's ability to respond sensitively and appropriately to the infant, affecting the developmental trajectory of the infant across the life span.

During the first 18 months of life a child constructs a lasting internal vision of what human relationships are, how they work, what to expect from them, and what to offer in return. What gets set in early life is one's deepest beliefs about human relationships. These determine how a person goes about learning, profiting from experience, using help, and parenting one's own children quoted by W. Schafer [49].

17.5 References

1. Fraiberg, S. (1977) *Every Child's Birthright: In Defense of Mothering.* Basic Books, New York.
2. Harris, D.B. (1957) *The Concept of Development.* University of Minnesota Press, Minneapolis, MN.
3. Freud, S. (1940/64) An outline of psycho-analysis, in *The Standard Edition of the Complete Psychological Works of Sigmund Freud,* **23** (ed. and trans. J. Strachey), Hogarth Press, London.

4. Freud, A. (1965) *Normality and Pathology in Childhood: Assessments of Development.* International Universities Press, Madison, WI.

5. Erikson, E. (1950) *Childhood and Society.* Norton & Co., New York.

6. Piaget, J. (1928) *The Child's Conception of the World.* Routledge & Kegan Paul, London.

7. Piaget, J. (1952) *The Origins of Intelligence in Children.* International University Press, New York.

8. Goldfarb, W. (1945) Effects of psychological privation in infancy and subsequent development. *American Journal of Psychiatry*, **102**, 18–33.

9. Spitz, R. and Wolf, K.M. (1946) Anaclitic depression: an inquiry into the genesis of psychiatric conditions in early childhood. *Psychoanalytic Study of the Child*, **2**.

10. Provence, S. and Lipton, R. (1962) *Infants in Institutions.* International Universities Press, New York.

11. Winnicott, D. (1965a) *The Family and Individual Development.* Basic Books, New York.

12. Phillips, A. (1988) *Winnicott.* Harvard University Press, Cambridge, MA.

13. Winnicott, D. (1965b) *The Maturational Processes and the Facilitating Environment.* International Universities Press, Madison, WI.

14. von Bertalanffy, L. von (1928/62) *Kritische Theorie der Formbildung (Modern Theories of Development).* Harper Torchbooks, New York.

15. von Bertalanffy, L. von (1950) The theory of open systems in physics and biology. *Science*, **3**, 23–29.

16. Sameroff, A.J. and Chandler, M.J. (1975) Reproductive risk and the continuum of caretaking casualty, in *Review of Child Development Research*, **4** (eds F.D. Horowitz, M. Hetherington, S. Scarr-Salapatek and G. Siegel), University of Chicago Press, Chicago, pp. 187–244.

17. Sameroff, A.J. and Emde, R. (1989) *Relationship Disturbances in Early Childhood: A Developmental Approach.* Basic Books, New York.

18. Bowlby, J (1969) *Attachment. Attachment and Loss*, Vol. **1**, Basic Books, New York.

19. Bowlby, J (1973) *Separation: Anxiety and Anger. Attachment and Loss*, Vol. **2**, Basic Books, New York.

20. Bowlby, J (1980) *Loss: Sadness and Depression. Attachment and Loss*, Vol. **3**, Basic Books, New York.

21. Bowlby, J (l979) *Bowlby: The Making and Breaking of Affectional Bonds*, Tavistock, New York.

22. Ainsworth, M. (1973) The development of infant-mother attachment, in *Review of Child Development Research*, Vol. 3 (eds B. Caldwell and H. Ricciuti), University of Chicago Press, Chicago, pp. 1–94.

23. Bretherton, I (1985) Attachment theory: retrospect and prospect, in *Growing Points of Attachment Theory and Research. Monographs of the Society for Research in Child Development*, **50** (eds I. Bretherton and E. Waters), 3–35.

24. Egeland, B. and Farber, E. (1984) Infant-mother attachment: factors related to its development and changes over time. *Child Development*, **55**, 753–71.

25. Stern, D. (1977) *The First Relationship: Infant and Mother.* Harvard University Press, Cambridge, MA.

26. Stern, D. (1985) *The Interpersonal World of the Infant: A View from Psychoanalysis and Developmental Psychology.* Basic Books, New York.

27. Stern-Bruschweiler, N. and Stern, D. (1989) A model for conceptualizing the role of the mother's representational world in various mother-infant therapies. *Infant Mental Health Journal*, **10**, 142–56.

28. Fraiberg, S. and Adelson, E. (1977) An abandoned mother, an abandoned baby. *Bulletin Menninger Clinic*, **41**, 162–180.

29. Stern, D. (1995) *The Motherhood Constellation: A Unified View of Parent-Infant Psychotherapy*. Basic Books, New York.

30. Fonagy, P., Steele, H. and Steele, M. (1991) Maternal representations of attachment during pregnancy predict the organization of infant-mother attachment at one year of age. *Child Development*, **62**, 891–905.

31. Fraiberg, S. (ed.) (1980) *Clinical Studies in Infant Mental Health*. Basic Books, New York.

32. Conger, R.D., Belsky, J. and Capaldi, D.M. (2009) The intergenerational transmission of parenting: closing comments for the special section. *Developmental Psychology*, **45**, 1276–83.

33. Lieberman, A. and Pawl, J. (1993) Infant-parent psychotherapy, in *Handbook of Infant Mental Health* (ed. C. Zeanah, Jr), Guilford Press, New York.

34. Stern, D. (2004) *The Present Moment in Psychotherapy and Everyday Life*. W.W. Norton, New York.

35. Ainsworth, M., Blehar, M., Waters, E. and Wall, S. (1978) *Patterns of Attachment: A Psychological Study of the Strange Situation*. Erlbaum, Hillsdale, NJ.

36. Main, M (1995) Attachment: overview, with implications for clinical work, in *Attachment Theory: Social, Developmental, and Clinical Perspectives* (eds S. Goldberg, R. Muir and J. Kerr), Analytic Press, Hillsdale, NJ, pp. 407–74.

37. Papousek, M (in press) Resilience, strengths and regulatory capacities: hidden resources in developmental disorders of infant mental health. *Infant Mental Health Journal*.

38. McDonough, S.C. (2004) Interaction guidance: promoting and nurturing the caregiving relationship, in *Treating Parent-Infant Relationship Problems* (eds A.J. Sameroff, S.C. McDonough and K. Rosenblum), Guilford Press, New York. pp. 79–96.

39. Conway, M.A. and Pleydell-Pearce, C (2000) The construction of autobiographical memories in the self-memory system. *Psychological Review*, **107**, 261–88.

40. Fitzgerald, H.E. and Zucker, R.A. (2006) Pathways of risk aggregation for alcohol use disorders, in *The Crisis in Youth Mental Health: Issues for Families, Schools and Communities* (eds H.E Fitzgerald and R.A. Zucker), Praeger Press, Westport, CT, pp. 249–72.

41. Osofsky, J.D. (2002) The effects of exposure to violence on infants, in *Infant Development: Ecological Perspectives* (eds H.E. Fitzgerald, K. Karraker and T. Luster), Routledge/Falmer, New York, pp. 253–72.

42. Emde, R. (1989) The infant's relationship experience: developmental and clinical aspects, in *Relationship Disturbances in Early Childhood* (eds A.J. Sameroff and R.N. Emde), Basic Books, New York, pp. 33–51.

43. Howe, M.L. and Courage, M.L. (1997) The emergence and early development of autobiographical memory. *Psychological Review*, **104**, 499–523.

44. Harley, K. and Reese, E. (1999) Origins of autobiographical memory. *Developmental Psychology*, **35**, 1338–48.

45. Trevarthen, C. (1980) The foundations of intersubjectivity: development of interpersonal and cooperative understanding in infants, in *The Social Foundations of Language and Thought* (ed. D. Olson), W.W. Norton & Co., New York.

46. Trevarthen, C. (1993) The self born in intersubjectivity: the psychology of an infant communicating, in *The Perceived Self* (ed. U. Neisser), Cambridge University Press.
47. Weatherston, D. (2000) The infant mental health specialist. *Zero to Three*, **21** (2), 3–10.
48. Weatherston, D. and Tableman, B. (2002) *Infant Mental Health Services: Supporting Competencies/Reducing Risks*. Michigan Association for Infant Mental Health, Southgate, MI.
49. Schafer, W, (1991) Root causes of juvenile delinquency. *The Infant Crier*, **55**, p. 2.

18

Welcoming a stranger: cultural and social aspects of parenting

Nathalie Zajde and Catherine Grandsard

University of Paris 8

18.1 Introduction

The birth of a child is an event that by nature is always uncertain. Who is this new arrival? What is its potential? What effect will it have on its parents, its grandparents, brothers and sisters, its society? What future will it have? How will it take its place in life? Under what conditions? All human societies without exception develop procedures to conceptualize these questions and to provide answers: the ways of announcing and monitoring the pregnancy, for example, as well as childbirth, naming the child, the official declaration of its existence, the care that it needs, and more. Most of the time all these procedures are perceived as obvious: though they may need to be learned by new parents, they need not be discussed or explained. However, some babies, on account of their clear problems to get a foothold in the world, remind us of the both indispensable and strictly cultural nature of such practices and their infinite diversity. This is the case of Jimmy,[1] whose story teaches us that it is not enough to be born to become human . . .

---

[1] To ensure confidentiality, all first names and family names have been changed.

Parenthood and Mental Health: A Bridge between Infant and Adult Psychiatry   Sam Tyano, Miri Keren, Helen Herrman and John Cox
© 2010 John Wiley & Sons, Ltd

18.2 Jimmy

Little Jimmy does not stay seated. He crawls around on the floor. He slips under our chairs, like a snake or a fish. He seems very much at ease. But when you try to touch him or pick him up, he screams and struggles. Communicating with him seems impossible. He is one-and-a-half years old. The nursery where he was placed in foster care a week after he was born can no longer keep him, he is no longer a baby. He worries the professionals. Where will he go? His parents are not even 20 years old. They separated before his birth. His mother suffers from serious psychological problems. She had to be hospitalized a first time during the pregnancy, and again for an unspecified time a few days after the birth. His father is a carefree young man, with neither a regular income nor a home. Nevertheless, responsible adults within the family are claiming Jimmy.

Unfortunately, they are in deep disagreement and are arguing over who should have care of the child. On one side, Mrs Dillon, the maternal grandmother, who hails from Guadeloupe but lives in Paris, claims that, as mother of the mother, she is the one to whom the judge should award the child. On the other hand, the father's older sister, Mrs Lemba, the paternal aunt from the Congo, who has lived in Paris for over 20 years, claims that she is the one who can best look after this child, on account of the psychological problems from which Jimmy's mother and maternal grandmother suffer. Further, in accordance with Bakongo customs, the aunt feels that she should care for the child of her brother who is too young to look after him himself. And French social and educational institutions are also ready to take in the child.

Before handing down her decision, the judge hearing the case ordered an ethnopsychiatric examination at the Centre Georges Devereux to obtain the input that would help understand and improve the situation. The Centre Georges Devereux[2] is a clinical psychology research centre run by a team of clinical psychologists and multi-ethnic and multilingual teachers and researchers from the University of Paris 8, Saint-Denis. It is located in Paris and was established in 1992 by Prof. Tobie Nathan, founder of clinical ethnopsychiatry, and of the first ethnopsychiatry department, set up in 1979 at the Avicenna Hospital in Bobigny, France, in the psychiatric ward headed by the late Prof. Lebovici.

18.3 Ethnopsychiatry

Ethnopsychiatry is a branch of psychology whose aim is to study therapeutic practices and understand their underlying intelligence and rationality, whatever:

1 The cultural contexts with which they are associated;

2 The conceptual matrices they carry;

3 The ontological and social choices that they lay claim to or activate;

4 The procedures they employ to achieve change.

Thus, in the words of Tobie Nathan, ethnopsychiatry is interested in all therapeutic techniques, whether scientific – from the general world of universities and science – or

---

[2] http://www.ethnopsychiatrie.net

popular – claimed by particular groups, by social, cultural or religious communities, and practiced and passed on by healers [1].

In this approach, research data is collected within two types of settings:

- Ethnopsychiatric therapy sessions – in this case the researchers take on clinical responsibility for their patients, who are there because they suffer from psychological problems that are largely resistant to traditional treatment; and

- In the field, among therapists, psychiatrists, psychologists, healers, priests, rabbis, shamans and other types of practitioners.

18.4 Ethnopsychiatric therapy sessions

Sessions bring together around the patient, for about three hours, his or her relatives and anyone else of the patient's choice, a group of psychologists, psychiatrists, nurses, social workers, ethnologists and linguists. Professionals form a multi-ethnic and multilinguistic group from different cultural backgrounds, educated at Western universities. At least one ethnoclinical mediator (or cultural broker) takes part in each ethnopsychiatric session. This is usually a psychologist of the same origin as the patient. The ethnoclinical mediator acting as go-between speaks the patient's language fluently, and knows and can explain to the other participants the particular cultural and religious aspects, the systems of kinship and parenting, theories of misfortune and sickness, and the therapeutic practices of the patient's culture. During the sessions with Jimmy, three languages were spoken, Guadeloupe Creole, Lingala and of course French.

The patients and professionals sit in a circle. They listen to Jimmy's story as told by the childcare worker responsible for him. Both sides of the family are represented and can contribute whenever they so wish. Everyone listens attentively. The problems had started well before the birth of the child.

18.5 Treatment

During the case presentation by one of the nursery professionals in charge of the child, the ethnoclinical mediator from the Centre Georges Devereux, a woman from the Congo, catches Jimmy by an arm, lifts him up above her, shakes him up and down, then takes him by the other arm and repeats the same movement. Jimmy shows no signs of objection, and on the contrary seems rather to like it. She blows into his ears and eyes, the way African midwives do with infants. Then she lies Jimmy on his back facing her, goes down on her knees and stares intently into his eyes – Jimmy stares back, as though hypnotized. The mediator, referring to the ancestral guardian spirits of Jimmy's family, which she identifies as hippopotamuses, speaks to Jimmy in Lingala,

So you don't want to stay with us? You don't love your parents? You prefer to go back to the hippopotamuses? Well, you're wrong! Take a look, there are good people here! France is a beautiful country, your parents, your aunt, your grandmother are very good people. They love you. You should stay. You'll see you'll like it here! *Mbutu Jimmy*, old Jimmy, stay with us, we beg you!

The first true contact with a strange child who has come from elsewhere, the first attempt to get close has been successful. It appears as though Jimmy is thinking it over. Perhaps he will agree to become part of the world of humans. On condition . . . on condition that humans negotiate his arrival, his presence in their world. On condition that they let him live among them. On condition that responsible humans identify who he is, why he has come, and offer him the place he deserves. His parents are much too young to understand. They do not know how to find the solutions to the complex difficulties that despite themselves they have contributed to creating.

18.6 Psychotherapy and diplomacy

The ethnopsychiatric session, a clinical locus that takes responsibility for patients by also welcoming their values, languages, their world, culture, gods, invisible beings and other 'social attachments' [2, 3, 4] is an uncommon setting. It is a locus for both psychotherapy and diplomacy, because mediation between different worlds and diplomacy have in recent decades become essential elements in the work of clinical psychologists in major cities.

Paris, like all contemporary metropolises, is a multicultural city, with populations stemming from hundreds of different origins. It is also a permanent melting pot. In fact those known as 'second generation', born to immigrant parents, or who arrived very young to live in France, quite naturally get involved, marry and have children with other young people from different backgrounds. They have in common the French language, living in France, mostly having French identification papers and having had the same sort of education. They have learned to read and write in the public school system, in the same language that conveys particular social and cultural values and concepts. And lastly, they share the experience of living, working and aging in France, and think of their children and grandchildren also as French citizens, future children of the French Republic. Thus these young people receive a double heritage, that of the home of their parent's social and cultural circle, and that of school. When they in turn start a family, without having given it any prior thought, they are sometimes caught up by the convictions and values strictly from the world of their family, especially when problems arise [5].

Marriage, pregnancy, the arrival of a child are events that very often summon up family and ancestral cultural values at odds with those of the society in which children of immigrants live, in our case French society. Thus in the case of a child from a mixed marriage of 'second generation' parents, three different social and cultural worlds face off against each other, each with its own meaning and values for marriage, family and children. Psychologists' clinical work in the context of ethnopsychiatric sessions necessarily includes an element of negotiation between these different worlds, mediation on behalf of the child. It requires that for each situation one redefines the concepts of 'family', 'parent' and 'parenting'. The definitions of parenting and upbringing held by each cultural group necessarily include specific ontological and ecological propositions.

In the case of little Jimmy, the situation was made even more complicated because of his double origin and triple cultural-membership, French, Guadelopean and Congolese. The issue at stake in the referral by the children's court judge of the child and which the ethnopsychiatric session must address, could be rendered by the question, *to whom does the child belong?* [3]. This question interests us insofar as it lets us get to the complex reasons underlying conflicts and the misunderstandings [7] between the two sides of the family.

Both belong to cultural universes in which children are profoundly attached to their families in specific ways, based on custom, that are objective but always negotiable.

18.7 The conflict between the two families

Mrs Lemba (the older sister of Jimmy's father) and Mrs Dillon (Jimmy's maternal grand-mother) are today sworn enemies, not willing to speak to each other and waging war over custody of the child, though they were not always enemies. They got to know one another when the young people, the future parents, started their relationship. Then they got on very well. Mrs Dillon found in Mrs Lemba a friend who brought her some comfort in her distress.

In fact, for a very long time Mrs Dillon had been having serious problems in her own marriage, so much so that during the pregnancy her daughter had to leave home and move in with Mrs Lemba to escape the violence between her parents. Mrs Dillon accused her husband, also from Guadeloupe like herself, of attacking her with witchcraft. She explained that for several years he had been training to become a sorcerer-healer, and as part of the process, to acquire the 'gift', he had applied sorcery against his wife, the person nearest to him. Mrs Dillon suffered greatly physically, was exhausted, depressed, highly disturbed and ill, and had opened up to Mrs Lemba.

The latter was heavily involved in an Evangelical church – she was married to the minister of that church – and made herself especially available to listen as much as Mrs Dillon needed, praying for her whenever possible. Mrs Lemba tried to get Mrs Dillon to come to her church, telling her it would be a place where she would be welcome and receive good care, but Mrs Dillon never agreed. The ties of friendship between Mrs Dillon and Mrs Lemba became impossible and even became reversed. Mrs Lemba understood that Mrs Dillon was expecting her to make use of Congolese sorcery to counteract the sorcery of Mr Dillon, which she absolutely refused to do. On her part, Mrs Dillon became angry with Mrs Lemba, feeling abandoned and betrayed in her friendship, when she realized that Mrs Lemba was refusing to take any non-Christian action and considered her a sinner for wanting to use sorcery. Mrs Dillon even hinted that Mrs Lemba would link up with Mr Dillon to harm her and take actions against her daughter – a malign partnership that was the source of the young mother's psychiatric decompensation.

18.8 Sorcery: from the Antilles to the Congo

Sorcery is the action of causing harm using complex, logical, technical, specific and always hidden procedures [3]. It exists both in the Antilles and in the Congo. Nevertheless, its techniques, motives, procedures and withdrawal are all strictly local. In other words, sorcery in the Antilles and that practised in the Congo are in fact very different and are each part of a distinctive social and cultural context. Sorcery practice does not follow the same rules and is not controlled in the same way. Nevertheless, if the actions and practices of sorcery remain culturally defined, in a Western urban context both practitioners and clients come from all kinds of different backgrounds.

Sorcery in the Antilles generally has a double origin, African and French, imported by the slaves and their white masters. While treating of malign and diabolical beings, they very often fit into Christianity. In other words, most *gadezafés* – a Guadeloupe Creole word meaning literally 'to look into matters', namely a 'healer' – are in fact practising Christians. The initiation of a healer, as Mrs Dillon made clear with respect to her husband, often takes place to the detriment of a close family member, who might be the spouse, a child or parent. It is a matter of acquiring the gift of influence and action over the world, in return for the sacrifice of someone dear. This logic behind how to acquire powers is not exclusive to the Antilles, but is generally shared by a number of African, Asian, American and European cultures. A common way of referring to it is to say that one 'gives' a person (i.e. to the group of sorcerers) in order to acquire powers.

Congolese sorcery is based on ancestral practice, related to lineage, ethnicity, specific regions and gods. It is strongly fought by the Catholic, Protestant and Evangelical churches, which are expressly and utterly opposed to it. Yet in the field, users often move from one world to another, from Christian areas to those of *nganga* (healers) and *ndoki* (sorcerers). Even within churches, the boundaries between these worlds can be porous, because they hold, for example, duly initiated *nganga* who have also become pastors, or where, as happens not infrequently, the members of one church accuse those of another of continuing to practise witchcraft, *kindoki,* under cover of Christianity.

18.9 Pentecostal churches in the Congo

In the last 30 years, evangelical and Pentecostal churches in central Africa have enjoyed considerable growth. Especially in major cities, they have become extremely well-attended places of worship, and have enjoyed similar success in Western capitals where there is heavy immigration. They are all at once meeting places, social and religious places and places for healing. They are openly presented as alternatives to sorcery and traditional healing, against which they fight fiercely, at least officially.

18.10 Misunderstanding no. 1

Mrs Dillon and Mrs Lemba have experienced a deep cultural misunderstanding. Each one translated in her own way what the other said, and when they realized that they were not getting satisfaction, they turned against each other.

When talking to Mrs Lemba about the sorcery her husband was practising against her, Mrs Dillon clearly expected her friend to react and help her by acting in a similar manner (Antillean sorcery neutralized by Congolese counter-sorcery). This was all the more so since Mrs Lemba was African, and in Antilles culture Africans generally have the reputation of being stronger than Antilleans in this field. This reputation is based on a double concept: on the one hand a good number of Antillean sorcery practices originated in Africa, and on the other hand, African sorcery is particularly alive, varied and employed at every level of society [8]. Because she didn't live up to Mrs Dillon's expectations by practising sorcery against the latter's husband, Mrs Lemba was suspected by Mrs Dillon of acting against her and her daughter; the deterioration of Mr Dillon's behavior towards his wife, her daughter's mental illness and separation from Jimmy's father were all signs that fed her suspicions. We should note that in a negative world such as that of sorcery, as in the context of any war or serious conflict, no one can remain uninvolved or neutral. Hence, Mrs Lemba, brought fully up to date by Mrs Dillon, in the logic of a social environment in which sorcery truly exists, cannot claim neutrality or to be well-meaning. In a world where sorcery prevails, if she refuses to act against her husband, this means she is acting as his accomplice.

From Mrs Lemba's perspective, fully involved in the Pentecostal church to the point of having married its deacon, going there every day for prayer and taking part in the life of her church, she logically assumed that if Mrs Dillon had confided in her, it was to help her find grace, divine blessings and protection within the church. When she realized that Mrs Dillon not only did not want to come to pray with her but was also demanding that she engage in actions of sorcery against Mr Dillon, Mrs Lemba started thinking her counterpart was seeking to achieve only one thing, to get her to stray from the true path and to plunge her into sorcery, something from which she had always fled. Mrs Lemba, who is around 40 years old, has been in France for about 20 years. She came to France for treatment following a serious car accident in Brazzaville in which she almost lost her life. Having been saved, Mrs Lemba had vowed to be an irreproachable Christian. Following Christian thinking, she interprets Mrs Dillon's demands and accusations as attempts by the Devil to get her to deviate from the true path, precisely what she is fighting against with all her strength.

18.11   The Bakongo kinship and parenting system

According to Bakongo tradition, as the oldest sister, Mrs Lemba is responsible for all her brothers and sisters. In France, her status is that of mother to them, which her siblings all acknowledge. After she arrived in France, Mrs Lemba was instructed by her own mother, who stayed in the Congo, to take in her younger brothers and sisters. Hence, the responsibility has become hers to ensure their health and to handle their problems as though she were their real parent. Since her arrival in France some 20 years ago, Mrs Lemba has never returned to her country. Last year she married a Bakongo man like herself, who holds the position of deacon in the church where she is a member. Mrs Lemba has no children.

Since the placement of Jimmy in foster care, Mrs Lemba has always been heavily involved in the child's situation, worrying constantly about his condition and his needs, going regularly to the nursery, acting like a mother, as is required by Bakongo custom. Since Jimmy's father was too young, he let his older sister handle this new situation. He was not prepared to cope with the problems that appeared with the arrival of his child, major problems requiring in-depth knowledge of the Bakongo kinship system, and also of the status of strange, foreign children. Jimmy's father does not yet have the ability needed to negotiate an agreement with the family of his son's mother, which not only is not Bakongo but on top of that has a lot of problems of its own.

18.12   Misunderstanding no. 2

Mother-centrism in the Antilles

Society in the Antilles by tradition is matricentric, in other words, it is matrilineal in terms of place of residence and who takes charge of the children. In fact, the most widespread, stable family model in the Antilles – doubtless drawn from the regulations of the notorious

Black Codes[3] – is made up of a mother and a maternal grandmother, even a maternal great-grandmother, who bring up the children, often born of different fathers. In Antillean Creole, these women are referred to as *potomitan*, the central post that supports a house [9]. The children have their father's name, refer to him in terms of origin and filiation, are often very close to him, but live with their mother and maternal grandmother, who bring them up [10]. It is with this frame of reference in mind that Mrs Dillon claims guardianship of Jimmy. An Antillean saying goes, 'Your husband is not family', in other words, an Antillean marriage is not a union between two families. It does not lead to a contract that would define the terms and conditions of the permanence of a given lineage. To whom the child belongs is not a question. The child is naturally brought up by its mother or maternal grandmother. The father's family will practically never claim it.

However, in this case, Jimmy's father is not Antillean but Congolese; he has an older sister acting as his mother and claiming his child.

Bakongo matrilineality

The Bakongo are matrilineal. In other words, children are tied to the maternal side of their family. The child knows its biological father, lives with him when he lives as a married man with the mother, but it is his maternal uncles who are responsible for bringing him up, his health, his development, his education, his very existence. From the mother's side, the child thus inherits goods, ancestors, functions, and religious and family obligations. This system remains balanced so long as matrilineal Bakongo marry among themselves.

Jimmy finds himself in a unusual situation since his mother is not a Bakongo but an Antillean woman who, as such, is not part of the matrilineal kinship system. Since, on the one hand, the mother is lacking and, on the other hand, the child's father's family is very present, we find ourselves in an uncommon situation, from a Bakongo point of view, in which it is the father's family, in effect the elder sister – the representative in France of the child's grandmother and great-uncles – who is obligated to bring up the child.

18.13 To whom does the child belong?

That is the question which unites all the players involved in this treatment situation, the judge who ordered the ethnopsychiatric session, the social and educational professionals, the psychologists, and of course Jimmy's relatives. That is the question every African parent asks when a child is born into a family with problems or in an unusually complicated situation [11]. To answer this question, we have to ask a second question, its corollary, 'Where does this child come from?'

18.14 Back to the treatment

'So you don't want to stay with us? You don't love your parents? You prefer to go back to the hippopotamuses?'

---

[3] 'Black Code' (*Code Noir*), issued in March 1685 by Louis XIV, 'Black Code or collection of edicts, declarations and decrees concerning Negro slaves in America', containing 60 clauses that legislated the life of slaves in the French Antilles.

This is how the mediator had started the human interaction with little Jimmy. Through these words, she let him know that she understood he was connected to his ancestors while also trying to convince him to become human. According to Bakongo psychological and psychiatric theories – also very widespread in a number of African cultures [12, 13, 14, 15, 16, 17] – even if they look the part, in fact certain children are not the children of humans, but rather the children of non-humans, such as spirits, ancestors, gods and others. Nevertheless, under certain conditions they can become human. These children belong to another world. They are born among humans, but they are a kind of messenger from a parallel and invisible world. Generally, if they are born into a human family and cause a lot of trouble and suffering, it is because they have been sent to remind the family of the need to renew the initial alliance established by the human founders of the family or lineage between themselves and their non-human doubles. This initial alliance is what has allowed the family, the lineage, the ethnic group to exist. These 'doubles' can be ancestors, spirits, animals or others. The work of a therapist consulted by a family is to identify who the child is, who has sent it and what the invisible world is asking of the family in order for the child to become fully theirs and agree to enter and remain in the strictly human world.

18.15   Identifying baby Jimmy

'You should stay. You'll see you'll like it here! *Mbutu Jimmy,* old Jimmy, stay with us, we beg you!'

Jimmy, who was born of a Bakongo father and a foreign woman, has a special status, which in Lingala is called *Mwana mbuta.* Within the paternal lineage such a child is considered a 'chief child'. He is someone who is extremely important. It is often said of this sort of child that it is an ancestor who has returned or who is dedicated to bringing riches or power to the family [12, 13, 14, 15]. In any case, it is very important that this sort of child be honored and treated with deference, because it has come to protect the father's lineage. Such children are often entrusted to one of their father's sisters or their husbands. In this case, and in accordance with custom, Jimmy should have been placed in the care of Mrs Lemba and her husband, who for Jimmy would then have become *Tata Nsakila,* meaning 'spiritual father' in Lingala. Because of the important place Jimmy has in his paternal family, he should be called *Mbutu Jimmy,* which translates as 'old Jimmy'. One would thereby address him with the respect owed to an elder.

18.16   Epilogue

Unlike Mrs Lemba, Mrs Dillon almost never came to see her grandson at the nursery. Terribly affected by her own marital problems and by her daughter's mental illness, she quickly withdrew her claim of guardianship of the child before the judge. She also clearly stated her disappointment with Mrs Lemba's categorical refusal to use Congolese sorcery to help her. The main reason for her friendship with the family of her daughter's boyfriend, she explained, had precisely been this hope. In the end, Mrs Dillon stepped out of little Jimmy's life. The child was awarded to Mrs Lemba by ruling of the judge. After a few weeks living with his paternal aunt, little Jimmy had acquired the behavior and ability to communicate of a child of his age.

18.17 Conclusion

Each year, dozens of cases such as Jimmy's are referred to the Centre Georges Devereux. These cases remind us of a self-evident fact: no child comes into the world without having been previously conceptualized by the group it belongs to. Indeed, there is no such thing as a 'naked' human being. Every person belongs to a cultural world with notions about pregnancy, birth, childhood; a cultural world that shapes that person by bringing her up according to ways and ideas that have been culturally and socially defined. In every society, parenting practices and procedures are based on theories. In so-called Western societies, these practices are based on ideas developed and validated by experts in the realm of academia before being adopted by the rest of society. In so-called traditional societies, childbirth and upbringing practices are based on theories developed and validated by practitioners, midwives, healers, thinkers, chiefs, priests, who have all undergone a long and rigorous training, though rather more secretly.

These different concepts are directly linked to the existential projects of the societies and cultures to which they belong. They involve definitions of what it is to be human, of how humans are shaped, what motivates them, their raison d'être and what allows them to exist; in other words, definitions of the human essence but also of where and with whom humans live. Hence, in every culture and society, the definition of a human being is intrinsically linked to the society's definition of itself, within which that human being leads his life.

The concept of child is necessarily linked to specific procedures. It is through actions, behaviors and words conceived to influence that the child is formed to become a human adult invested with an identity. Thus, in many so-called traditional societies these procedures always involve culturally organized traumatic experiences, most often in the form of specific ancestral rituals performed at different stages of an individual's life (birth, weaning, puberty, marriage, birth of a child, etc.) [18]. Often involving fear, intellectual confusion, and some measure of physical pain, these rituals are designed both to shape and strengthen the personal and social identities of a society's members. As such, they are major stakes in a cultural group's survival and future, therefore constantly evolving in response to various influences and needs.

In a globalized world where, on account of mass migration, people end up living in multicultural metropolises, childcare today requires of psychological, medical and social professionals to be knowledgeable of specific cultural practices and to acquire special skills in negotiating between different worlds [19].

18.18 References

1. Nathan, T. (1998) Georges Devereux and clinical ethnopsychiatry www.ethnopsychiatrie. net.
2. Nathan, T. (2001) *Nous ne sommes pas seuls au monde*, Les empêcheurs de penser en rond, Seuil.
3. Nathan, T. (2007) *À qui j'appartiens?* Les empêcheurs de penser en rond, Seuil.
4. Latour, B. (1999) Factures/fractures: from the concept of network to the concept of attachment. *Res*, special issue on Factura, **36**, 20–31. Available online: http://www. bruno-latour.fr/articles/article/76-FACTURE-GB.pdf.

5. Nathan, T. (1993) Figures culturelles de la guerre des sexes. Conflits de personnes, conflits de familles, conflits de cultures. *Informations sociales*, **3**.

6. Devereux, G. (1968) L'image de l'enfant dans deux tribus : Mohave et Sedang, *Nouvelle Revue d'Ethnopsychiatrie*, **4**, 1985, 109–20.

7. Pury S. de (1998) *Traité malentendu. Théorie et pratique de la médiation interculturelle en situation clinique.* Synthélabo, Les empêcheurs de penser en rond, Paris.

8. Geschiere, P. and Fisiy, C. (1995) *Sorcellerie et politique en Afrique.* Khartala, Paris.

9. Rolle-Romana, V. (1999) Psychotherapie d'antillaises ensorcelées. Doctoral thesis in psychology, University of Paris.

10. Gracchus, F. (1979) L'Antillais et la question du père. *CARE*, **3**.

11. Nathan, T. and Hounkpatin, L. (1996) *La parole de la forêt initiale.* Odile Jacob, Paris.

12. Bonnet, D. (1981) Le retour de l'ancêtre, *Journal des Africanistes*, **51** (1–2), 133–49.

13. Collomb, H. (1974) L'enfant qui part et qui revient ou la mort du même enfant, in *L'enfant dans la famille* (eds J. Anthony and C. Koupernik), Masson, Paris, 354–62.

14. Lallemand, S. (1978) Le bébé-ancêtre mossi, in *Systèmes de signes, Hommage à G. Dieterlen*, Hermann, Paris, pp. 307–16.

15. Nathan, T. (1985) 'L'enfant-ancêtre', *Nouvelle Revue d'Ethnopsychiatrie*, **4**, 7–8.

16. Nathan, T. and Moro, M.R. (1989) Enfants de djinné. Evaluation ethnopsychanalytique des interactions précoces, in *L'évaluation des interactions précoces entre le bébé et ses partenaires* (eds S. Lebovici, P. Mazet and J.P. Visier), Eshel, Geneva, pp. 307–39.

17. Zempleni, A. and Rabain, J. (1965) L'enfant Nit-Ku-Bon. Un tableau psychopathologique traditionnel chez les Wolof et les Lebou du Sénégal. *Psychopathologie Africaine*, **1** (3), 329–441; in *Nouvelle Revue d'Ethnopsychiatrie* (1985), **4**, 9–41.

18. Zajde, N. (1998) Traumatismes, in *Psychothérapie*, (eds T. Nathan, A. Blanchet, S. Ionescu and N. Zajde), Odile Jacob, Paris.

19. Grandsard, C. (2005) *Juifs d'un côté. Portraits de descendants de mariages mixtes entre juifs et chrétiens.* Les empêcheurs de penser en rond, Seuil, Paris.

19

Filicide: parents who murder their child

Sam Tyano[1] and John Cox[2]

[1]Tel-Aviv University, Israel
[2]University of Gloucestershire, UK

Clinical vignettes

A 4-year-old girl has disappeared for two months, and was found dead in a suitcase at the bottom of a river. Father admitted to have killed her, mother is suspected to have asked to do so.

A 3-year-old boy has been drowned by his single-parent mother. Until then, this boy filled the mother's world. She had planned to commit suicide, but did not do it.

A 1-year-old infant girl was killed and hidden in a forest by her father. Parents are divorced. 'I knew this would be the solution for all my problems,' he said.

19.1   Introduction

The interdiction against killing one's own child is not a universally shared value.

The first published 'near-filicide' of our ancestor Abraham, who was ready to sacrifice his son Isaac, was the ultimate proof of his unconditional commitment to God. But God did not allow it to happen . . .

To most Western minds, the thought of a parent killing his or her child evokes a deep sense of horror and outrage, as it is viewed as a betrayal of the assumption that parental

Parenthood and Mental Health: A Bridge between Infant and Adult Psychiatry   Sam Tyano, Miri Keren, Helen Herrman and John Cox
© 2010 John Wiley & Sons, Ltd

love is one of the tenets of civilization. Therefore, parental and especially maternal filicide is regarded as a crime committed by 'crazy' people. While reviewing the literature, it turns out that many societies have practised infanticide, including those in Greece, China, Japan, India, Brazil, England, Italy and France, among others. Infanticide has been the most widely used method of population control during much of human history [1] and fully reviewed by Brockington [2]. Reasons for infanticide include the desires to control the size and composition of the family, maximize reproductive success and ensure social stability [3].

Culture-bound priorities, still in the early twenty-first century, give legitimization for filicide [4]. For instance, in parts of Northern India, adults prioritize the well-being of family rather than the survival of individual members [5]. In some societies, infants with visible deformities and twinships are legitimately killed [3, 6]. Female gender is also a culture-bound risk factor for infanticide [7]. Some societies, such as in rural parts of India, seem to prefer sons, but the reasons behind this preference is economic: 'Too many girls, too much dowry' [8]. Culture-bound beliefs, such as that evil spirits that can grab the souls of newborns, may make infanticide a legitimate act, as it has been described in Bolivia [9]. Other common reasons for killing infants were social, such as family size and poverty. These authors found that both communities of their sample gave legitimization to infanticides that were the result of biological and social reasons. Killing infants for social reasons only was rarely justified.

While the rationale for engaging in infanticide varies widely by culture, commonalities emerge, especially among less-industrialized places. Contrary to current Western thinking and studies (that will be reviewed below), filicide is not always an unpredictable crime committed by mentally ill parents: Oberman [4] showed that parents who commit filicide often cannot raise children under the circumstances dictated by their specific position in place and time.

Besides the cultural and socio-economic motives, little is known about the circumstances and factors that lead to filicide, and this lack of knowledge makes prevention difficult. While it is obvious that filicide is one of the rare conditions where prevention is the *only* treatment, this lack of knowledge is especially bothering.

In this chapter we will first review the empirical data available nowadays, continue with some psychodynamic possible explanations, and end with clinical implications.

19.2 Prevalence of filicide among Western societies

A recent survey in the United States [10] reported that homicide was the fourth leading cause of death among children from ages one to years, and the third one among children from ages five to fourteen years. The first year of life is the most prone. Among children and adolescents, homicides are most likely to occur in the first year of life; the second peak is during later adolescence [11]. Abuse and felicide are on the same spectrum: more than 80% of homicides in very young children were actually fatal child abuse.

Among those under the age of five years, 61% were killed by their own parents, half by their mothers (30%) and half by their fathers (31%). The majority of homicides of children older than three years are committed by a person unrelated to the child.

The conclusion of these statistics is that filicide is a real problem, and that the first three years are critical for early detection of infants at high risk.

Early detection necessitates knowing the risk factors.

19.3 Filicide and the child's age

Already before 1970, Resnick [12] suggested differentiating between *neonaticide* (within the first 24 hours of life) , *infanticide* (within the first 12 months of life) and filicide (older children), because he found different parental characteristics according to the age of the murdered child, such as neonaticide being typically committed by young, poor and unmarried mothers with little or no prenatal care. A more recent review [13] replicated these findings, and added a high frequency of denied or concealed pregnancy (in spite of the fact that these mothers tend to live with their own parents) among maternal perpetrators of neonaticide.

Among mothers who committed *infanticide*, young age, non-employment and high frequency of psychiatric disorders have been described [14].

19.4 Filicide and parent's gender

Among the murdered children under five years of age in the USA, in the last quarter of the twentieth century, 61% were killed by their parents, equally by mothers and fathers (30% by mothers, 31% by fathers). Twice as many fathers as mothers committed filicide-suicide [13]. In a Quebec sample [15], paternal filicide has been found more common than maternal filicide after the age of one year (neonaticide is very rarely committed by fathers, and most infanticides are committed by mothers).

Despite these findings, paternal filicide has attracted limited research, and is even less well understood than maternal filicide. Also, there were investigated retrospectively 60 cases of male parent filicides, that had led to 77 deaths [15]; 23% of the children were under the age of one year, 26% between one and five years, 22% between six and ten years, and 29% were more than ten years old. Siblings were murdered in 23% of the cases. Of the homicides committed by fathers, 60% were followed by suicide, especially in the instances involving multiple sibling victims. At the time of the filicide, 18% of the sample also killed their spouses.

The most common means of homicide was the use of a firearm (34%), followed by beating (22%). The use of knife, strangulation, blunt instrument, intoxication and drowning were much less common, in decreasing order. Recent rupture of the marital relationship had happened in 40% of the cases, family violence was indicated in 40% of the cases, but drugs and/or alcohol use were uncommon.

The presence of severe psychopathology was observed in 60% of the fathers: major depression (52%), schizophrenia and other psychoses (10%), and acute substance intoxication (5%). Fathers are often perpetrators of fatal-abuse filicide, with a childhood history of abuse, especially in paternal filicides involving infants under the age of one year. These fathers are rarely psychotic.

Retaliating filicides are rare among mothers, and typically reflect personality disorders with a high incidence of suicide attempts.

19.5 Parental motivations for committing filicide: at the psychiatric level

The major motivational factors for filicide have been classified, as follows [16, 17, 18, 19, 20]:

(a) Mental illness

(b) Retaliation

(c) Rejection of an unwanted child

(d) Mercy killing

(e) Chronic abuse that lead to accidental death (i.e. the 'shaken baby' syndrome).

Empirical studies have made clear the fact that in most cases of filicide, *multiple factors* act together at causing the parent to kill his or her own child [21, 22]. These include financial difficulties, social isolation, single motherhood, work-related stress, housing problems, a childhood of abuse and/or trauma, marital problems and jealousy, alcohol abuse, physical illness, depression, mood disorders, psychosis.

Filicidal parents who are not defined as mentally ill

Neonaticide is caused mostly by this group of mothers, usually very young mothers who cannot cope with social stress factors [14, 23, 24]. The absence of mental illness, as defined by the law, meaning psychosis or affective disorder, does not imply the existence of a healthy personality. As has been shown [25], there is a high rate of *personality disorders*, with very low ego organization, among these mothers who commit neonaticide. Similarly, among 16 cases of neonaticide [26], nearly all of the women reported symptoms of *belle indifference*, depersonalization, dissociative hallucinations and intermittent amnesia at delivery. Most of the cases were preceded by denial of pregnancy. 56% of Spinelli's sample [26] had a history of sexual abuse. Accidental filicide, i.e. fatal abuse, is more frequent among parents with personality disorders and intense psychosocial stress at the time of the fatal abuse, than among parents with psychosis and depression [23].

Filicidal parents who are defined as mentally ill

In a review from the late 1960s of the world psychiatric literature, a high frequency of depression, psychosis, prior use of psychiatric services and suicidality was found [12].

Among 57 mothers admitted to a forensic psychiatric hospital, after having been found not competent to stand trial, researchers [27] identified two groups of women, based on the age of the murdered child, with different motivational profiles: the *neonaticidal mothers were mostly psychotic and socially deprived, while the filicidal mothers were mostly depressed, with a history of childhood abuse and self-directed violence, and a high frequency of suicide attempts following the murder.* As Stanton [23] has reported in her six interviewed mentally ill filicidal mothers, these women perceived their murder act as altruistic or as an extension of suicide, were intensely involved in mothering their child, had no extreme external stressors, but were over-whelmed by the mental illness, and regretted the killing.

Filicide–suicide, a relatively rare situation, has been reported as being committed more frequently by fathers than by mothers (twice as many times), and mostly due to altruistic and acutely psychotic motives, with a past history of depression or psychosis [13]. Older children were more often victims than infants in their cohort of 30 filicide–suicide families.

19.6 Parental motivations for committing filicide: at the psychodynamic level

Obviously, only a minority of parents who become psychiatrically ill and/or have environ-mental stressors kill their child. Similarly, most of the parents who experienced neglect and/ or abuse in their own childhood do not kill their children, in spite of their deficient parenting skills. Therefore, one must try to comprehend the phenomenon of filicide as a complex one, where psychodynamic factors should be included in the constellation of risk factors identified in individuals at risk for filicide [28]. We put aside here filicidal acts legitimized by culture-bound norms.

The individual, non-cultural, filicidal act is at the ultimate point of violence. Still, violence is not a unitary phenomenon: various core complexes, motives and fantasies need to be explored [29]. Two broad conceptual categories of psychopathic versus psychotic parents result from the empirical data on the filicidal parents' characteristics. Among the psychopathic, narcissistic, retaliatory individuals, the aim is sadistic [30]. The child was never really wanted, and is killed either as an accidental result of severe abuse, or in the parent's deliberate vengeance towards his/her spouse. This group of parents, *though psychologically disturbed, but not mentally ill* [28], are typically found guilty of murder.

In the second group of parents, who suffer from schizophrenia, bipolar disorder or psychotic depression, the violence is very different in nature: it is self-preservative, aimed at protecting the self and/or the child from perceived threat [31]. There is a suggestion of a distinction between two types of psychotic women [32]:

1 The *disorganized* type, characterized by extreme personality fragmentation that is the *combined result of a biologically based chronic mental illness and a destructive early environment (such as severe neglect and abuse)*. Their crime is the result of bizarre acting-out, where the infant is not perceived as human, but rather as a lifeless part-object into which the mother projects unwanted, threatening parts of her fragmented ego.

2 The *organized* type, distinguished by a premorbidly more integrated ego (reflected in quite good educational achievements, work and interpersonal functioning), that becomes temporarily but severely fractured. The crime is organized into 'logic', though pathological and distorted. The childhood history is less chaotic than in the disorganized group but, based on Kunst's sample of filicidal mothers [32], all the women had a history of intrafamilial sexual abuse and depressed, inconsistent maternal care. Unlike the first group, these filicidal mothers are *very invested in their child, but in a pathological way:* they look to their children to be for them *objects of transformation, of repair of themselves*

[33]. Such women seek for a mother in their own child. Again, the filicidal act comes when *environmental stresses,* such as marital stress or separation, severe financial problems, poor support, *combine with the mother's psychological vulnerability,* and lead them to feel increasingly alienated from the world around. The unbearable anxiety turns into depression, and fantasies of ultimate annihilation, where the child is entrapped, because of the mother's enmeshed, undifferentiated relationship with him or her. It is in that state of mind that these mothers start to build 'the' plan. A mother's statement, illustrates this catastrophical dynamic very well: 'I didn't kill my son, I killed myself' [31, p. 36].

This distinction of the two groups of women is important; both in terms of understanding better the phenomenon of filicide, and in planning for intervention. Indeed, in Kunst's experience [32], the organized group women are often treatable patients who can use psychotherapy to understand the core complex and fantasies that led them to commit the crime.

19.7   Characteristics of the child at risk for filicide

A study which took place in Japan [14] found not only a high frequency of psychiatric disorders among murder mothers, but also a high frequency of physical anomalies among the child victims. This is consistent with the well-known link between physical handicap and child abuse.

It has also been shown that perpetrator gender correlated with victim gender: fathers are more likely to kill boys, and mothers tend to kill girls [34].

19.8   Clinical implications

As reviewed above, a significant proportion of both maternal and paternal filicide perpetrators suffer from depression and/or psychosis, except in the neonaticide cases. Personality disorders, especially borderline personality disorder, are also frequent in both fathers and mothers. Additional risk factors, for both, include life stressors, social isolation and history of abuse in childhood. Fathers rarely commit neonaticide; filicidal fathers are more likely to be abusive to their children, and tend to commit suicide after the filicidal act.

A recent Finish study [35] has compared the psychiatric and personality profiles of homicide and filicide offenders. They did *not* find that the filicide offenders had significantly more mental illness and more serious psychopathology than the other homicide offenders. One of the significant differences was in the level of psychopathy: filicide offenders were not psychopaths, and suicide attempts at the scene of the murder were much more frequent. Filicide offenders showed signs of emotional dysfunction, with major difficulties in handling everyday difficulties, similar to domestic batterers.

Early detection

The knowledge of motivating factors causing a parent to kill a newborn, a toddler or an older child, is a prerequisite for any early intervention planning. The above reported data imply, for instance, that a psychotic mother is at heightened risk of killing her newborn, especially if other factors add to the burden of motherhood, such as being a single parent, having a low IQ and a history of drug abuse. For these women, there is a specific need for social and psychiatric support during pregnancy and the first year of life. The same stands for teenage, isolated and poor first mothers. Psychiatrists also need to remember that a very depressed woman may be at risk of killing an older child, especially if she has other risk factors.

Thoughts of infanticide should be directly probed by general practitioners and other health professionals, among non-psychotic post-partum depressed mothers, because they tend to spontaneously disclose their suicidal thoughts, but not their infanticidal ones [36].

In spite of the high proportion of child homicides committed by fathers, the tendency to overlook filicidal risk among men is still high; the possibility of homicidal tendencies in depressed fathers, especially when suicidal ideation is present, should be assessed systematically. Almost half of the filicidal women and men had had previous contact with health professionals before the time of offence [15].

To date, the most effective early detection is still a case-by-case approach, which necessitates a high degree of vigilance and general awareness of homicidal risk. The findings of the above-cited Finnish study [35] suggest that prevention of filicide is not the task of psychiatry alone, but health care and society must work together.

Existing programs

In the USA and other Western countries, programs usually center on

1 Developing comprehensive reproductive health programs, including giving access to family planning and abortion.

2 Improvement of social support networks.

3 Targeting at risk families, such as those with high levels of domestic violence.

4 Clinical interventions.

5 Legal sanctions.

One of the evidence-based efficient interventions is home visitation by trained nurses during pregnancy and the first two years of life, which reduced rates of child abuse and neglect among first-born children of unmarried adolescents of low socio-economic status [37].

These programs do not necessarily fit other places of the world.

19.9 Conclusion

'The eye sees only that which the mind is prepared to comprehend', has brilliantly enounced Henri Bergson, French philosopher and recipient of the Nobel Prize for Literature in 1927. The central task for those who seek to eliminate filicide is first to understand the lives of those who commit this crime, and the unspoken messages conveyed by their society and culture. It is important also to recognize the serious nature of perinatal mental disorder, and its link to abnormal personality and to consequent relationship problems with the parent and infant, and to plan risk reduction strategies in primary and secondary services where staff are trained in infant and perinatal psychiatry.

19.10 References

1. Harris, M. (1997) *Cannibals and Kings: the Origins of Cultures*. Random House, New York.
2. Brockington, I. (1996) *Infanticide in Motherhood and Mental Health*. Oxford University Press, pp. 430–68.
3. Mull, D.S. and Mull, J.D. (1987) Infanticide among the Tarahumara of the Mexican Sierra Madre, in *Child Survival: Anthropological Perspectives on the Treatment and Maltreatment of Children* (ed. N Scheper-Hughes), Dordrecht, Holland, Reidel, pp. 113–34.
4. Oberman, M. (2003) Mothers who kill: cross-cultural patterns in and perspectives on contemporary maternal filicide. *International Journal of Law and Psychiatry*, **26**, 493–514.
5. Miller, B. (1981) *The Endangered Sex: Neglect of Female Children in Rural North India*, Cornell University Press, Ithaca.
6. Larme, A.C. (1997) Health care allocation and selective neglect in rural Peru. *Social Science and Medicine*, **44**, 1711–23.
7. Fuse, K. and Crenshaw, E.M. (2006) Gender imbalance in infant mortality: a cross-national study of social structure and female infanticide. *Social Science and Medicine*, **62**, 360–74.
8. Diamond-Smith, N., Luke, N. and McGarvey (2008) 'Too many girls, too much dowry': son preference and daughter aversion in rural Tamil Nadu, India. *Culture, Health, and Sexuality*, **10**, 697–708.
9. De Hilari, C., Condori, I. and Dearden, K.A. (2009) When is deliberate killing of young children justified? Indigenous interpretations of infanticide in Bolivia. *Social Science and Medicine*, **68**, 352–61.
10. Hatters-Friedman, S., McCue Horwitz, S. and Resnick P.J. (2005) Child murder by mothers: a critical analysis of the current state of knowledge and a research agenda. *American Journal of Psychiatry*, **162**, 1578–87.
11. Overpeck, M.D., Brenner, R.A., Trumble, A.C., Trifiletti, L.B. and Berendes, H.W. (1998) Risk factors for infant homicide in the United States. *New England Journal of Medicine*, **329**, 1211–16.
12. Resnick, P.J. (1969) Child murder by parents: a psychiatric review of filicide. *American Journal of Psychiatry*, **126**, 325–34.
13. Hatters-Friedman, S., Hrouda, D.R., Holden, C.E., Noffsinger, S.G. and Resnick, P.J. (2005) Filicide-suicide: common factors in parents who kill their children and themselves. *Journal of American Academy of Psychiatry and the Law*, **33**, 496–504.
14. Haapasalo, J. and Petaja, S. (1999) Mothers who killed or attempted to kill their child: life circumstances, childhood abuse, and types of killing. *Violence and Victims*, **14**, 219–39.
15. Bourget, D. and Gagné, P. (2005) Paternal filicide in Québec. *Journal of the American Academy of Psychiatry and the Law*, **33**, 354–60.
16. Gagné, P. (2002) Maternal filicide in Quebec. *Journal of American Academy of Psychiatry and the Law*, **30**, 345–51.
17. Resnick, P.J. (1972) Infanticide, in *Modern Perspectives in Psycho-Obstetrics* (ed. J.G. Howells, Oliver & Boyd, Edinburgh, pp. 410–31.

18. d'Orban, P.T. (1979) Women who kill their children. *British Journal of Psychiatry*, **134**, 560–71.

19. Pitt, S.E. and Bale, E.M. (1995) Neonaticide, infanticide and filicide: a review of the literature. *Bulletin of the American Academy of Psychiatry and the Law*, **23**, 375–86.

20. Farooque, R. and Ernst, F.A. (2003) Filicide: a review of eight years of clinical experience. *Journal of the National Medical Association* **95**, 90–94.

21. Saisto, T., Salmela-Aro, K., Nurmi, J.E. and Halmesmaki, E. (2001) Psychosocial disappointment with delivery and puerperal depression: a longitudinal study. *Acta Obstetricia et Gynecologoca Scandinavica*, **80**, 39–45.

22. Schwartz, L.L. and Isser, N.K. (2000) *Endangered Children: Neonaticide, Infanticide and Filicide*. CRC Press, New York.

23. Stanton, J., Simpson, A. and Wouldes, T. (2000) A qualitative study of filicide by mentally ill mothers. *Child Abuse and Neglect*, **24**, 1451–60.

24. Bourget, D., Grace, J. and Whitehurst, L. (2007) A review of maternal and paternal filicide. *Journal of the American Academy for Psychiatry and the Law*, **35**, 74–82.

25. Putkonen, H., Collander, J., Honkasalo, M.L. and Lonnqvist, J. (1998) Finnish female homicide offenders 1982–1992. *Journal of Forensic Psychiatry*, **9**, 672–84.

26. Spinelli, M.G. (2001) A systematic investigation of 16 cases of neonaticide. *American Journal of Psychiatry*, **158**, 811–13.

27. Kirscher, M.K., Stone, M.H., Sevecke, K. and Steinmeyer, E.M. (2007) Motives for maternal filicide: results from a study with female forensic patients. *International Journal of Law and Psychiatry*, **30**, 191–200.

28. Papapietro, D.J. and Barbo, E. (2005) Commentary: toward a psychodynamic understanding of filicide—beyond psychosis and into the heart of darkness. *Journal of the American Academy of Psychiatry and the Law*, **33**, 505–8.

29. Perelberg, R.J. (1995) A core phantasy in violence. *International Journal of Psycho-Analysis*, **76**, 1215–31.

30. Glasser, M. (1986) Identification and its vicissitudes as observed in the perversions. *International Journal of Psycho-Analysis*, **67**, 9–16.

31. Fonagy, P., Target, M. (1995). Understanding the violent patient: the use of body and the role of the father. *International Journal of Psycho-Analysis*, **76**, 487–501.

32. Kunst, J.L. (2005) Fraught with the utmost danger: the object relations of mothers who kill their children. *Bulletin of the Menninger Clinic*, **66**, 19–38.

33. Bollas, C. (1987). *The Shadow of the Object*, Columbia University Press, New York.

34. Rodenburg, M. (1971) Child murder by depressed parents. *Canadian Psychiatric Association Journal*, **16**, 41–49.

35. Putkonen, H., Weizmann-Henelius, G., Lindberg, N. *et al.* (2009) Differences between homicide and filicide offenders: results of a nationwide register-based case-control study. *BMC Psychiatry*, **9**, 27doi.

36. Barr, J.A. and Beck, C.T. (2008) Infanticide secrets: qualitative study on postpartum depression. *Canadian Family Physician*, **54**, 1716–17.e5.

37. Olds, D., Henderson, C.R., Chamberlin, R. and Tatelbaum, R. (1986) Preventing child abuse and neglect: a randomized trial of nurse home visitation. *Pediatrics*, **78**, 65–78.

20

Maternal postnatal mental disorder: how does it affect the young child?

John Cox[1] and Joanne Barton[2]

[1]Keele University, Staffordshire, UK
[2]North Staffordshire Combined Healthcare NHS Trust, UK

'Recently, when I was in an up-country hospital in Tanzania, I was shown a marasmic baby, aged 11 months, with his mother. Understandably, but I think wrongly, all the emphasis was being placed on trying to get extra protein into the baby, when in fact the mother had plenty of milk but was extremely depressed.' [1]

'I enjoyed my pregnancy and I enjoyed having him, it was the greatest thing I have ever experienced until I came home. And then I thought, God I don't want you . . . I have been sad before and I have been unhappy, but never felt like after I had Thomas, to the point where I just didn't want to live any more.' [2]

20.1 Introduction

Childbirth in all cultures is a stressful psychosocial transition, and for many first-time mothers a 'rite of passage'. Thus in some traditional and modern societies special names are given to the mental disorders that occur at this time, such as *Amakiro* (Uganda) and puerperal psychosis. Childbirth is generally expected to be a joyful event, yet for some

Parenthood and Mental Health: A Bridge between Infant and Adult Psychiatry   Sam Tyano, Miri Keren, Helen Herrman and John Cox
© 2010 John Wiley & Sons, Ltd

mothers the birth of an infant is an overwhelming stressor and is associated with disabling anxiety and depression, or with another serious mental disorder. Changing patterns of family life and the diminished status of childbearing in many modern societies can increase stress and cause 'cultural confusion'. It can also lead to breaks in the transmission of parenting knowledge between generations [3, 4].

It is important therefore to consider the effect of such stress and the impact of mental illness on the care of the developing infant. A severe perinatal mental disorder, especially when characterized by delusional ideas and marked behaviour disturbance, is however only rarely treated by appropriately trained health professionals and the impact on the infant is seldom fully assessed. The modern management of perinatal psychiatric disorders must therefore routinely include assessment of the impact of such disorders on the infant in the short and long term [5], and yet also take fully into account the positive coping potential of the parents and the infant, which can ameliorate an otherwise very adverse outcome.

A mother with a sub-threshold disorder, such as minor depression or mild phobic anxiety, may not be referred to a specialist mental health service or be treated adequately in primary care and many such distressed mothers are dismissed as the 'worried well'. Yet their condition may adversely affect bonding, impair development of the infant and can progress to a more severe mental disorder. It is not uncommon, for example, for parents who present with their disturbed child to a child psychiatrist, to describe an untreated postnatal mental disorder that commenced immediately after delivery.

A postnatal mental illness of any severity may affect *all* aspects of child development and increase vulnerability to abuse and neglect. Furthermore associated risk factors for mental disorder may also compromise the child's outcome. Women with mental disorders, for example, are more at risk of unplanned pregnancies, single parenthood, social disadvantage, substance misuse, poor uptake of antenatal care, relapse of their illness following birth, and are more likely to have their children taken into care. These factors each represent a much-increased risk for poor child outcome [6].

However, some children have a good outcome despite their parents having mental disorder and lead healthy undamaged lives. An assessment therefore of both risk and protective factors is thus fundamental to any consideration of child outcome and to establishing the optimal relationship between mother and child. This mother–child relationship is bi-directional so that disruption in either direction affects outcome.

Some effects of a postnatal mental disorder on the infant can be generalized across a range of conditions, while some diagnoses (such as depression, schizophrenia and eating disorders) are also associated with particular risks and effects.

20.2 Postnatal mental illness: immediate effect on parenting

Parenting involves the provision of a safe environment for the infant, attendance to physical needs, appropriate age-related stimulation and the establishment of a secure relationship. This complicated task, which involves attachment and attunement as well as the specific provision of food and safety, can be adversely affected by a new-onset postnatal mental disorder, or by a long standing illness, such as schizophrenia, substance misuse, rapid cycling bipolar illness or depression with onset during pregnancy.

The immediate adverse effect of these mental disorders on the infant may be caused by symptoms such as *delusional beliefs* that the baby is a dangerous voodoo baby or is bewitched; mood *disturbances,* such as severe anxiety or very low mood, which reduces self esteem and impairs the mother's coping ability; and negative *cognitions,* such as excessive guilt or obsessional doubt, which may cause the mother to withdraw from her infant.

Furthermore, some mothers with a psychotic disorder, such as puerperal mania or an undifferentiated psychosis, are unable to care in a safe manner for their baby because they are *too disorganized*, are preoccupied with psychotic ideas and are intentionally or accidentally risking the life and livelihood of the baby.

Postnatal depression

Primary care workers, whether in low or high income countries, can be alerted to the likelihood that the mother may have a unipolar non-psychotic depression by one or more of the following observations:

- Complaints of fatigue, being very worried, low mood or severe sleep difficulties.

- Somatic symptoms, such as headache and abdominal pain without obvious cause, are complained of.

- Excessive fearfulness that the health worker will be critical of her mothering ability and might take the baby from her.

- Preoccupation with minimal feeding difficulties and excessive worry about weight gain. The mother provides less structure and discipline for her infant and is often irritable and angry with the baby and with other family members. The mother may seek advice from a community perinatal service because her baby is crying excessively or is positing.

Such depression, which affects at least 10–13% of postnatal mothers, commonly has an onset within a month of childbirth but can also be continuous with a depression present before birth, which may be exacerbated by the stresses of immediate motherhood, including feeding difficulties, and by severe postnatal blues [7].

The cardinal symptoms of a depressive disorder, using international criteria, can then subsequently be elicited by clinical interview and include depressed mood, lack of interest and pleasure in doing things, sleep difficulties and self-blame – usually lasting for at least two weeks. These symptoms will each adversely affect the ability of the mother to be attuned to her baby and particularly her ability to synchronize her communications with her infant [8]. She may be withdrawn or excessively over-stimulate the baby. In at least 15% of mothers with postnatal depression, the onset of this disorder is during pregnancy and the effect of antenatal depression and of severe stress on the fetus and subsequent child development is a subject of much contemporary research and controversy.

The risk of suicide in bipolar patients and of infanticide in women with a psychotic illness, whether of sudden onset after delivery or as a continuation of symptoms present in pregnancy, must always be carefully assessed. The psychological disturbance and symptoms experienced by mothers during the course of *psychotic illnesses* (both established and first-episode) are potentially highly disruptive to their adjustment to pregnancy and motherhood and to their availability to parent.

Anxiety disorders

Generalized anxiety disorder, post-traumatic stress disorder, obsessive compulsive disorder (OCD) etc. may occur de novo or be exacerbated during pregnancy. In such illnesses the fetus or baby may be the focus of anxieties and concerns. Thus in acute onset obsessive compulsive disorder, the obsessional thoughts may be about the baby and include distressing thoughts of harming the baby, inclusion of the baby in repetitive washing routines and the need for excessive cleanliness [9]. Anxious mothers who are preoccupied with their anxiety will be unavailable for their infants, which may compromise the attachment relationship [10].

Personality disorder

Maternal *personality disorder* represents a different kind of threat to parenting, particularly in terms of the persistence of the disorder and the impact on the mother's capacity to develop and sustain relationships. The evidence base in this area is limited, but the impact of the disorder will be on the mother's conceptualization of her role as a parent and her ability to adjust to her pregnancy and prepare for the arrival of her baby. Postnatally she may be unable to form a relationship with her child or to parent [11].

20.3   Mother–infant relationships

It is essential to consider the emerging relationship between mother and child from the mother's perspective and in particular to examine disorders of this process. Disorders of a mother's relationship with her infant are common and can result in the mother rejecting her infant [12]. Children are then at risk of abuse and neglect, and there is evidence of a later detrimental effect on the child's cognitive functioning [13]. The neurobiology of parent–infant relationships and behavior has been explored with studies describing the neurohormonal and neuro-anatomical basis of parents' responses to children [14].

20.4   Risk and resilience

While the focus of this chapter is on the impact of maternal mental health on parenting, it is important to recognize that children are not passive in their relationship with their parents or caregivers. Some children whose mothers are mentally ill during their infancy do well.

What allows some children to flourish whilst others in similar situations fail to thrive is not well understood. The concept of resilience however is increasingly recognized to be important in determining child outcome. From birth children are recognized to have different temperamental styles. This may be important in how the infant responds to adversity, including maternal mental illness.

Thomas *et al.* [15], in the New York Longitudinal Study, described nine characteristics of infant temperament, including: activity level, rhythmicity of biological functions, quality of mood, approach or withdrawal from new experiences, persistence and ease of adapt-ability. They found that some of these characteristics clustered together and they identified three patterns of infant temperament:

- *Difficult*   biologically irregular, withdraw from new situations, adapt poorly, have negative mood and intense reactions;

- *Easy* positive mood, biological regularity, mild intensity, adaptable and react positively to new situations; and

- *Slow to warm up* initial withdrawal, slow adaptation and mild intensity.

Infants with easy temperaments were found to have the best outcome and were least likely to develop mental health problems later in life.

Infant temperament may thus facilitate – or not – the development of a robust relation-ship/attachment. The infant's response to its mother in turn imparts an effect on the mother's subsequent behaviour. Infants with 'difficult' temperaments (who are difficult to soothe and who do not feed or sleep well) may undermine maternal self-confidence, which in turn affects the way they feel towards their infant.

Child temperament may be an important component of resilience. Work is ongoing to operationalize resilience, measuring it in terms of achievement against a range of global markers of outcome [16]. It is also important to think about what maternal factors may contribute to an overall resilience for vulnerable mothers and infants.

The range of potential risk and resilience factors (paternal mental illness, family and community factors) is huge and a full discussion is beyond the scope of this chapter (for a review see Zeanah [17]). The intention of the authors was to highlight the importance of considering resilience in the assessment of any family affected by parental mental illness.

20.5   Infant outcome and child development

Maternal mental illness is known to be associated with poor child outcome by potentially adversely affecting all aspects of child development, physical, social, emotional, behavioural and cognitive.

Poor interaction between mother and child, as may occur in perinatal mental illness, is associated with poor physical health outcomes for children [18]. A study by O'Brien *et al.* revealed that there was twice the rate of depression in a controlled community sample of mothers of children presenting with non-organic failure to thrive [19]. The work of Patel, Rahman and colleagues in the developing world highlights the observation of Hugh Jolly, quoted at the beginning of this chapter, by showing that perinatal depression is associated with illness and growth impairment in infants [20, 21]. Robust antenatal and postnatal screening programmes are essential to alert health-care professionals to any child at risk both in utero and postnatally. Clinicians have a responsibility to identify children who are failing to thrive and to put in motion appropriate interventions through child protection and safeguarding processes [22].

Maternal mental illness may compromise the physical development of the fetus and infant in a number of ways. The effects of drugs and alcohol on the developing fetus are explored in Chapter 23 of this book. Recognized effects include fetal alcohol syndrome and drug withdrawal states in the perinatal period. Addicted mothers are less focused on preparing for their baby. They often neglect themselves and do not attend for antenatal care, putting the unborn child at risk. Associated environmental and psychosocial factors may also be important to the outcome of the child, and effects may depend on other vulnerability factors.

Maternal eating disorders can threaten the physical well-being of the fetus, with an increased risk of the baby being small for dates. In the postnatal period the mother may have a distorted image/perception of the baby, be excessively controlling [23] and be concerned that the baby is too fat with consequent risks of feeding difficulties and failure to thrive [24]. Mothers with eating disorders may find feeding their children difficult; in turn their children are at risk of developing eating problems.

Maternal mental illness thus represents a risk to a child's social, emotional and behavioral development, through the effects of illness on her ability to meet her child's needs. Such needs are complex and multifaceted and change over time. Infants are entirely dependent and the mother has to ensure that her child is fed and kept warm and safe. She also has a crucial role in facilitating other aspects of her child's development. By responding to her child's emotional state, for example soothing the child when distressed, the mother fulfills an important role in helping her child differentiate between the range of arousal states. This is recognized to be important in the early development of higher-order executive functions [25, 26].

There are links between maternal postnatal depression and adverse infant/child cognitive outcome. The mechanism for this association is through impaired mother–infant interaction [13]. Recurrent maternal depression and especially antenatal depression [27], may be particularly detrimental in the longer-term outcome of children who have an increased likelihood of depression and antisocial behavior in adolescence.

20.6 Child mental health problems

Children of mothers affected by mental illness are at increased risk themselves of developing mental disorders. Up to one third of children of parents affected by mental illness will develop emotional or behavioral problems [28]. The mechanism for this is complex but will involve an interaction between genetic predisposition and environmental influences. At this stage however, we do not understand the complexity of this interaction. Not every child whose mother has a mental illness will become mentally ill or present with emotional or behavioral problems.

There is evidence however to link specific psychiatric disorders with particular child mental health outcomes; for example maternal smoking and substance misuse are linked with child behavioral problems [29]. There is a potential link between exposure to alcohol *in utero* and the development of alcohol misuse in later life [30]. Maternal eating disorders are associated with child feeding disorders, problems regulating food intake and eating difficulties [24]. Stress in the later stages of pregnancy is associated with emotional and behavioural problems in the child [31].

20.7 Child abuse and neglect

Parents in general instinctively protect their children and very few parents set out deliberately to harm or neglect their offspring. Children of parents who have a mental illness are at increased risk of abuse and neglect [32]. Most mentally ill mothers and fathers do not intend to harm their children. Instead their illness compromises their ability to meet the needs of their child. An important role for professionals working with parents affected by mental illness is to be aware of the impact of mental illness on parenting capacity and to advocate for parents' rights for appropriate support to allow them to continue in their parenting role. This must be balanced against an assessment of the possibility that because of their illness, parents may physically or emotionally neglect and abuse their children. Child sexual abuse may occur in the context of a parental mental illness. Rarely a mentally ill mother may murder her child. See Chapter 19 for a detailed discussion of infanticide.

Because parental mental health problems are consistently identified as a risk factor for recurrent maltreatment [32], it is essential that professionals working with parents with mental health problems are aware of the potential for neglect and abuse and know about child protection and safeguarding procedures [22]. In Factitious Illness by Proxy (FIP) a mother, or a carer looking after other people's children, present a child as ill by fabricating symptoms, or by inducing symptoms in the child that can be life-threatening.

The capacity of a mentally ill mother to care for her child must always be examined as part of assessment. In some instances it is obvious that a mother is unable to provide for the needs of her child and that the child is at risk. In such circumstances we rely heavily on other family members to care for the child until the mother is well enough to take over once again.

Being 'Looked After or Accommodated' by social services and being cared for by another family are risk factors for mental health problems in children and young people. We must also recognize that having a child accommodated has adverse effects on mothers.

20.8 Family aspects

Maternal mental illness has an effect on the whole family. Equally, the response of the family to the mother's illness may be important in her recovery. It is thus often necessary, in our experience, to consider the role of extended family and close friends as part of an assessment of risk and resilience. Depending on the nature and severity of maternal mental illness, her roles and responsibilities as a parent may have to be taken over to varying degrees by other people: father, other family members, friends or professionals. This is often associated with disruption for all concerned and there may be increased levels of stress, conflict and discord [33, 34].

Thus grandparents, siblings and family friends may have to take on childcare responsibilities and this can be associated with negative effects on their own mental health [35]. Looking after young children can be stressful for grandparents who had not anticipated such a role and who may themselves have age-related problems and limits on their coping capacities.

Such family members may also take on responsibilities for caring for the ill mother. Older children who take on the role of carer for an ill mother, as well as looking after siblings, are particularly vulnerable [36].

The implications of a postnatal mental illness for other family members can also be an additional burden for the mother herself. Many mothers, for example, think of themselves as a burden and so feel guilty about the impact of their illness on their family. Also, many such mothers struggle with their loss of role. In a study by Boath *et al.*, the verbatim comments from fathers whose partners had postnatal depression [37], vividly underline the severe stress within the family, the fathers' need for support and the possibility that they may require specific treatment for depression or substance misuse.

It is not known how many relationships break up within three months of childbirth as a consequence of mental disorder, nor what effect this disruption has on the infant and older siblings. It is likely however, from our clinical experience, that these disengagements are not only common but can be reversed if there is prompt treatment available to both parents, and if a family approach, which includes the infant and any older siblings, is undertaken.

20.9 Considering the child in the management of maternal mental illness

One aim of therapy is to restore the parent to normal day-to-day functioning, which will then facilitate their parenting. Increasingly it is recognized, however, that it is important to consider the outcome of the child in its own right and the specific needs of the child must be identified and addressed in any management plan. Some interventions have been developed with the aim of promoting positive child outcome; however there continues to be a paucity of evidence about the effect of routine treatment in terms of child outcome. The measurement of child outcome in the perinatal period is difficult and frequently this is confined to physical measurements e.g. growth. More research is needed to identify indicators of infant mental health. As children get older, their outcome can be described in terms of their social, emotional and behavioral adjustment and cognitive function.

Assessment

The information presented earlier in this chapter and elsewhere in this book, about the potentially detrimental effect on child outcome of maternal perinatal mental illness, highlights the need for early identification and intervention. In order to achieve this, there is a need for all staff involved in perinatal services to be aware of the range of maternal mental health problems and risk factors for the child. Early identification must be followed by the implementation of appropriate interventions, which include therapies that focus on mother–child interaction. There is a great need for more robust mental health screening programs in the perinatal period.

An excellent example of a mechanism for the early identification of maternal mental illness is to be found in postnatal depression, where the use of the Edinburgh Postnatal Depression Scale [38] by primary care workers offers opportunities to identify mothers vulnerable to serious illness. Unfortunately there is a lack of specifically validated measures for screening for other mental health problems, particularly in the antenatal period. Mothers who have severe mental illness will usually be identified, but even in such cases some children will be at risk if, because of their illness, mothers do not take up available ante- and postnatal care.

As mentioned above, the measurement of child outcome in the early neonatal period is often limited to physical parameters, such as birth weight and the achievement of milestones, etc. It is clear however that a key outcome is the quality of parent–child interaction and it is possible to make some assessment of this. A range of measures is currently available including self-report, structured interviews and observational schedules e.g. the Parenting Stress Index (PSI) [39], The Parent–Child Early Relational Assessment (PCERA) [40] and the HOME Inventory (Home Observation for the Measurement of the Environment) [41]. The Adult Attachment Interview [42] explores the adult's experience of attachment and may be relevant in view of the importance of the parent's experience of being parented.

These tools provide a considerable amount of information about parent–child relationships. Unfortunately their use, in the main, is restricted to research because they are impractical to use in the clinical setting. These measures are, in general, lengthy and time-consuming to both administer and score. Also there is often a need for training in their use. Self-report measures have much to recommend them in terms of their usefulness and simplicity of administration etc. They also however have limitations, particularly in relation to objectivity, which can be influenced by maternal mood. There is an urgent need for the development of clinically useful assessment tools which can be used by the range of professionals working in perinatal services.

As the child gets older, other measures become available e.g. the Bayley Infant Development Scale [43], which looks at cognitive development and the Strengths and Difficulties Questionnaire [44], which includes both parent and teacher reports of child emotional and behavioral adjustment.

Treatment

When a mother is mentally ill, she is the focus of treatment. It is often assumed that if the mother's mental illness is treated, she will then be able to attend to her infant's needs and all will be well. The evidence base describing the effect of maternal treatment on child outcome, both in the short and longer term, is however limited. There is a need therefore for child outcome, across a range of domains of functioning, to be included when assessing the effect of treatment of maternal mental illness. It is important that research addresses this, but also that clinicians consider child outcome as part of their routine assessment of treatment effectiveness. From the information presented in this chapter, it is clear that it is important for treatment to include some consideration of the promotion of the mother–child relationship and to address any detrimental effect on this resulting from the mother's illness.

The range of treatments for maternal mental illness is described elsewhere in this book (see Chapter 34). The pharmacological treatment of maternal mental illness is complex, and it is important that clinicians prescribing treatment for pregnant women, or any woman of childbearing age, are aware of any potential adverse effects on the fetus and that any risks are discussed in full. In addition to any known teratogenic effects, it is important to consider the potential psychological aspects of pharmacotherapy for the mother. Mothers are often concerned about the effect of any medication on their unborn child and will later raise concerns about any difficulties their child might have being the result of something they did or a medication they took during pregnancy. Concerns about potential harm to the fetus must also be set against the potential harm of not treating the mother.

A range of interventions are available to promote mother–child relationships and these are fully discussed in Chapter 14. There is, however, little information available from systematic reviews or randomized controlled trials, specifically in relation to the use of such interventions in mothers with a moderate to severe perinatal mental illness. Most of the evidence describing effectiveness of interventions relates to specific community programs for disadvantaged mothers, or those with depressive symptoms detected by screening questionaires.

Interventions include baby massage and interaction coaching. Residential treatments for expectant mothers with substance misuse problems have been shown to improve the physical outcome of babies in terms of their birth weight and length. [45]. There is also evidence that adding attachment-based parenting interventions into such programs improves parent–child relationships [46].

The role of large-scale intensive home-visiting programs in the promotion of the well-being of children born into adverse circumstances has been explored in a number of early intervention/prevention projects. The majority of these programs include a component of 'parent training'. There is evidence of positive benefit in terms of maternal mental health and mother–child interaction [47]. These programs do provide support of parental (especially maternal) mental health on a large scale.

The parent–infant psychotherapies described in Chapter 34 aim to work with parents to develop their reflective capacities, so that they can observe and reflect on their infant's emotional life and follow their lead. Video feedback has been shown to improve mother–child interaction in mothers with bulimia [48].

As mentioned earlier, it is not always safe for a child to remain with a mother with severe mental disorder. It is therefore essential that staff across a range of specialties and professions, who work with parents and children, are aware of their responsibilities in terms of child protection. Many mothers are aware of the effect of their illness on their parenting and are concerned about this, feeling guilty that they are failing their children. While it may be necessary for a child to be removed from a seriously ill mother, it is important to remember that parenting remains important and to look for ways to support mothers with this. Mothers describe their efforts to maintain meaningful relationships with their children, even when they have been separated [49]. The aim is always to try to return a child to his/her mother, but this will require close attention to the mother's response to the separation and feelings of guilt.

20.10 Conclusions

Perinatal mental illness is complex and has the potential to adversely affect parents and children across multiple domains of functioning. This would suggest a need for a multi-disciplinary approach to management. There are, however, few specialist multidisciplinary perinatal mental health services and very little comparative evaluation data describing their effectiveness. In the absence of specialist services, it is essential that, in day-to-day clinical practice, child mental health services develop close working relationships with their colleagues in adult mental health, so that collaborative working can take place where parents are affected by mental health problems. Work to identify effective models of service delivery, incorporating liaison between child and adult mental health services, must now be a priority. We are however very mindful of the fact that in many countries the support and care of parents with mental health problems is provided (if at all) by generic community workers. This highlights the importance of a global training agenda around parental mental health.

As 15–30% of adult mental health patients are parents, and at least 13% of mothers experience perinatal mental illness, it is remarkable that so little joint working takes place routinely. In many adult mental health services there is no routine or reliable collection of information about or assessment of dependent children. There is a pressing need for further evaluation of the effectiveness of interventions on child outcome, both in the short and long term.

This chapter has focused mostly on the immediate impact of perinatal mental illness on the infant and other family members. While some perinatal mental health problems are short-lived, in some cases they may be indicative of longer-term ill health and enduring psychopathology. The potential longer-term effects of this on the child beyond the perinatal period must therefore be considered. It is equally important to assess and identify potential resilience factors for vulnerable children and to be mindful that a child who is exposed to perinatal mental illness and whose early development is thereby potentially compromised, may have positive experiences later on which promote well-being.

20.11 References

1. Jolly, H. (1975) Published discussion, p. 44, following Cox, J.L. (1975) Psychiatric morbidity and child birth: a preliminary report on a prospective study from Kasangati Health Centre, in: *The Child in the African Environment: Growth, Development and Survival*. East African Literature Bureau.
2. Holden, J. (1988) A randomised controlled trial of counselling by health visitors in the treatment of post natal depression. MPhil thesis, Edinburgh University.
3. Cox, J.L. (1996) Postnatal mental disorder – a cultural approach. *International Review of Psychiatry*, **8**, 9–16.
4. Cox, J.L. (1999) Postnatal mood disorders in a changing culture; a transcultural European and African perspective. *International Review of Psychiatry*, **11**, 103–11.
5. Barton, J. (2009) Postnatal mental illness, children and the family, in *Modern Management of Perinatal Psychiatric Disorders* (eds C. Henshaw, J. L. Cox and J. Barton), Gaskell Press, London.
6. Hall, A. (2004) Parental psychiatric disorder and the developing child, in *Parental Psychiatric Disorder: Distressed Parents and Their Families* (eds M. Göpfert, J. Webster and M.V. Seeman), Cambridge University Press.
7. Henshaw, C., Foreman, D. and Cox, J.L. (2004) Postnatal blues :a risk factor for postpartum depression. *Journal of Psychosomatics Obstetrics and Gynaecology*, **25**, 267–72.

8. Tronick, E.Z. and Weinberg, M.K. (1997) Depressed mothers and infants: failure to form diadic states of consciousness, in *Postpartum Depression and Child Development* (eds L. Murray and P.J. Cooper), Guildford Press, London, p. 54.

9. Abramowitz, J.A., Moore, K., Carmin, C., *et al.* (2001) Acute onset of obsessive-compulsive disorder in males following childbirth. *Psychosomatics*, **42**, 429–31.

10. Henshaw, C., Cox, J.L. and Barton, J. (2009) *Modern Management of Perinatal Psychiatric Disorders*, Gaskell Press, London.

11. Hobson, R.P., Patrick, M., Crandell, L. *et al.* (2005) Personal relatedness and attachment in infants and mothers with borderline personality disorder. *Developmental Psychopathology*, **17**, 329–47.

12. Brockington, I.F. (2004) Postpartum psychiatric disorders. *Lancet*, **363** (9405), 303.

13. Murray, L., Hipwell, A. and Hooper, R. (1996) The cognitive development of 5-year old children of postnatally depressed mothers. *Journal of Child Psychology and Psychiatry*, **37**, 927–35.

14. Swain, J.E., Lorberbaum, J.P., Kose, S. *et al.* (2007) Brain basis of early parent-infant interactions; psychology, physiology, and in vivo functional neuroimaging studies. *Journal of Child Psychology and Psychiatry*, **48** (3–4), 262–87.

15. Thomas, J.M., Chess, S. and Birch, H.G. (1968) *Temperament and Behaviour Disorders in Children*. New York University Press, New York.

16. Daniel, B. (2006) Operationalizing the concept of resilience in child neglect: case study research. *Child Care Health Development*, **32**, 303–9.

17. Zeanah, C.H. (2005) *Handbook of Infant Mental Health*, 2nd edn, Guilford Press, New York.

18. Mantymaa, M., Puura, K., Luoma, I. *et al.* (2003) Infant-mother interaction as a predictor of child's chronic health problems. *Child Care Health and Development*, **29**, 181–91.

19. O'Brien, L.M. *et al.* (2004) Postnatal depression and faltering growth: a community study. *Pediatrics*, **113**, 1242–47.

20. Patel, V., Rahman, A., Jacob, K.S. *et al.* (2004) Effect of maternal mental health on infant growth in low income countries: new evidence from South Asia. *British Medical Journal*, **328**, 820–23.

21. Rahman, A., Harrington, R. and Bunn, J. (2002) Can maternal depression increase infant risk of illness and growth impairment in developing countries? *Child Care Health and Development*, **28**, 51–56.

22. Hall, D. and Williams, J. (2008) Safeguarding, child protection and mental health. *Archives of Diseases in Childhood*, **93** (1), 11–13.

23. Stein, A. *et al.* (2001) Influence of psychiatric disorder on the controlling behaviour of mothers with 1-year old infants. *British Journal of Psychiatry*, **179**, 157–62.

24. Park, R.J., Steiner, R. and Stein, A. (2003) The offspring of mothers with eating disorders. *European Child and Adolescent Psychiatry* (Suppl. 1), **12**, 110–19.

25. Kopp, C.B. (1982) Antecedents of self-regulation: a developmental perspective. *Developmental Psychology*, **18**, 199–214.

26. Barton, J. (2003) The effect of modifying maternal expressed emotions on outcome of preschool hyperactivity. PhD thesis, University of Glasgow.

27. Pawlby, S., Hay, D.F., Sharp, D. *et al.* (2009) Antenatal depression predicts depression in adolescent offspring: prospective longitudinal community-based study. *Journal of Affective Disorders*, **113** (3), 236–43.

28. Rutter, M. and Quinton, D. (1984) Parental psychiatric disorder: effects on children. *Psychological Medicine*, **14**, 853–80.

29. Wasserman, G.A., Liu, X., Pine, D.S. *et al.* (2001) Contribution of maternal smoking during pregnancy and lead exposure to early child behavior problems. *Neurotoxicology and Teratology*, **23**, 13–21.

30. Alati, R., Al Mamun, A. and Williams, G.M. (2006) In utero alcohol exposure and prediction of alcohol disorders in early adulthood: a birth cohort study. *Archives of General Psychiatry*, **63** (9). 1009–16.

31. O'Connor, T.G., Heron, J., Golding, J., *et al.* (2003) Maternal antenatal anxiety and behavioural/emotional problems in children: a test of a programming hypothesis. *Journal of Child Psychology and Psychiatry*, **44**, 1025–36.

32. Hindley, N. Rachmandani, P.G. and Jones, D.P.H. (2006) Risk factors for recurrence of maltreatment: a systematic review. *Archives of Diseases in Childhood*, **91**, 744–52.

33. Hanley, J., Cox, J.L. and Taylor, B. (2007) A critical analysis of videotapes on postnatal depression. *Contemporary Nurse*, **24** (1), 52–64.

34. Oates, M.R., Cox, J.L., Neema, S. *et al.* (2004) Postnatal depression across countries and cultures; a qualitative study, in *Transcultural Study of Postnatal Depression (TCS PND): Development and Testing of Harmonised Research Methods* (eds M.N. Marks, M.W. O'Hara, N. Glangeaud-Freudenthal *et al.*). *British Journal of Psychiatry*, **184** (suppl. 46).

35. Göpfert, M.V., Webster, M. and Seeman, M.V. (eds) (2004) *Parental Psychiatric Disorder: Distressed Parents and Their Families*. Cambridge University Press.

36. Aldridge, A. and Becker, S. (2003) *Children Caring for Parents with Mental Illness: Perspectives of Young Carers, Parents and Professionals*. Policy Press, Bristol.

37. Boath, E., Pryce, A.J. and Cox, J.L. (1998) Postnatal depression: the impact on the family. *Journal of Reproductive and Infant Psychology*, **16**, 199–203.

38. Cox, J. and Holden, J. (2003) Perinatal mental health: a guide to the Edinburgh Postnatal Depression Scale. Gaskell Press, London.

39. Abidin, R.R. (1986) *Parenting Stress Index Manual*, 2nd edn. Pediatric Psychology Press, Charlottesville, VA.

40. Clark, R. (1985) *The Parent-Child Early Relational Assessment. Instrument and Manual*. Department of Psychiatry, University of Wisconsin Medical School, Madison, WI.

41. Caldwell, B.M. and Bradley, R.H. (1978) *Manual for the Home Observation for Measurement of the Environment*. University of Arkansas, Little Rock.

42. George, C., Kaplan, N. and Main, M. (1996) Adult attachment interview protocol, 3rd edn. Unpublished manuscript. University of California, Berkley.

43. Bayley, N. (1993) *Bayley Scales of Infant Development*, 2nd edn. Psychological Corporation, San Antonio, TX.

44. Goodman, R. (1997) The Strengths and Difficulties Questionnaire: a research note. *Journal of Child Psychology and Psychiatry*, **38**, 581–86.

45. Little, B.B., Snell, L.M., van Beveren, T.T., *et al.* (2003) Treatment of substance abuse during pregnancy and infant outcome. *American Journal of Perinatology*, **20**, 255–62.

46. Suchman, N., Mayes, L. and Conti, J. (2004) Rethinking parenting interventions for drug dependent mothers: from behaviour management to fostering emotional bonds. *Journal of Substance Abuse Treatment*, **29**, 179–85.

47. Beeber, L.S., Holdithch-Davis, D., Belyea, M.J. *et al.* (2004) In-home intervention for depressive symptoms with low-income mothers of infants and toddlers in the United States. *Health Care Women International*, **25**, 561–80.

48. Stein, A., Woolley, H., Senior, R. *et al.* (2006) Treating disturbances in the relationship between mothers with bulimic eating disorders and their infants a randomized, controlled trail of video feedback. *American Journal of Psychiatry*, **163** (5), 899–906.

49. Savvidou, I., Bozikas, V.P., Hatzigeleki, S. *et al.* (2003) Narratives about their children by mothers hospitalized on a psychiatric unit. *Family Process*, **42**, 391–402.

21

Psychopathological states in the father and their impact on parenting

Michael W. O'Hara and Sheehan D. Fisher

University of Iowa, USA

21.1 Introduction

The literature on the parenting of mentally ill mothers is abundant, particularly that which addresses depressed mothers. Studies of mothers often begin during pregnancy and extend to the teenage years of their offspring. In stark contrast is the meager literature on the parenting of mentally ill fathers. There have been numerous reviews that point to this fact and call for more research on the link among psychopathological states in fathers, their parenting, and internalizing and externalizing disorders in their offspring [1, 2, 3]. These recommendations principally address several issues as they bear on fathers' psychopathology and parenting, and child outcomes. First, there have been very few studies of the relation between paternal psychopathology and child outcomes relative to the studies that have addressed maternal psychopathology and its relation to child outcomes [4, 5]. There have been very few studies of the parenting of fathers with mental illness [2]. Finally, there have been even fewer studies of paternal parenting as a mediator of the relation between paternal psychopathology and child outcomes, such as internalizing and externalizing disorders. For example, in a review of the relation between paternal depression and child psychopathology and father–child conflict, there were 17 studies that addressed paternal and child psychopathology and only six studies that addressed paternal depression and parenting and only one of these included toddler-aged children [6]. In sum, there is very little research on the parenting of mentally ill fathers and extremely little research on fathers' parenting of infants. As a consequence, this review briefly addresses issues of prevalence of common paternal psychopathology and what is known about the link between paternal psychopathology and child outcomes, particularly internalizing and externalizing symptoms. Next, we address how depressive symptoms, in particular, may affect parenting. In the next section we review the literature on parenting of infants and toddlers, middle-school-age children and adolescents. In this section we will also address the extent to which paternal parenting mediates the relation between paternal psychopathology and child outcomes for studies where these data are available. Finally, suggestions for future research are made.

21.2 Prevalence of psychiatric disorders in men

Recent World Health Organization data suggest that rates of psychiatric disorder vary across the world, ranging from a 12-month prevalence of 26.4% in the USA to below 10% in Nigeria, Japan and China [7]. Lifetime rates are, of course, much higher. Recent epidemiological studies have not reported separate rates for males and females, but older studies suggest that the 12-month and lifetime prevalence rate for 'any disorder' are similar for men and women [8]. The overall rates are probably somewhat lower for men for internalizing disorders such as depression and anxiety and they are higher for externalizing disorders such as substance abuse, intermittent explosive disorder and antisocial personality [9]. These epidemiological data suggest that children are commonly exposed to psychopathology in their parents; although the exposure to specific disorders does vary by gender of the parent.

Similar to studies that have estimated the prevalence of depression and anxiety disorders in the postpartum period for mothers, there have been several studies that have addressed the same question for fathers. Of course, these studies bear specifically on the exposure of infants to paternal psychopathology. In a very large study in the UK, 4% of fathers (compared to 10% of mothers) exceeded the 'depression' threshold on the Edinburgh Postnatal Depression Scale [10]. In a recent study in Australia, 3.2% of fathers (compared to 7.6% of mothers) met diagnostic criteria for generalized anxiety disorder or panic disorder [11]. These two studies suggest that the rates of depression and anxiety disorders in fathers during the postpartum period are somewhat less than half of what is typically found for mothers. In sum, exposure of infants to parental psychopathology early in life is significant. For example, with approximately 4 000 000 births each year in the United States approximately 150 000 infants are exposed to depressed fathers and about 128 000 infants are exposed to fathers suffering from anxiety disorders. Even more significant is the fact that depression is often present at the same time in new mothers and fathers, leaving the infant without a well parent to buffer the effects of a depressed mother or father's poor parenting [10].

21.3   Paternal psychopathology and child internalizing and externalizing problems

Two recent meta-analyses have addressed the relation between paternal psychopathology and child psychopathology [4, 6]. The results of these two meta-analyses suggest that the effect sizes for the relations between a variety of paternal psychopathologies and child internalizing and externalizing behaviors are small and comparable to that for mothers. For example, the mean effect size linking paternal depression and internalizing behaviors ($r = 0.14$, 31 studies) was nearly the same as the effect size linking maternal depression and internalizing behavior ($r = 0.16$, 78 studies) [4]. Similar findings were obtained for alcohol abuse and externalizing behaviors (fathers, $r = 0.16$, 32 studies; mothers, $r = 0.20$, 13 studies) [4]. Aggregating all diagnoses for mothers and fathers produced comparable results for internalizing problems (fathers, $r = 0.14$, 59 studies; mothers, $r = 0.18$, 94 studies) and externalizing behaviors (fathers, $r = 0.16$, 56 studies; mothers, $r = 0.17$, 90 studies) [4]. Further analyses revealed that maternal influence was most pronounced for younger children and paternal influence was most pronounced for older children. In sum, both maternal and paternal psychopathology are linked to important child behavior outcomes, and psychopathology in mothers and fathers may be differentially important across development, an effect perhaps moderated by changes in parenting responsibilities of mothers and fathers as the child develops from infancy through adolescence.

21.4   How depressive symptoms may affect parenting

There is little question that depressive symptoms interfere with social functioning and that interacting with one's child or adolescent is a key domain of social behavior. To what is a child likely to be exposed if his or her father is depressed? Depressed and anhedonic fathers may be sad and withdrawn and simply be unavailable to their children and take little pleasure in them. This may take the form of isolating behaviors such as watching television or spending excessive time at bars or pubs. The irritability that is common in depression may be associated with difficult social interactions with older children, who may believe that they are responsible for the difficult social interactions they have with a depressed father. Reduced energy and fatigue also diminish the likelihood that fathers will interact in a positive way with their children. Excessive feelings of guilt may lead depressed fathers to overindulge their children or be inconsistent in their discipline. Difficulties in concentrating, memory and decision-making may lead to poor parenting decisions in child care. Examples include leaving a child alone in a bath, not safety proofing a home, forgetting to put a child in a car seat, and leaving dangerous chemicals or medicines in reach of a young child. These potential parenting problems for a depressed father are only a sample of many that may occur and may have a negative impact on the child.

Disorders other than depression, such as substance abuse and antisocial personality, have their own related problems and may place children at risk for physical harm frequently because of the severe nature of the disability associated with these disorders. In sum, there is good reason to believe that the parenting of mentally ill fathers will be compromised by the symptoms they experience. Next we will consider the extant literature on the parenting of fathers with mental illness.

21.5 Paternal psychopathology and parenting

Studies that have addressed the impact of paternal psychopathology on parenting often include children whose ages span a wide range. Nevertheless, studies can be roughly categorized as those that address paternal parenting of infants and toddlers (up to 2 years of age), preschool and elementary-age children (3–12 years of age), and older children and adolescents (8–18 years of age). These groups do overlap but the vast majority of the children in each group do not overlap by age with children in the other age groups. Most of the literature to be reviewed addresses the parenting of depressed fathers and the vast majority of the studies index depression with a self-report measure. As a consequence, most findings in these studies are of the form 'higher levels of depressive symptoms are associated with some parenting behavior'. Alternatively, cut-off scores on self-report measures are used to categorize fathers as, for example, depressed or not depressed. Very little research has been conducted with fathers who have received clinical diagnoses. In sections, where terms such as 'depressed' or 'mentally ill' or 'psychopathology' are used, it is important to understand that they do not necessarily refer to clinical populations in the traditional sense but rather are used to indicate that fathers exceeded some threshold on a self-report measure.

Infants and toddlers

There appears to be only one study in which depressed and non-depressed fathers (based on self-report) were directly observed interacting with their 3- to 5-month-old infants [12]. Fathers were observed interacting with their infants and were rated on numerous behaviors including physical activity, head orientation, gaze, vocalizations, and game-playing, as well as parenting style, including positivity, intrusiveness and warmth in the interactions. There were no behavioral differences between depressed and non-depressed fathers. In fact, depressed fathers interacted significantly more positively with their infants than did depressed mothers [12].

In another study of depression in fathers, a voice recording of depressed fathers (based on self-report) was found to be less reinforcing (in a conditioned attention paradigm) to their 5- to 12-month-old infants compared to non-depressed fathers, a finding similar to that observed for depressed and non-depressed mothers [13]. For depressed and non-depressed fathers, their speech acoustics were not significantly different, so it was not entirely clear what accounted for the outcome differences between depressed and non-depressed fathers. Other studies of fathers and infants have relied on maternal report and found that depressed and alcohol- and drug-abusing fathers report lower engagement and more aggravation in their parenting than well fathers [14, 15]. Finally, in a study examining adherence to pediatric anticipatory guidance recommendations (based on self-report) among parents with 9-month-old infants there was only one significant association between adherence to recommendations and depression among fathers. Depression in fathers (based on self-report) was significantly related to the likelihood of a child being put to bed while awake (a positive behavior) [16]. In one of the few longitudinal studies, alcoholic fathers (based on self-report and interview) showed significantly less warmth in their observed interactions with their 2-year-old children than non-alcoholic fathers [17], but paternal warmth was not related to later child outcomes including self-regulation, social competence and externalizing behavior problems [17].

It is very difficult to draw any conclusions about the parenting of infants by mentally ill fathers because so little work has been done. The few studies do suggest that fathers may be distressed by their depression and experience aggravation with their infants, but there is little evidence for a negative impact on their parenting. The one study with alcoholic fathers does point to a clear behavioral deficit. Whatever the current findings, much more work needs to done to elucidate features of the parenting of mentally ill fathers with infants and toddlers and link them to important developmental outcomes.

Preschool and elementary-aged children

Among preschool and school-aged children the impact of paternal psychopathology is more striking than that for younger children. For example, in a recent study paternal depression (based on self-report) was significantly associated with father–child hostility (among 136 10-year-olds) in the context of laboratory based interactions [18]. Father–child hostility was derived from coding the frequency of behaviors such as anger, irritation, scolding, chastising and insulting behaviors over the course of about 17 minutes during which family members played games and later discussed both positive aspects of family life as well as conflict. Also, father–child hostility mediated the link between paternal depression and children's internalizing and externalizing behaviors [18].

In a large study of 449 fathers, paternal depression level was related to lax and over-reactive parenting, an association which was mediated by the types of attributions made by the father regarding causes (parent vs. child blaming) of child misbehavior [19]. Fathers who tended to blame themselves for child misbehavior were more likely to engage lax parenting; whereas fathers who blamed their child for misbehavior were more likely to engage in over-reactive parenting. In a study of Mexican–American fathers and their 10-year-old children, depressive symptoms were associated with decreased warmth (father and child report) and disciplinary consistency (father report) [20]. Finally, in a study of fathers of 4- to 12-year-old children diagnosed with ADHD, paternal inattention and impulsivity were associated with self-reports of lax parenting and observations of arguing during parent–child interactions [21].

Most of the research on the impact of paternal psychopathology on parenting of school-aged children has focused on depression in fathers and in every study depression was determined by a self-report measure rather than through diagnosis. In every study, higher levels of paternal depressive symptomatology were related to some deficit in parenting such as negative interactions or lax parenting or decreased warmth, leading to a negative emotional climate in the home. Importantly, one study [18] found that paternal behavior mediated significant relations between paternal depression and child outcomes.

Older children and adolescents

There is no clear demarcation across development in what constitutes optimal and impaired parenting of children. As a consequence, parenting of older children and adolescents is considered within this chapter. Moreover, as already noted, the literature on the parenting of mentally ill fathers is meager and the nature of parenting by mentally ill fathers of children across development is informed by a consideration of all of the available literature. Finally, as will become evident, the types of deficits that characterize the parenting of mentally ill fathers do not change substantially as their offspring age.

Among older children and adolescents most of the studies that have addressed paternal parenting have used father or adolescent report of parenting behaviors rather than direct observation. For example, in a study that evaluated adolescents' perception of their fathers' parenting, for boys (but not girls) there was a significant association between paternal depression and anxiety (based on self-report) and higher levels of conflict in their relationship and lower levels of acceptance and control in their parenting [22]. However, paternal depression and anxiety was significantly related to daughters' (but not sons) internalizing and externalizing behaviors. It was not clear whether paternal parenting mediated the relation between parenting and daughters' outcomes.

A recent large-scale study also examined the extent to which paternal parenting mediates the relation between paternal depression and child outcomes [23]. The investigators found that paternal depression (based on self-report) was significantly related to low nurturance, rejection, and less monitoring as reported by the adolescents. Moreover, paternal parenting was found to be a mediator of the relation between paternal depression and child internalizing and externalizing problems [23]. Another recent study, which used paternal reports of parenting, found a significant association (in a negative direction) between paternal depression and a composite measure that reflected autonomy, acceptance and firmness in parenting [24]. The researchers also found that paternal parenting mediated the relation between paternal depression and a composite measure of child adjustment (in a negative direction).

In a study of families with a depressed father or mother (based on self-report) or with no depressed parent, investigators directly observed parents and adolescents interacting [25, 26]. The investigators found that families with a depressed mother displayed less positivity and parent–child interactions that were more negative than that found in families with depressed fathers. However, families with depressed fathers showed a positivity suppression following a positive communication from another family member, a pattern that was not found in families with a depressed mother or no depressed parent. Moreover, families with depressed fathers demonstrated more impaired parent–child communication than families with a no depressed parent. The investigators also found that paternal communication (but not positivity suppression) was a moderator of the relation between paternal depression and depression in the child. Finally, in contrast to a similar study with younger children [19], there was no association between paternal depression (based on self-report) and negative attributions about the behavior of 14- to 18-year-old male and female adolescents (27).

In a study of fathers of anxious adolescents, there were no differences between anxious and non-anxious fathers (based on self-report) with respect to paternal control and rejection during laboratory-based parent–adolescent interactions [28]. Finally, in a large study of fathers with a variety of psychiatric disorders (clinical assessment based on interviews with fathers and mothers) there was no association between any individual disorder and paternal behaviors (reported by mothers and offspring) such as 'low affection toward the child' and 'poor communication with the child'; however, there was a significant association between the number of paternal psychiatric disorders and maladaptive parenting behaviors [29].

Similar to the case for younger children, depressed fathers show deficits in their parenting of older children and adolescents across most dimensions that investigators have studied. Interestingly, in the Bosco *et al.* [22] study, the association between paternal depression and parenting was evident only for boys in the sample. The correlations for the girls were non-significant and for the two of the three correlations much lower than the comparable ones for boys, suggesting that there may be an important gender effect.

21.6 Summary

Across the child's life span from infancy through adolescence, depressed fathers show evidence of suboptimal parenting. This finding is not evident in every study but it does characterize the vast majority of studies. Other forms of psychopathology such as anxiety disorders and substance abuse have been the subject of too few studies to draw any conclusions. What seems to come through most clearly in this research are two dimensions that reflect negativity/positivity and engagement/disengagement in parenting. Examples of these findings include:

- Father–child hostility [18];

- Decreased warmth [20];

- Relationship conflict, low acceptance and control in parenting [22];

- Low nurturance, rejection, less monitoring, low autonomy, acceptance and firmness in parenting [24]; and

- Positivity suppression [26].

These problems or parenting deficits are clearly linked to paternal depression symptoms described earlier in this chapter. Moreover, the evidence from studies in which parenting was evaluated as a mediator in the relation between paternal depression and child internalizing and externalizing behaviors suggests that problematic parenting in the context of depression is at least partially responsible for problematic child and adolescent behavior.

21.7 Research agenda

Research on the parenting of mentally ill fathers is still in its infancy. As noted earlier, the vast majority of the work has been conducted with 'depressed' fathers; however, depression has been indexed by a score on a self-report measure rather than through clinical assessment. Although it is useful to understand the relation between increasing scores on a self-report measure of depression and paternal parenting, findings from these studies do not necessarily generalize to populations of fathers who are experiencing the full syndrome of depression. It will be important to identify populations of fathers who are clinically depressed and include them in parenting studies. The same recommendation applies to anxiety disorders, substance use disorders, and other common forms of psychopathology experienced by men.

A completely barren area concerns the parenting of fathers with personality disorders (e.g. antisocial personality disorder). Personality disorders are chronic rather than episodic, which means that children are likely to be exposed to parenting by a father with a personality disorder from infancy until they leave home. Much like the case of depression, the symptoms of personality disorders almost guarantee a dysfunctional parenting style. In sum, there is a great need for studies of fathers who are experiencing clinical levels of common psychiatric disorders as well personality disorders.

Much of the research reviewed in this chapter points to suboptimal parenting on the part of depressed fathers. Only a subset of these studies relied on direct observation of fathers with their children. This was particularly true in the area of infancy. The nature of observational research with children will be quite different depending on the age of the child. Appropriate parenting also varies with the age of the child. Longitudinal studies would be very welcome, in that they would provide an opportunity to characterize the parenting, for example, of a depressed father from the child's infancy up through middle childhood or adolescence. Characterizing the parenting deficits of depressed or anxious or substance-abusing or personality disordered fathers should inform investigators as to the relative importance to child outcomes of paternal parenting behaviors across the span of infancy to adolescence. Understanding the particular deficits in parenting that characterize different types of paternal psychopathology will inform parenting interventions for fathers. It may be that different types of parenting inventions may be most useful depending upon whether a father is experiencing depression, anxiety, substance abuse, or a personality disorder. Alternatively, there may be no specificity to parenting deficits across different forms of paternal psychopathology, in which case the research task turns to identifying parenting deficits that are common across many different types of psychopathology. As a consequence, it will be necessary to carry out research that includes sufficient numbers of fathers with various disorders so as to be able to characterize similarities and differences in parenting across psychiatric disorders.

Over the past 20 years there has been a significant increase in research on the parenting of mentally ill fathers. Nevertheless, the sentiment expressed by Phares still holds – 'It is time that clinical researchers and clinical therapists stop serving as gatekeepers who prevent fathers' involvement in research and therapy' [1, p. 283]). Whether it is researchers and therapists, or funding agencies, or even fathers themselves, it is critical that clinical researchers more adequately study the ways in which mentally ill fathers parent their children and determine the extent to which this parenting affects the social and emotional development of their children so that new parenting interventions may be developed to assist mentally fathers in their role as parents.

21.8 References

1. Phares, V. (1997) Psychological adjustment, maladjustment, and father-child relationships, in *The Role of the Father in Child Development*, 3rd edn (ed. M.E. Lamb), John Wiley & Sons, Inc., New York, pp. 261–83.
2. Belsky, J. and Jaffee, S.R. (2006) The multiple dimensions of parenting, in *Developmental Psychopathology* (eds D. Cicchetti and D. Cohen), John Wiley & Sons, Inc., Hoboken, NJ, pp. 38–85.
3. Zahn-Waxler, C., Duggal, S. and Gruber, R. (2002) Parental psychopathology, in *Handbook of Parenting, Vol. 4, Social Conditions and Applied Parenting* (ed. M. Bornstein), Erlbaum, Mahwah, NJ, pp. 295–328.

4. Connell, A.M. and Goodman, S. (2002) The association between psychopathology in fathers versus mothers and children's internalizing and externalizing behavior problems: a meta-analysis. *Psychological Bulletin*, **128**, 746–73.

5. Cassano, M., Adrian, M., Veits, G. and Zeman, J. (2006) The inclusion of fathers in the empirical investigation of child psychopathology: an update. *Journal of Clinical Child and Adolescent Psychology*, **35**, 583–89.

6. Kane, P. and Garber, J. (2004) The relations among depression in fathers, children's psychopathology, and father-child conflict: a meta-analysis. *Clinical Psychology Review*, **24**, 339–60.

7. WHO World Mental Health Survey Consortium (2004) Prevalence, severity, and unmet need for treatment of mental disorders in the World Health Organization World Mental Health Surveys. *Journal of the American Medical Association*, **29**, 2581–90.

8. Kessler, R.C., McGonagle, K.A., Zhao, S. *et al.* (1994) Lifetime and 12-month prevalence of DSM-III-R psychiatric disorders in the United States: results from the national Comorbidity Survey. *Archives of General Psychiatry*, **51**, 8–19.

9. Kessler, R.C., Chiu, W.T., Demler, O. and Walters, E.E. (2005) Prevalence, severity, and comorbidity of 12-month DSM-IV disorders in the National Comorbidity Survey Replication. *Archives of General Psychiatry*, **62**, 617–709.

10. Ramchandani, P., Stein, A., Evans, J., O'Connor, T.G. ALSPAC study team. (2005) Paternal depression in the postnatal period and child development: a prospective population study. *Lancet*, **365**, 2201–5.

11. Matthey, S. (2008) Using the Edinburgh Postnatal Depression Scale to screen for anxiety disorders. *Depression Anxiety*, **25**, 926–31.

12. Field, T.M., Hossain, Z. and Malphurs, J. (1999) 'Depressed' fathers' interactions with their infants. *Infant Mental Health Journal*, **20**, 322–32.

13. Kaplan, P.S., Sliter, J.K. and Burgess, A.P. (2007) Infant-directed speech produced by fathers with symptoms of depression: effects of infant associative learning in a conditioned-attention paradigm. *Infant Behavior and Development*, **30**, 535–45.

14. Bronte-Tinkew, J., Moore, K.A., Matthews, G. and Carrano, J. (2007) Symptoms of major depression in a sample of fathers of infants: sociodemographic correlates and links to father involvement. *Journal of Family Issues*, **28**, 61–99.

15. Eiden, R.D. and Leonard, K.E. (2000) Paternal alcoholism, parental psychopathology, and aggravation with infants. *Journal of Substance Abuse*, **11**, 17–29.

16. Paulson, J.F., Dauber, S. and Leiferman, J.A. (2006) Individual and combined effects of postpartum depression in mothers and fathers on parenting behavior. *Pediatrics*, **118**, 659–68.

17. Eiden, R.D., Colder, C., Edwards, E.P. and Leonard, K.E. (2009) A longitudinal study of social competence among children of alcoholic and nonalcoholic parents: role of parental psychopathology, parental warmth, and self-regulation. *Psychology of Addictive Behaviors*, **23**, 36–46.

18. Low, S.M. and Stocker, C. (2005) Family functioning and children's adjustment: associations among parents' depressed mood, marital hostility, parent-child hostility, and children's adjustment. *Journal of Family Psychology*, **19**, 394–403.

19. Leung, D.W. and Slep, A.M.S. (2006) Predicting inept discipline: the role of parental depressive symptoms, anger and attributions. *Journal of Consulting and Clinical Psychology*, **74**, 524–34.

20. White, R.M.B., Roosa, M.W., Weaver, S.R. and Nair, R.L. (2009) Cultural and contextual influences on parenting in Mexican American families. *Journal of Marriage and the Family*, **71**, 61–79.

21. Harvey, E., Danforth, J.S., McKee, T.E. *et al.* (2003) Parent of children with attention-deficit/hyperactivity disorder (ADHD): the role of parental ADHD symptomatology. *Journal of Attention Disorders*, **7**, 31–42.

22. Bosco, G.L., Renk, K., Dinger, T.M. *et al.* (2003) The connections between adolescents' perceptions of parents, parental psychological symptoms, and adolescent functioning. *Journal of Applied Developmental Psychology*, **24**, 179–200.

23. Elgar, F.J., Mills, R.S.L., McGrath P.J. *et al.* (2007) Maternal and paternal depressive symptoms and child maladjustment: the mediating role of parental behavior. *Journal of Abnormal Child Psychology*, **35**, 943–55.

24. Du Rocher Schudlich, T.D. and Cummings, E.M. (2007) Parental dysphoria and children's adjustment: marital conflict styles, emotional security, and parenting as mediators of risk. *Journal of Abnormal Child Psychology*, **35**, 627–39.

25. Jacob, T. and Johnson, S.L. (1997) Parent-child interaction among depressed fathers and mothers: impact on child functioning. *Journal of Family Psychology*, **11**, 391–409.

26. Jacob, T. and Johnson, S.L. (2001) Sequential interactions in the parent-child communications of depressed fathers and depressed mothers. *Journal of Family Psychology*, **15**, 38–52.

27. Chen, M., Johnston, C., Sheeber, L. and Leve, C. (2009) Parent and adolescent depressive symptoms: the role of parental attributions. *Journal of Abnormal Child Psychology*, **37**, 119–30.

28. Bögels, S.M., Bamelis, L. and Bruggen, C. (2008) Parental rearing as a function of parent's own, partner's and child's anxiety status: fathers make the difference. *Cognition and Emotion*, **22**, 522–38.

29. Johnson, J.G., Cohen, P., Kasen, S. and Brook, J.S. (2004) Paternal psychiatric symptoms and maladaptive paternal behavior in the home during the child rearing years. *Journal of Child and Family Studies*, **13**, 421–37.

22

The impact of trauma on parents and infants

Joy D. Osofsky, Howard J. Osofsky and Erika L. Bocknek

LSU School of Medicine, New Orleans, USA

22.1 Introduction

A burgeoning scholarship demonstrates the significant effects of traumatic experiences for young children, predicting delays across domains of development [1, 2, 3]. Young children are traumatized by exposure to violence in their communities or homes [4, 5, 6], natural disasters [7], and abuse and neglect by caregivers [1, 8]. Trauma exposure occurs in many different settings including homes, schools and childcare centers, communities and even hospitals.

Although children who are exposed to trauma are at high risk for numerous poor outcomes, most children will be resilient following exposure to trauma, as resilience does not require something rare or special. Masten [9] describes resilience as 'ordinary magic'. The greatest threat to resilience in young children after exposure to traumatic events is the concomitant disruption or destruction of adaptive systems that typically provide nurturance and protection for children. When parents are exposed to trauma, their own experiences of fear, helplessness and hopelessness may impair their ability to provide the protection children need to feel secure [2, 10].

Young children depend on parents and other adults in their environment for support and, therefore, when traumatic events occur, it is crucial to support adults so that they can work to nurture their children and restore adaptive systems for them [11]. For this reason,

Parenthood and Mental Health: A Bridge between Infant and Adult Psychiatry   Sam Tyano, Miri Keren, Helen Herrman and John Cox
© 2010 John Wiley & Sons, Ltd

a multisystemic approach to intervention is often effective in ameliorating symptoms of trauma in young children and their families [12]. Given the need to support both young children and their caregivers after traumas, early identification of risk and implementation of interventions greatly improves the likelihood of positive outcomes. Yet, identification of traumatic exposure and risk factors may be difficult, especially in young children where developmental issues play an important role. In this chapter, we will describe work with traumatized, abused and neglected young children which focuses on prevention and early intervention to minimize risk and increase potential. We will first focus on the problem of abuse and neglect and then on other traumatic exposure, particularly that with which we have been dealing since Hurricane Katrina.

22.2 The problem of abuse and neglect

Worldwide, approximately 40 million children less than 15 years of age are abused [13]. Often physical violence in the home is accompanied by psychological violence such as insults, name-calling and other types of emotional abuse [14]. Only 25 countries have prohibited the use of corporal punishment in the home [15], and cross-cultural research indicates that children in poor health, females, unwanted children, and children born in conditions of rapid socio-economic change are at higher risk for maltreatment [16].

Every year, in the USA, approximately one million cases of child abuse and neglect are substantiated [17]. Forty-five percent of these children are under the age of 5, comprising the largest percentage of maltreated children. Studies conducted in China [18], Australia [19] and Italy [20] similarly demonstrate that young children may be at higher risk for maltreatment as compared to older children. In 2006, more than 100,000 children under the age of 3 entered the child welfare system in the USA [21]; children under the age of 5 are the largest cohort entering the system as 43% of all children entering the system are birth to age five [22]. Not only do infants and toddlers make up almost one half of all admissions into the child welfare system in the USA but, once they are in care, young children remain longer and are more likely to be abused and neglected [8]. Lengthy stays in out-of-home care are particularly detrimental to young children who lack a meaningful understanding of 'temporary' versus 'permanent' [23]. Further, there is greater vulnerability for young children as a result of maltreatment. Children under age 4 account for 79% of child fatalities, and children under age 1 account for 44% [18]. Worldwide, the statistics are similar with the highest child homicide rates occurring among children, ages 0–4 [24].

Research shows that children who suffer maltreatment have multiple poor outcomes including developmental delays, physical health problems and emotional delays [25, 26, 27]. Developmental delays are four to five times greater for abused than non-abused children with, not unexpectedly, a much higher incidence of behavioral problems and risk for mental health problems [28, 29]. Data indicate that one in five children who have been abused or neglected have a diagnosable mental health disorder [30]. Similar comprehensive data are not available for very young children in specific, but research consistently demonstrates notable symptomatology among maltreated young children including dysregulation and impairment in stress response systems [31, 1]. The youngest children may in fact be at even higher risk than their older counterparents for developmental and emotional problems, with one study [32] estimating that rates of such problems occurred in 76–92% of their sample of children ranging in age from birth to 60 months old.

Children who are exposed to domestic violence may be particularly vulnerable for psychological consequences as the very people who are supposed to protect them contribute to their vulnerability [33]. Indeed, specific risks to young children who experience abuse and neglect include the trauma of the violence itself and the disruption of the attachment system, a crucial component of early development. Compounding family stressors include poverty, mental illness and substance use, which often predict abuse potential, and unmet medical needs, which are often co-morbid with abuse and neglect among young children [34]. As they grow older, these children are at higher risk than non-abused children for problems in school and behavioral problems including increased aggression, depression and disruptive and risk-taking behaviors. Alarmingly, half of all children who are maltreated experience such problems.

Significant increases in child protection referrals worldwide have compelled child welfare systems in many countries to consider best policy and practice for intervention [35]. Researchers in the UK discuss the importance of adopting a systemic approach to intervention by noting the high risk for recidivism, particularly among parents of young children [36]. In Australia, scholars advocate cross-sectoral partnerships as a key component of successful child welfare prevention and intervention service provisions [37].

Work that the first author has done in juvenile courts in North America with abused and neglected children and their families provides the opportunity for intervention and systems change with the objective of breaking intergenerational cycles of abuse and neglect affecting maltreated infants and young children [38, 39, 40]. Frequently, young children who are abused and neglected as they grow older repeat the neglectful and abusive patterns, resulting in intergenerational abuse and neglect. The Miami Court Team Project, a collaborative effort between Judge Cindy Lederman, Dr Joy Osofsky and Dr Lynne Katz, has provided an opportunity for establishing an effective, evidence-based early intervention program. The project, which has been extended to other jurisdictions in North America, includes training for judges, lawyers and other court personnel, providing helpful information about the science of early childhood development. Emphasis is placed on increasing judges' knowledge about trauma and the related effects on development as they make decisions that influence the lives of children coming into their courts because of abusive or neglectful parents. This approach provides judges in juvenile and family courts with additional information about developmental needs of infants and toddlers and the value of evaluations and services to provide more information to help in their decision-making about the best interests of the young child. The judges' decisions can help break the intergenerational cycle of trauma that these children experience and give both the parents and children a chance for a healthy, safe, nurturing future. The project involves coordination of the different systems and agencies that impact on young children who are in court settings due to abuse and neglect which works best with the leadership and convening power of the judge. Finally, the program includes intensive evidence-based training for mental health and outreach providers and implementation of clinical and parenting components.

Outcome data and clinical reports from the program demonstrate a significant decrease in future abuse, increase in successful reunifications and permanency for the children, improved functioning of parents, enhanced developmental outcomes, and satisfaction with parenting. Significant improvements result if the different components of a quality system are implemented collaboratively in a court system [40, 41, 38, 42]. As anticipated, positive outcomes are more likely if the parents referred to the program are able to comply with their case plan goals with the support of a coordinated provider response. For such a program to be successful, it is crucial to build capacity through collaborative efforts with the courts and training of professionals to help them gain expertise in infant and early childhood mental health, health, early intervention, child welfare and early childhood education.

22.3   Other trauma exposure in young children

The manifestation of traumatic exposure in young children is a function of age and developmental phase and is strongly influenced by the child's limited perceptual, cognitive and linguistic abilities [10]. Post-traumatic stress disorder (PTSD), including re-experiencing, avoidance and hyperarousal, has been shown to occur in young children in varying degrees and form with manifestations that are somewhat different from those of older children [43, 44]. For example, young children re-experience the traumatic event, but are more likely to show their reactions through changes in play, new fears, regressive behaviors and frightening nightmares. Young children are also likely to engage in avoidant behaviors similar to older children. Young children can become withdrawn, emotionally restricted and numb, and lose interest in play. Young children may demonstrate regression, reverting to behaviors from an earlier development stage, such as thumb sucking and clinging; regression may include the loss of previously acquired self-care, language, or motor skills [44]. Symptoms of increased arousal may be manifested through exaggerated startle responses, irritability, hypervigiliance and physiologic deregulation [43]. Following a trauma, preschoolers are more likely to engage in irritable, impulsive and aggressive behaviors.

The Diagnostic Classification System for young children (DC:0-3R) was developed in an effort to help mental health and other professionals enhance their ability to prevent, diagnose and treat mental health problems in infants, toddlers and young children [45]. To aid in understanding and diagnoses, crosswalks are available to DSM-IVR and ICD-9 (e.g. [46, 47, 48]).

For over a decade, the LSUHSC child trauma team and the Louisiana State University Health Sciences Center (LSUHSC) Harris Center for Infant Mental Health have provided trainings, extensive evidence-based evaluations, and prevention and intervention services for young children exposed to trauma. Beneficial results have been found in children's development and functioning, through our work strengthening the relationship between child and caregiver. In our extensive work with young children and families traumatized by Hurricane Katrina, we have found considerable increases in post-traumatic stress symptoms among young chidren as well as increases in parents asking for help for their children. Infants and toddlers' reactions to trauma resonate with those of their caregivers [10], further emphasizing the importance of systemic interventions such as Child Parent Psychotherapy [49, 50]. Parents' unresolved responses to trauma prevent their ability to provide support and protection for their children [51], a particular concern in traumatized populations. The parent–child relationship is the most important context for healthy early development, particularly in the context of risk, when predictable and loving care provided by a parent to his or her child buffers the effects of stressors and vulnerabilities [50].

In the first year following Hurricane Katrina, parental reports on the National Child Traumatic Stress Network Hurricane Assessment and Referral Measure [52] indicated that 35% of young children had symptoms sufficient to meet the cut-off for referral for further evaluation and/or mental health services. Many parents also requested services for their children and themselves. Outreach training programs and collaborative services provided in re-opening schools, preschools, Head Start, Early Head Start, and childcare programs were well received and helpful in reducing symptoms, supporting developmental growth, and meeting family and caregiver needs. Yet, as expectable, considerable needs remained in the most devastated areas of the region in years 2 and 3, given the extent of the devastation and complexities of the recovery.

22.4 Lessons learned

For prevention and early intervention, it is essential to raise awareness by providing immediate and ongoing education and training about trauma and the effects on infants and young children to service providers across systems that serve young children and their families. This education and training is applicable in a wide variety of settings including young children who have been traumatized by abuse and neglect, community violence, domestic violence, war, as well as nature disasters, all of which impact not only on the young child but also impact their caregivers and the community. The goal is to work toward the development of a coordinated system that focuses on social, emotional, and behavioral well-being for children under 6 years of age. From a preventive mental health perspective, child and family mental health needs are a crucial component of child-serving systems.

Scholars in many countries such as New Zealand, Finland and Japan identify the importance of mental health and wellness among infants and toddlers in the context of healthy caregiving relationships, noting how significant the early years are to lifespan mental health and wellness [53, 54, 55]. However, at present, at least in the USA, children under age 6 are seldom identified by primary care providers or childcare providers as needing mental health services, with a concomitant scarcity of referrals to mental health programs. The stigma associated with mental health problems and the fear of 'labeling' children at such a young age are powerful reasons for this situation, as is limited knowledge about the developmentally grounded mental health needs of infants and young children. These obstacles can be addressed by providing more accessible consultation, assessment, prevention, and therapeutic services in ecologically acceptable settings, including homes, childcare centers, schools, family resource centers and community centers.

It is also crucial to recognize that intervention and services will be most effective by addressing the parent–child relationship. Research underscores the cross-cultural implications of the attachment relationship [56, 57]. Focus must be placed both on the young child's symptoms, behaviors, or regulatory problems and the parent or caregiver, so that the relationship which is so crucial for healthy development will be strengthened. The work of our programs with traumatized young children are strength-based, emphasizing resilience rather than weaknesses and problems [9]. By emphasizing resilience in development, we also follow Selma Fraiberg's important perspective that 'working with young children is a little bit like having God on your side!'

It is essential to learn ways to prevent difficulties by intervening as early as possible, during the prenatal period when risk is identified, in newborn nurseries with nurses and hospital visits, and through active, consistent home-visiting programs. Pediatricians and health-care providers need to be educated on 'red flag' behaviors indicating possible trauma exposure in pediatric clinics and emergency rooms in order to refer young children who may be traumatized or need mental health evaluation and services. By focusing on the needs of our most vulnerable citizens, young children, we can prevent human tragedy and also save immeasurable human and financial costs for the repair and rehabilitation that may be needed for traumatized children later in their lives.

22.5   References

1. Dozier, M., Manni, M., Gordon, M.K. *et al.* (2006) Foster children's diurnal production of cortisol: An exploratory study. *Child Maltreatment*, **11** (2), 189–97.
2. Osofsky, J.D. (1995) The effects of exposure to violence on young children. *American Psychologist*, **50** (9), 781–88.
3. Osofsky, J.D. and Fenichel, E. (1994) *Caring for Infants and Toddlers in Violent Environments: Hurt, Healing, and Hope.* Zero to Three Press, Richmond, VA.
4. Bogat, G.A., DeJohnge, E., Levendosky, A.A. *et al.* (2006) Trauma symptoms among infants exposed to intimate partner violence. *Child Abuse and Neglect: The International Journal*, **30** (2), 109–25.
5. Levy-Shiff, R., Hoffman, M.A. and Rosenthal, M.K. (1993) Innocent bystanders: Young children in war. *Infant Mental Health Journal*, **14** (2), 116–30.
6. Vig, S. (1996) Young children's exposure to community violence. *Journal of Early Intervention*, **20** (4), 319–28.
7. Osofsky, J.D., Osofsky, H.J. and Harris, W. (2007) Katrina's children: Social policy considerations for children in disasters. *Social Policy Reports*, **21**, 3–19.
8. Wulczyn, F., Hislop, K. and Harden, B. (2002) The placement of children in foster care. *Infant Mental Health Journal*, **23**, 454–75.
9. Masten, A.S. (2001) Ordinary magic: Resilience processes in development. *American Psychologist*, **56** (3), 227–38.
10. Osofsky, J.D. (ed.). (2004) *Young Children and Trauma: Intervention and Treatment.* Guilford Press, New York.
11. Masten, A.S. (9 June 2009) *Trauma and Resilience in Children: Practical Lessons.* NCTSN Learning Center. Accessed at http://learn.nctsn.org.
12. Appleyard, K. and Osofsky, J. D. (2003). Parenting after trauma: Supporting parents and caregivers in the treatment of children impacted by violence. *Infant Mental Health Journal*, 24 (2), 111–125.
13. World Health Organization (2001) *Prevention of Child Abuse and Neglect: Marking the links between human rights and public health.* Geneva: World Health Organization.
14. United Nations Committee on the Rights of the Child (2006) Convention on the Rights of the Child. Accessed 17 February 2010 at http://www.unhchr.ch/tbs/doc.nsf/0ac7e03e4fe8f2bdc125698a0053bf66/6545c032cb57bffc12571fc002e834d/$FILE/G0740771.pdf.
15. Global Initiative to End all Corporal Punishment of Children (2009) Ending legalised violence against children: Global report 2009. Accessed 17 February 2010 at http://www.endcorporalpunishment.org/pages/pdfs/reports/GlobalReport2009.pdf.
16. Finkelhor, D. and Korbin, J. (1988) Child abuse as an international issue. *Child Abuse and Neglect: The International Journal*, **12** (1), 3–23.
17. Report from US Department of Health and Human Services Administration on Children, Youth, and Families (2005) Washington, DC.
18. So-kum Tang, C. (1998) The rate of physical child abuse in Chinese families: A community survey in Hong Kong. *Child Abuse and Neglect: The International Journal*, **22** (5), 381–91.

19. Broadbent, A. and Bentley, R. (1997) *Child Abuse and Neglect Australia 1995–96 (Child Welfare Series No. 17)*. Australian Institute of Health and Welfare, Canberra, Australia.

20. Bardi, M. and Borgognini-Tarli, S. M. (2001). A survey on parent-child conflict resolution: Intrafamily violence in Italy. *Child Abuse and Neglect: The International Journal*, 25 (6), 839–853.

21. Center for Family Policy and Research (2009) State of Child Welfare in America. Accessed 31 March 2009 at http://mucenter.missouri.edu/statechildwelfare09.pdf.

22. U. S. Department of Health and Human Services (2008) Child welfare outcomes 2002–2005: Report to Congress. Accessed 17 February 2010 at http://www.acf.hhs.gov/programs/cb/pubs/cwo05/cwo05.pdf.

23. American Academy of Pediatrics Committee on Early Childhood, Adoption and Dependent Care (2000) Developmental Issues for Young Children in Foster Care. *Pediatrics 105* (5), 1146.

24. World Health Organization (2006) Global estimates of health consequences due to violence against children: Background paper to the UN Secretary-General's study on violence against children. Accessed 31 March 2009 at http://www.violencestudy.org/IMG/pdf/English.pdf.

25. Chernoff, R., Combs-Orme, T., Risley-Curtiss, C. *et al.* (1994) Assessing the health status of children entering foster care. *Pediatrics*, **93** (4), 594–601.

26. Dale, G., Kendall, J.C. and Stein-Schultz, J. (1999) A proposal for universal medical and mental health screenings for children entering foster care, in *The Foster Care Crisis: Translating Research into Policy and Practice* (eds P.A. Curtis, G. Dale and J.C. Kendall), University of Nebraska Press, Lincoln, NE, pp. 175–92.

27. Hochstadt, N.J., Jaudes, P.K., Zimo, D.A. and Schachter, J. (1987) The medical and psychosocial needs of children entering foster care. *Child Abuse and Neglect: The International Journal*, **11** (1), 53–62.

28. Dore, M. (2005) Child and adolescent mental health, in *Child Welfare for the Twenty-First Century: A Handbook of Practices, Policies, and Programs* (eds G. Malon and P. Hess), Columbia University Press, New York, pp. 148–72).

29. Leslie, L., Gordon, J.N., Lambros, K. *et al.* (2005) Addressing the developmental and mental health needs of young children in foster care. *Developmental and Behavioral Pediatrics*, **26** (2), 140–51.

30. Mills, C., Stephan, S.H., Moore, E. *et al.* (2006) The president's new freedom commission: Capitalizing on opportunities to advance school-based mental health services. *Clinical Child and Family Psychology Review*, **9**, 149–61.

31. DeBellis, M.D. (2005) The psychobiology of neglect. *Child Maltreatment*, **10** (2), 150–72.

32. Halfon, N., Mendonca, A. and Berkowitz, G. (1995) Health status of children in foster care: The experience of the Center for the Vulnerable Child. *Archives of Pediatric and Adolescent Medicine*, **149** (4), 386–92.

33. Koenen, K.C., Moffitt, T.E., Caspi, A. and Taylor, S. (2003) Domestic violence is associated with suppression of IQ in young children. *Development and Psychopathology*, **15**, 297–311.

34. Vig, S., Chinitz, S. and Shulman, L. (2005) Young children in foster care: Multiple vulnerabilities and complex service needs. *Infants and Young Children*, **18** (2), 147–60.

35. Parton, N. and Mathews, R. (2001) New directions in child protection and family support in Western Australia: A policy initiative to re-focus child welfare practice. *Child and Family Social Work*, **6** (2), 97–113.

36. Biehal, N. (2007). Reuniting children with their families: Reconsidering the evidence on timing, contact, and outcomes. *The British Journal of Social Work, 37* (5), 807–823.

37. Tomison, A.M. and Wise, S. (1999) *Community-based Approaches in Preventing Maltreatment.* Melbourne, Australia: National Child Protection Clearinghouse Issues Paper Published by the Australian Institute of Family Studies.

38. Lederman, C.S. and Osofsky, J.D. (2008) A judicial-mental health partnership to heal young children in juvenile court. *Infant Mental Health Journal,* **29**, 36–47.

39. Osofsky, J.D. and Lederman, C. (2004) Healing the child in juvenile court, in *Young Children and Trauma: Intervention and Treatment* (ed. J.D. Osofsky), Guilford Press, New York, pp. 221–41.

40. Osofsky, J.D., Kronenberg, M., Hammer, J.H. *et al.* (2007) The development and evaluation of the intervention model for the Florida infant mental health pilot program. *Infant Mental Health Journal,* **28**, 259–80.

41. Lederman, C. and Osofsky, J.D. (2004) Infant mental health interventions in juvenile court: Prevention for the future. *Psychology, Public Policy, and the Law,* **10**, 162–77.

42. Osofsky, J.D. & Lederman, C. (2006) Healing the Child in Juvenile Court. In J.D. Osofsky (Ed.), *Young Children and Trauma: Intervention and Treatment* (pp. 221–232). New York: The Guilford Press.

43. Blank, M. (2007). Posttraumatic stress disorder in infants, toddlers, and preschoolers. *BC Medical Journal, 49* (3), 133–138.

44. Lieberman, A. and Knorr, K. (2007) The impact of trauma: a developmental framework for infancy and early childhood. *Psychological Annals,* **June**, 416–22.

45. Zero to Three (2005) *Diagnostic Classification of Mental Health and Developmental Disorders of Infancy and Early Childhood: Revised edn (DC: 0-3 R).* Author, Washington, DC.

46. Maine DC 0-3 Committee. (2004) *Crosswalk for DC 0-3 to ICD-9 Diagnosis Coding.* Author, Augusta, ME.

47. Michigan Department of Community Health. (2007) *Crosswalk between Diagnostic Classifications 0-3, ICD 9 CM and DSM IVR.* Author, Lansing, MI.

48. Oklahoma Healthcare Authority Behavioral Sciences Department. (2008) *Oklahoma's crosswalk for DC: 0-3R and ICD-9-CM.* Oklahoma City, OK: Author.

49. Lieberman, A.F. and Van Horn, P. (2004) *Don't hit my mommy: A manual for child parent psychotherapy with young witnesses of family violence.* Zero to Three Press: Washington, D.C.

50. Lieberman, A.F. and Van Horn, P. (2008) *Psychotherapy with Infants and Young Children: Repairing the Effects of Stress and Trauma on Early Attachment.* Guilford Press, New York.

51. Fraiberg, S., Adelson, E. and Shapiro, V. (1975) Ghosts in the nursery: A psychoanalytic approach to the problems of impaired mother-infant relationships. *Journal of the American Academy of Child Psychiatry,* **14**, 378–421.

52. National Child Traumatic Stress Network (2005) *Hurricane Assessment and Referral Tool for Children and Adolescents.* [Electronic version]. Accessed 15 September 2005 at http://www.nctsnet.org/nctsn_assets/pdfs/intervention_manuals/referraltool.pdf.

53. Hirose, T., Teramoto, T., Saitoh, S. *et al.* (2007) Preliminary early intervention study using nursing child assessment teaching scale in Japan. *Pediatrics International,* **49** (6), 950–58.

54. Mäntymaa, M., Puura, K., Luoma, I. *et al.* (2004) Early mother–infant interaction, parental mental health and symptoms of behavioral and emotional problems in toddlers. *Infant Behavior and Development,* **27** (2), 134–49.

55. Masoe, P. and Bush, A. (2009) A Samoan perspective on infant mental health. *Pacific Health Dialog*, **15** (1), 150–84.

56. Rothbaum, F., Kakinuma, M., Nagaoka, R. and Azuma, H. (2007) Attachment and amae: Parent-child closeness in the United States and Japan. *Journal of Cross-Cultural Psychology*, **38** (4), 465–86.

57. Van Ijzendoorn, M.H. and Sagi, A. (1999) Cross-cultural patterns of attachment: Universal and contextual dimensions, in *Handbook of Attachment: Theory, Research, and Clinical Implications* (eds J. Cassidy and P.R. Shaver), Guilford Press, New York, pp. 713–34.

23

Substance problems: bridging the gap between infant and adult

Ilana Crome

Keele University Medical School, UK

23.1 Introduction

Background

It is widely acknowledged that the preschool years are the launching pad for emotional, cognitive, social and physical potential. While this period can be bursting with opportunities, for some it is clouded by vulnerability to stressful factors, which may persist if not recognized and rectified as early as possible. The UK Government has placed considerable emphasis on reducing health inequalities.

One example of stress is the use of substances by parents. Over the last two decades substance use in young people of childbearing age has become increasingly commonplace, although the effects on babies and children were documented centuries ago [1, 2]. Use may be obvious, but it may also be hidden. In the worst-case scenario, substance misuse can kill both the mother and baby and leave families and communities facing emotional and social deprivation. Many live with varying degrees of general and specific psychological and physical effects directly and indirectly related to substance misuse. Certain young women may find themselves especially vulnerable to the use and impact of substances, but ignorance about the benefits of treatment coupled with stigma, prejudice and fear of services deter them from seeking treatment. Bridging the gap between need and improved outcome is essential.

Parenthood and Mental Health: A Bridge between Infant and Adult Psychiatry   Sam Tyano, Miri Keren, Helen Herrman and John Cox
© 2010 John Wiley & Sons, Ltd

What is a drug?

In the context of this chapter, the term 'drug' will be used to cover psychoactive substances that can affect mood, cognition, perception and consciousness itself. Licit substances, such as alcohol and nicotine, and illicit substances, including central nervous system depressants such as opiates and opioids (e.g. heroin and methadone), stimulants (e.g. cocaine, crack-cocaine, amphetamine and ecstasy) and cannabis, LSD, khat and magic mushrooms are included. Street use and non-compliant use of prescription drugs such as benzodiazepines and non-compliance in the use of over-the-counter preparations such as codeine-based products (e.g. cough medicines, decongestants) are also involved. The use of combinations of licit and illicit substances, prescribed and over-the-counter medications, which may result, is known as polypharmacy or polydrug misuse. Patients may borrow, share or steal drugs, may not report all the medications they are using, may use outdated medications, or may inadvertently take substances that interact. Patients may intentionally use medications for purposes other than those intended. Lack of judgement, limited awareness of the effects of drugs, no funds to purchase suitable medications, confusion about medication regimes and inappropriate storage of drugs due to disorganized lifestyle can be dangerous for children living in a household where substances are consumed.

What is addiction?

In order to decide what treatment options are most appropriately matched to severity, it is vital to distinguish non-dependent substance misuse from dependent (addictive) use. Three of the following criteria are required to make a diagnosis of dependence (or addiction) for both the International Classification of Diseases (ICD 10) [3] and the Diagnostic and Statistical Manual of the American Psychiatric Association (DSM IV) [4]:

- Compulsion or craving, i.e. a strong desire to take the substance
- Tolerance, i.e. needing more of the substance to get the same effect
- Difficulties in controlling the use of substances
- A withdrawal symptom when substance use is reduced or stopped
- Relief of withdrawal by substance use
- Persistent use, despite evidence of harmful consequences
- Neglect of interests and an increased amount of time taken to obtain the substance or to recover from its effects.

23.2 The prevention and policy framework

Tension exists between the need to protect the child and the desire to attract families into supportive treatment and it is difficult to find the right balance. The policy context demonstrates that there are many potential preventive and treatment 'interventions', including medical, psychiatric, socio-economic and political measures. Some may be implemented before the substance misuser ever experiences a 'problem', for example education and advice, increased price of alcohol or reduction in the supply of drugs. For some the intervention has to come at a crisis point.

Since 2004 in the UK there have been a range of policy initiatives that partially or directly focus on the needs of the pregnant substance misuser and her family and that recognize that the substance misuser functions in a social network. For example, the new Drugs Strategy in the UK [5] focuses on families and communities, following a range of other influential policy documents published by the government and other agencies, related to substance misuse, pregnancy, families and children, including involving the 'voices' of children, carers and families of substance-misusing women. Readers are referred to books and reviews that provide more detail [1, 2, 6, 7].

23.3 Epidemiology: the magnitude of the problem

Background

In the UK, it has been estimated that up to 1.3 million children are affected by alcohol problems and approximately 300 000 live in households where one or both parents have serious drug problems [8, 9, 10].

Substance use in young women

Prevalence rates vary substantially in different countries and regions and in different ethnic groups [6]. Definitions of substance use, techniques for screening assessment and diagnosis, and the time frame under consideration (e.g. lifetime, previous year or previous month usage) may differ. Studies may be conducted in the general population or in a range of clinical settings (e.g. obstetric, psychiatric, primary care), which affects the findings.

Illicit drug use

Use starts early. Approximately one third of 15-year-olds admit to illegal drug misuse in the past year and a quarter continue to use on a monthly basis.

While 7% of females aged 16 to 59 reported use of any illicit drug in the past year in 2006/2007, in the 16–24 age group use of 'any drug' was 24% or 1.5 million [11]. Men more commonly report use, and from 1998 to 2006/2007 the use of any drug in the past year by males and females decreased. Young people between 20 and 24 years old use approximately twice as many Class A illicit drugs as 16- to 19-year-olds. Fortunately, there are some recent indications that drug use is declining [12]. However, international studies confirm that about one fifth to one quarter of women in younger age groups have used illicit drugs in the past year.

Alcohol

Around 25% of the UK population drink above safe recommended limits, but abstention rates are consistently higher among women than men. The UK has a relatively low abstention rate (14%, compared with 38% in the USA) [6]. However, drinking among young women is increasing and the consumption of many is in excess of the sensible drinking benchmarks. The proportion of women drinking above the weekly benchmark of 14 units has nearly doubled, from 10% in 1988/1989 to 17% in 2002/2003, yet there has only been a 1% increase among men. Among young women aged 16 to 24, this has more than doubled from 15% in 1988/1989 to 33% in 2002/2003 and rates of heavy alcohol use have increased by 50% [13, 14].

Nicotine

There was a fall in the overall prevalence of cigarette smoking between 1998/1999 and 2004/2005 from 28% of people aged 16 and over to 25%. However, in 2004/2005, 26% of men and 23% of women were cigarette smokers, narrowing the gender gap. It is higher among 20- to 24-year-olds than in any other age group in Great Britain. In 2004, 7% of boys aged 11 to 15 in England were regular smokers (that is, they usually smoked at least one cigarette a week), compared with 10% of girls. This has obvious implications for the future.

Substance misuse in pregnancy

Illicit drug use

Several US and Australian studies have reported on substance use in pregnancy. The American National Pregnancy Health Survey found that 5.5% of pregnant women were using any illicit drug, consistent with another US study that showed 5.2% of pregnant women to be using illicit drugs and an Australian survey that reported any illicit drug use in 6% of pregnant women (for details of sources, see Crome and Ismail [2] and Crome and Kumar [6]).

Alcohol

Alcohol exposure varies from 2% to 25% depending on stage of pregnancy, definition of exposure, diagnostic classification and method of assessment. A recent Swedish study reported 'risky' use of alcohol during the first six weeks of pregnancy at 15% [15], while a Norwegian study demonstrated similar findings: binge drinking was reported in 25% during the first six weeks of pregnancy [16]. The behavioral risk factor surveillance system survey in the USA reported that approximately 10% of pregnant women aged 18 to 44 used alcohol and approximately 2% engaged in binge drinking (five or more drinks on one occasion) or frequent use of alcohol (seven or more drinks per week) [17].

Moreover, an Australian national survey revealed that 47% of pregnant and/or breastfeeding women were using alcohol up to six months post-partum [18].

Nicotine

In industrialized countries, between 20% and 30% of pregnant women report smoking [19]. Although studies have demonstrated that anything between 10% and 50% of pregnant smokers quit at some stage during pregnancy, in the UK an estimated 27% of pregnant women continue to smoke throughout pregnancy [20]. While up to a quarter of women who smoke before pregnancy are likely to stop before their first antenatal visit without professional help, a further 10% are likely to stop following their first antenatal visit. However, the majority of those who do not quit prior to becoming pregnant continue to smoke.

The time course of substance misuse in pregnancy

That up to 15% of women may be using alcohol, about 5% may be using illicit drugs and 27% may continue to smoke during pregnancy is confirmed by a recent report in the USA [21]. While many women reduced their use of alcohol, cigarettes and illicit drugs in the third trimester, a sizable proportion were past-month users of alcohol (19%), cigarettes (21%) and marijuana (4.6%) in the first trimester and one in seven women used cigarettes in the second and third trimesters. In addition, many women resumed their substance use rapidly after childbirth. Within the first three months of the child's life five times the number of women were drinking (32%), ten times were binge drinking (10%), 1.5 times were smoking (20%) and 2.5 times (3.8%) were using marijuana as compared with during the third trimester. By 18 months, cigarette use was almost as high as pre-pregnancy use, as was alcohol use. This has important ramifications for screening and detection in obstetric units and for future treatment.

Mortality

The mortality associated with alcohol and drugs is between 9 and 16 times higher than in the general population [22]. Injecting drug users have a mortality rate that is 12 to 22 times greater than that of their peers (see Crome *et al.* [1]) and age-standardized alcohol-related death rates for women aged 25 to 44 have tripled over the last 30 years [7].

Substance misuse is a very strong predictor of completed suicide In England and Wales: 33% of inpatient suicides have a history of alcohol misuse and 30% a history of drug misuse, while 41% of suicides in the community have a history of alcohol misuse and 28% a history of drug misuse [23].

The Confidential Enquiry into Maternal Deaths in the UK (2000–2002), which looked into all deaths up to one year from delivery, reported that 8% were caused by substance misuse [24]. The most recent report (2003–2005) stated that deaths related to substance misuse have more than doubled [25].

23.4 Health and welfare: context and consequences

Why do people use?

There are a host of 'reasons' why people use substances: because they like the positive effects, for curiosity, because of boredom, to improve mood, or to get intoxicated. With more regular use, dependence may develop, sometimes very rapidly (e.g. cocaine, nicotine) and then substance use controls withdrawal symptoms. Psychiatric co-morbidity may lead to initiation or continuation of use. Influences such as availability, price, social acceptability, religious and cultural diversity, legal regulation and implementation of criminal justice policies have a bearing on the type of substance used, route and level of use and effect. In an extensive review of risk factors in young drug users, the most consistent evidence revolved around family interaction [26].

Parental discipline, family cohesion and parental monitoring were important predictors. Some aspects of family structure, e.g. siblings of a similar age, parental divorce and having young parents, were associated with substance misuse, as were peer pressure and drug availability. The prenatal environment (e.g. maternal substance use during pregnancy and at birth), as well as genetic factors, may interrupt attachment processes. Improving the general social environment of children and supporting parents may be effective strategies to prevent substance misuse in young people [27].

Physical health effects on the mother and father

The effect of substances on the physical and psychological health of the mother is well documented and is beyond the scope of this chapter, so some key considerations will be highlighted [28, 29, 30]. It is necessary to establish whether recent substance use (including the type, quantity, route and time course of use) may have an overt or covert physical and psychological symptomatology. Even where the incidence of serious adverse effects is low, the unpredictability of these events makes the health consequences significant.

Some of the negative impact may be acute and may present as a medical emergency, e.g. confusion, or even coma, as a result of intoxication. Some may be cumulative, e.g. cancer as a result of smoking tobacco or drinking alcohol. Crack-cocaine use may result in cardiovascular incidents such as hypertension, tachycardia, cardiac failure and myocardial infarction, and smoking crack-cocaine may result in bronchitis and pulmonary edema. Injecting and sharing drug equipment (opiates, cocaine, amphetamines) may lead to infections and transmission of blood-borne viruses (HIV, hepatitis C) and bacterial infections (tetanus, staphylococcus aureus). Trauma may occur as a result of alcohol intoxication (falls, accidents, violence). Intravenous drug users are at increased risk of cellulitis, phlebitis, thrombosis, endocarditis, septicemia, septic osteomyelitis and, importantly, difficult intravenous access. Overdose (whether intentional or accidental) and other forms of self-harm are strongly associated with substance misuse, as discussed earlier. Liver and gastrointestinal disorder, deficiency syndromes, infertility, and bone and muscle disease are some of the physical complications of alcohol misuse.

Psychological effects

Substance misuse can lead to virtually every psychological symptom and psychiatric disorder, or alternatively may result from psychological symptomatology or disorder. Anxiety, depression, psychosis, paranoia, traumatic stress disorder, confusional states, delirium tremens, cognitive impairment, impulsivity, aggression and disinhibition, eating disorders and personality disorder are related to substance misuse. Co-morbid conditions might constitute up to 75% of some clinical populations [31]. Females are more likely to report a co-morbid psychiatric condition (especially depression or borderline personality disorder), while males are more likely to suffer from antisocial personality disorder [32]. Patients with co-morbid conditions have poorer prognoses, encounter greater difficulty in accessing appropriate support and are more costly to treat than those with a single diagnosis because of their associated physical and social problems [33]. This is has serious consequences for the pregnancy and for the family.

Withdrawal syndromes

Once the individual has become dependent on a substance, a specific withdrawal syndrome will develop if access to the substance is withdrawn. This is often associated with craving and results in further substance use to curtail the unpleasant effects of withdrawal. In its most severe form, alcohol withdrawal leads to delirium tremens, which may occasionally be fatal. Withdrawal from stimulants leads to depression and even to suicidal behavior. Withdrawal from sedative hypnotics may lead to a confusional state, even if the dose is quite low. Infants may suffer from neonatal withdrawal after delivery.

Impact of the development of dependence

Using record linkage methodology, Burns *et al.* confirmed that births in drug misusers (opioids, stimulants or cannabis) occurred in women who were younger, had a higher number of previous pregnancies, were indigenous, smoked heavily and were not privately insured [34]. These women also presented later to antenatal services and were more likely to arrive at hospital without having been booked in. Neonates were more likely to be premature and to be admitted to the neonatal intensive care unit and special care nursery.

Behaviors associated with substance misuse, such as drug-seeking and a preoccupation with obtaining substances to the extent that other interests and obligations (e.g. family, occupational and social roles) are neglected, result in social disintegration. Therefore, the social context, whether predisposing to substance misuse or consequential, cannot be ignored. Parents with chronic drug addiction spend considerable time and attention on accessing and using drugs, which reduces their emotional and actual availability for their children. A chaotic lifestyle, homelessness, social isolation, deprivation, criminal activity, victimization, abuse, violence, unsafe sex, sexual exploitation, sexual abuse and prostitution may ensue. These difficulties can lead to disengagement from families, communities and services [35].

This combination of sometimes erratic and volatile behaviors does not make for the optimal environment in which to conceive or raise a child. Despite this, substance misusers should not automatically be stereotyped as poor parents. Services prefer to work together to retain the integrity of the family if this is feasible, by engaging the family in treatment and support.

Health of the fetus, neonate and infant

Miscarriage, ectopic pregnancy, preterm labour, antepartum hemorrhage and placental abruption are recognized features when expectant mothers are substance misusers. Babies may have congenital abnormalities, restricted growth, be still born, and experience fetal distress and sudden unexplained death. Neurodevelopmental delay may occur.

Opiates, stimulants, alcohol and sedative-hypnotics may lead to neonatal withdrawal syndrome, which may necessitate admission to a special care baby unit. Gastrointestinal disturbances, high-pitched cry, irritability, hyperactivity and hyper-reflexia, feeding and sleeping disturbance, autonomic hyperactivity, and convulsions characterize the neonatal abstinence syndrome.

If mothers smoke cigarettes, babies may be born prematurely, have intrauterine growth restriction and be of low birth weight, small for gestational age with a small head circumference, and have digital abnormalities, cardiac septal defects, oral clefts and cyanotic episodes, while cannabis use may lead to shorter gestation and low birth weight. Cocaine leads to placental abruption, growth restriction, cerebral infarction and neonatal necrotizing enterocolitis, and methamphetamine leads to growth restriction, while opiates produce growth restriction, preterm delivery, and preterm rupture of membranes.

Alcohol may lead to abortion, fetal distress, microcephaly, growth restriction, orofacial clefts, low APGAR scores, cognitive dysfunction, poor visual acuity, and behavioral and neurodevelopmental abnormalities. A specific syndrome (i.e. fetal alcohol syndrome [FAS]) may be found in 0.5–3.0 births per 1000 in the US population, although worldwide the estimate is 0.33 per 1000 live births. If FAS is combined with alcohol-related birth defects then the number rises to 10 per 1000 births or 1% of all births. Stratton *et al* [36] have developed detailed diagnostic criteria.

In a 14-year follow-up study, Streissguth *et al.* [37] identified dose response effects of prenatal alcohol exposure on neurobehavioural attention, speed of information processing and learning function at 14 years. There is no conclusive evidence of adverse effects on either growth or IQ at levels of consumption below 120 g (15 units) per week. However, Day and Richardson [38] note a linear relationship between growth and alcohol use below one drink a day. Nonetheless, despite lack of certainty regarding the immediate, short- and long-term effects of alcohol on the fetus and later development, it is recommended that women be careful about alcohol consumption in pregnancy and limit themselves to no more than one standard drink per day [39]. This contrasts with the UK Department of Health, which advised that women should not drink during pregnancy [40], though 'the minimum safe levels' of drinking during pregnancy have not been established [40, 41].

Longer-term development

Since substance use in parents is frequently associated with mental, physical and social problems, it sometimes impossible to disentangle whether these undesirable effects are a direct result of the substances or are due to the difficulties related to social adversity. Long-term developmental neurocognitive, physical and psychosocial effects resulting from *in utero* exposure to opioids and other drugs are poorly understood. Children of mothers who smoke display ADHD [42] and, in one study, exhibited five-month delay in reading, mathematics and general ability [43]. There is some evidence that prenatal cocaine use is associated with specific cognitive impairment at 4 years old. Prenatal exposure to cannabis is a significant predictor of intelligence test performance at age 6 [35, 44].

The adolescent pregnant substance misuser

Given the escalation of substance use in young women over the last decade, particular concerns revolve around the teenage pregnant substance misuser, who may be at grave risk of psychosocial disadvantage. Her background may feature substance-misusing parents, family disharmony, traumatic early life events such as bereavement and abuse, mental illness and self-harm, poor education, unstable accommodation and criminal justice involvement [45].

23.5 Assessment and treatment: uniting families

Practitioners working with substance misusers need not only to be aware of the relationship of a history of substance misuse to presenting physical or psychological problems, but also of the fact that this combination of disorders results in poorer treatment compliance and outcome.

Screening and assessment

A cornerstone of treatment intervention is assessment of the nature and extent of substance misuse in the mother and father, so that problems can be recognized and support provided. Substance misuse is rarely a 'stand alone' issue – it tends to come embedded in a social matrix, which requires a coordinated response.

There are a variety of instruments, some of which have been modified for and/or tested in pregnant substance misusers, but nothing can substitute for a detailed history. The CAGE questionnaire, Alcohol Use Disorders Identification Test (AUDIT) and the TWEAK questionnaire have been identified as optimal for use in antenatal settings [46]. The AUDIT-C (a brief version of the AUDIT) [47] and the T-ACE (a modified version of the CAGE questionnaire) [48] have proved useful in pregnancy. The use of biological markers, though helpful in the detection of alcohol use in pregnancy, requires more development [49].

Assessment and the relationship to intervention: getting it right

This general protocol is adapted from one developed for nicotine dependence and is a useful way to formulate the assessment process because it translates into specific management plans [50].

Phase 1 – Ask

- Ask all patients about all substance use and misuse.

- Differentiate between substance use, harmful use and dependence.

- Conceptualize assessment as ongoing.

- Record the information.

- Be aware of, and sensitive to, the ambivalence substance-misusing patients may feel.

- Be non-judgemental and act in a non-confrontational way, since this can be a powerful determinant of both the extent to which relevant information is elicited and engagement with the therapeutic process.

Phase 2 – Assess

- Assess the degree of dependence.

- Educate patients about the effects of substances.

- Inform mothers and fathers about withdrawal symptoms.

- Make some assessment of the level of motivation or 'stage of change' at which the patient may be.

- Suggest what the 'goals' may be for a particular patient at a particular stage (e.g. abstinence or harm reduction).

- Negotiate treatment choices and appropriateness (e.g. pharmacological interventions, the need for referral or admission to specialist services).

- Clinical manifestations of the condition may impair the history-taking process (e.g. neurocognitive dysfunction).

- Follow an assessment schedule.

Phase 3 – Advise

- Continue the assessment within a brief five- to ten- minute 'motivational interviewing' framework.

- Provide the patient with the opportunity to express their anxieties and concerns.

- Offer personalized feedback about clinical findings, including physical examination and laboratory tests.

- Outline and discuss the personal benefits and risks of continued substance use, e.g. drinking and 'safe' levels of drinking.

- Provide self-help materials (e.g. manuals).

Phase 4 – Assist

- Provide support and positive expectations of success.

- Acknowledge loss of confidence and self-esteem as a result of failed attempts.

- Suggest that, if the goal is abstinence, a 'quit date' be set, so that the patient can plan accordingly (e.g. get rid of any alcohol or drugs in the house) and safely (is it safe to stop drinking abruptly or not?).

- Work through a range of alternative coping strategies, including the identification of cues that might help distract the patient.

Phase 5 – Arrange

Be prepared to refer or organize admission to a specialist or appropriate unit if the patient:

- is in severe withdrawal, or is likely to develop severe withdrawal, including delirium tremens;

- is in unstable social circumstances;

- is severely dependent;

- has a severe comorbid physical and/or psychiatric illness, including suicidal ideation;

- is using multiple substances;

- has a history of frequent relapse.

Psychological interventions and treatment of psychiatric conditions: rebuilding the rift between parents and child

There are various treatment options, the choice of which depends on the nature and extent of the problem and which approach may appear more appropriate and suitable for a particular drug user. These include non-directive counseling and cognitive behavioral, family, group, individual, motivational enhancement and social network behavioral therapies. Motivational enhancement has become very popular and evidence is accumulating about its benefits and cost-effectiveness [1, 28, 29, 35, 51, 52].

There is a vast literature on the benefits of psychological therapies for substance misusers in general. National Institute for Health and Clinical Excellence (NICE) guidelines and health technology assessments have been undertaken or are being developed on both substance misuse and pregnancy (see http://www.nice.org.uk/) and the reader can access the wealth of evidence online.

Psychiatric disorder

In the most comprehensive review to date, Tiet and Mausbach [53] considered both psychological and pharmacological treatments for substance misuse in association with depression, anxiety, schizophrenia, bipolar disorder and severe mental illness. Fifty-nine studies met the standards for inclusion, of which 36 were randomized controlled trials. There was not clear evidence of superiority of any intervention over the comparison treatment for both psychiatric disorder and substance misuse and treatments were not replicated. However, the review did demonstrate that effective treatments for psychiatric conditions tended to reduce psychiatric symptomatology and effective treatments for substance misuse tended to reduce substance use. The value of 'integrated' treatment was not substantiated [33].

Strengthening families

Recent studies that focus on the effectiveness of active support for families and developing social skills and competence in parents and children are of relevance (see Academy of Medical Sciences review [27]). The Iowa Strengthening Families Program [54] and Preparing for the Drug Free years [55] are examples. These programs are introduced before substance misuse has commenced and should promote positive parenting by raising parental awareness regarding the child's needs, supporting joint activities between parent and child, enhancing educational opportunities and care facilities for children, acting as a catalyst to encourage supervision by parents, and identifying high-risk children so that help is available for parents.

23.6 Specific interventions for pregnant substance misusers

The following section summarizes the relatively few studies that have been undertaken specifically on pregnant substance misusers. It is important to note that studies focus on the treatment of the mother rather than that of the father.

Illicit drug use

Opiates/opioids

Methadone treatment as part of a comprehensive package of care for pregnant heroin users has been shown to improve birth outcomes and maternal psychosocial function [56].

Cocaine

A study on pregnant indigent women using crack pointed to improved treatment retention when specialized interventions were provided [57].

Alcohol

Brief interventions lasting about an hour have been recommended as the first step in approaching people with mild-to-moderate alcohol problems. Pregnant women are generally motivated to change their behaviors and only infrequently have severe alcohol problems [58]. A trial for early alcohol treatment in women of childbearing age demonstrated a significant treatment effect when two 15-minute physician-delivered counseling sessions were provided. Both seven-day alcohol use and binge drinking were reduced at 48 months [59].

In a recent study, 304 pregnant women were assigned either to receive a single session of a brief intervention or to be in a control group. Results indicated that the women with the highest levels of drinking had the greatest reductions in drinking when they received the brief intervention, the effects of which were much greater when a partner participated [60].

The Protecting the Next Pregnancy Project intervenes with women who were identified as drinking during their last pregnancy so as to reduce alcohol use during future pregnancies. Women not only drank significantly less than those in a control group during their later pregnancies, they also had fewer low birth weight babies and fewer premature deliveries [58]. Moreover, children born to women in the brief intervention group had better neurobehavioral performance at 13 months when compared with control group children.

A randomized clinical trial using a motivational intervention in women exposed to alcohol and at risk of pregnancy has promising findings, though follow-up was only for one month [61].

Nicotine

Pregnant women should be advised of the harms associated with substances, including those related to second-hand and environmental smoke. Support should also be given to those patients who have managed to quit spontaneously. A meta-analysis of 64 trials involving 20 931 women showed that a smoking cessation program in pregnancy reduces the proportion of women who continue to smoke, as well as low birth weight and preterm births [19]. However, the studies could not detect reductions in perinatal mortality or in very low birth weight. Smoking interventions resulted in a 20% reduction in preterm births and low birth weight and an absolute difference of 6% in the proportion continuing to smoke in late pregnancy. The use of contingency management, a voucher-based incentive scheme, promoted abstinence for 24 weeks post-partum [62]. There were barriers to implementation of effective interventions in terms of medical settings (e.g. lack of trained personnel to undertake interventions) and the impact of partner substance misuse [63].

23.7 Pharmacological treatments for pregnant substance misusers

Detailed coverage of specific treatment regimes and the supporting evidence is beyond the scope of this chapter. However, many guidelines may be consulted (see http://www. nice.org.uk/) [64, 65]. Several NICE guidelines are under development for alcohol dependence and substance misuse and mental illness.

Pharmacological treatments may be used for stabilization, detoxification, reduction, maintenance and relapse prevention, in addition to treatment for psychiatric disorder or physical problems [64, 66]. Most of these treatments can be administered in the community with close supervision, but some patients may need to be admitted to hospital or to a rehabilitation unit. These decisions are clinically complex, especially in the pregnant user, and are related to degree of dependence, polysubstance misuse, social stability, medical contra-indications and support network. The treatment must be individualized to the patient's needs. The benefits must, where possible, be weighed against the potential risks, which the patient, partner and family must appreciate. Currently, 'good practice' must encompass prescribing within a comprehensive care plan.

Pharmacotherapies are available to treat a variety of situations, such as:

- Emergencies, e.g. overdose, fits, dehydration, hypothermia, delirium tremens.
- Detoxification and withdrawal syndromes, e.g. lofexidine, methadone, buprenorphine, chlordiazepoxide.
- Substitution, e.g. methadone, buprenorphine, nicotine replacement therapy.
- Relapse prevention, e.g. naltrexone, acamprosate, disulfiram.
- Treatment of vitamin deficiency.
- Co-morbid psychiatric disorders, e.g. depression, anxiety, psychosis.
- Co-morbid physical disorders, e.g. HIV, hepatitis C, diabetes, hypertension.

Illicit drug use

Opiates/opioids

Methadone treatment as part of a comprehensive package of care for pregnant heroin users has been shown to improve birth outcomes and maternal psychosocial function [2, 61]. However, although methadone has been used safely for many years, it lacks a licence for this use in the UK, and the risks must be explained to parents. If possible, detoxification should be avoided in the first trimester and carried out very cautiously in the third. Methadone maintenance treatment improves outcomes in that it decreases illicit opioid use, maternal mortality and morbidity, criminality, drug-seeking behavior, prostitution, sexually trans-mitted diseases and incidence of obstetric complications. It increases fetal stability and ensures improved compliance with obstetric care [67].

At this stage it is not clear whether there is any advantage in using buprenorphine rather than methadone, but a number of small-scale studies have been undertaken [68, 69, 70, 71]. The most recent study reported that buprenorphine is not inferior to methadone on neonatal abstinence syndrome and neonatal and maternal safety in the second trimester of pregnancy. However, despite considerable progress in engaging and retaining pregnant substance users in treatment, illicit use and its subsequent complications should not be downplayed [72] and, therefore, the use of contingency management as an adjunct has been promoted [73]. In the USA, buprenorphine is advantageous as it can be dispensed by prescription, rather than at federally certified methadone clinics [74].

Stimulants and cannabis

There is no evidence that substitution is effective and safe for stimulants and there is no pharmacotherapy for cannabis.

Alcohol

There is no research data available specifically for pregnancy. Good practice involves in-patient admission for detoxification so that the mother can be carefully monitored, since severe withdrawal is potentially fatal. Treatment with benzodiazepines should probably be kept to a minimum. If an alcohol-dependent mother delivers while in withdrawal, the fetus may suffer from withdrawal symptoms. Vitamin B (thiamine) replacement should be considered to avert Wernicke-Korsakoff's syndrome. Since there is no information about the safety or effectiveness of acamprosate, disulfiram and naltrexone in pregnancy, it is advisable not to prescribe these medications.

Nicotine

Clinical trials in non-pregnant smokers indicate that forms of nicotine replacement therapy (NRT) such as nicotine gum, patches, inhalers and nasal sprays are similar in efficacy and that they double quit rates compared with placebos [75]. A recent study has shown that cigarette smoking during pregnancy poses a greater risk than nicotine alone [76]. NICE approves the use of NRT in pregnancy, so long as the patient seeks a medical recommendation [77]. The lowest dose necessary should be prescribed so as to avoid harm to the fetus. The formulation that best suits the patient should be chosen and pharmacotherapy should be initiated as early as possible during the pregnancy, once it is clear that psychosocial treatments are not effective. On the basis of Benowitz and Dempsey's review [76], NRT should be used in combination with behavioral therapy. Therefore, although NRT is likely to be safer than smoking, a study is underway to produce direct evidence and investigate effectiveness [78]. There are no trials of bupropion in pregnancy and it is best avoided at present, as advised by NICE.

23.8 Catalysing change by implementation of research: service models

Since women who are at risk of poor health outcomes are least likely to approach services, integration of agencies can promote entry. While these include the health services (including addiction, child and adolescent and adult psychiatry, general medicine, obstetrics, pediatrics, midwifery, health visitors and others), these are not the only agencies. Other statutory agencies, such as social services (for education, training, employment, housing), criminal justice and the voluntary sector, are essential components [35]. A collaborative network should be activated through a common strategy so that duplication and, most importantly, gaps are avoided. Though protocols and pathways, conforming to NICE guidelines where feasible and encompassing national policies (e.g. the Children's and Young People's National Service Framework), must allow for flexibility, this arrangement must also be sustainable and inherently developmental. Therefore, resources for staffing, facilities and training are key features, which are not optional but vital.

A triage or stepped approach has been conceptualized to manage multiprovider, multi-agency and multidisciplinary services. Universal services would be provided for those at low risk, such as early booking, regular assessment and education and support about parenting skills, child development and health lifestyles, including substance use, diet and exercise. At the next level, specific advice for smoke-free homes and support for smoking cessation and assessment and treatment for drug and alcohol problems would be provided. Other specialist medical antenatal and social care, for example, for teenagers or those with mental health needs and physical illness (e.g. diabetes) would be initiated. For those at the highest risk of complex problems, intensive highly specialized care would be coordinated, which might include in-patient admission for alcohol detoxification or arrangements for rehabilitation. Peer volunteers and user involvement should allow individual, cultural, socio-economic and behavioral considerations to be taken into account. More cohesive families and safer communities are likely to result.

23.9 Conclusion

Nowadays, some degree of substance misuse in pregnancy is to be expected. Many of the factors that predispose to or emanate from substance misuse are also related to adversity and poor outcomes for infants, parents, families and communities. However, if substance misuse is detected early and treated collaboratively in a multidisciplinary context, interventions are likely to have a ripple effect far beyond the mother or father. At stake is the chance to mitigate the range of inequalities, allowing the child normal attachment and the potential for development.

Key messages

- Substance use in pregnancy is to be expected.

- Substance use is associated with considerable morbidity and mortality, as well as social adversity and inequalities.

- Substance misusing parents are not necessarily poor parents.

- Effective interventions are available for most forms of substance misuse.

- Improving resources for this often marginalized group must include training professionals.

- Services should be coordinated in a multidisciplinary and multi-agency framework.

- Despite the tension between child protection and supporting parents, every effort must be made to deliver effective interventions to families so that inequalities are minimized and normal attachment is maximized.

- More research on specific innovative interventions delivered at vulnerable periods during pregnancy and up to at least two years postnatally is required.

23.10 References

1. Crome, I., Ghodse, H., Gilvarry, E. *et al.* (2004) *Young People and Substance Misuse.* Gaskell, London.
2. Crome, I.B. and Ismail, K.M.K. (in press) Substance misuse in pregnancy, in *De Swiet's Medical Disorders in Obstetric Practice*, 5th edn (eds R. Powrie, M. Greene and W. Camann), Blackwell Publishing, Oxford.
3. World Health Organization (1992) *International Classification of Diseases 10 (ICD-10).* World Health Organization, Geneva.
4. American Psychiatric Association (1994) *Diagnostic and Statistical Manual IV.* American Psychiatric Association, Washington DC.
5. HM Government (2008) *Drugs: Protecting Families and Communities – The 2008 Drugs Strategy.* COI, London.
6. Crome, I.B. and Kumar, M. (2007) Epidemiology of drug and alcohol use in young women. *Seminars in Fetal and Neonatal Medicine*, **12**, 98–105.
7. Henshaw, C., Cox, J. and Barton, J. (2009) *Modern Management of Perinatal Psychiatric Disorders.* RCPsych Publications, London.
8. Prime Minister's Strategy Unit (2004) *Alcohol Harm Reduction Strategy for England.* Cabinet Office, London.
9. Advisory Council on the Misuse of Drugs (ACMD). (2003) *Hidden Harm.* Home Office, London.
10. Advisory Council on the Misuse of Drugs (ACMD). (2007) *Hidden Harm – Three Years On: Realities, Challenges and Opportunities.* ACMD, London.

11. Murphy, R. and Roe, S. (2007) *Drug Misuse Declared: Findings from the 2006/07 British Crime Survey* (Home Office Statistical Bulletin 18/07). Home Office, London.

12. Frisher, M., Martino, O., Crome, I. *et al.* (2009) Trends in drug misuse recorded in primary care in the United Kingdom from 1998 to 2008. *Journal of Public Health*, **31**, 69–73.

13. Office for National Statistics (2003) *General Household Survey 2003*. Office for National Statistics, London.

14. Office for National Statistics and Department of Health (2004) *Statistics on Alcohol, England 2004*. Office for National Statistics and Department of Health, London.

15. Magnusson, A., Goransson, M. and Helig, M. (2005) Unexpectedly high prevalence of alcohol use among pregnant Swedish women: failed detection by antenatal care and simple tools that improve detection. *Journal of Studies on Alcohol*, **66**, 157–64.

16. Alvik, A., Heyerdahl, S., Haldorsen, T. *et al.* (2006) Alcohol use before and during pregnancy: a population based study. *Acta Obstetrica et Gynecologica Scandinavica*, **85**, 1292–98.

17. Centers for Disease Control and Prevention (CDC). (2008) Behavioral Risk Factor Surveillance System. At http://www.cdc.gov/brfss (accessed 20 July 2009).

18. Turner, C., Russell, A. and Brown, W. (2003) Prevalence of illicit drug use in young Australian women: patterns of use and associated risk factors. *Addiction*, **98**, 1419–26.

19. Lumley, J., Oliver, S.S., Chamberlain, C. *et al.* (2004) Interventions for promoting smoking cessation during pregnancy. *Cochrane Database of Systematic Reviews*, **4**. Art. No. CD001055. DOI: 10.1002/14651858.CD001055.pub2.

20. Owen, L.A. and Penn, G.L. (1999) *Smoking and Pregnancy: A Survey of Knowledge, Attitudes and Behaviour, 1992-1999*. Health Education Authority, London.

21. National Survey on Drug Use and Health (NSDUH) (2009) Substance Use Among Women During Pregnancy and Following Childbirth. At http://www.oas.samhsa.gov/2k9/135/PregWoSubUse.htm (accessed 21 July 2009).

22. Wilcox, H.C., Conner, K.R. and Caine, E.D. (2004) Association of alcohol and drug use disorders and completed suicide: an empirical review of cohort studies. *Drug and Alcohol Dependence*, **76S**, S11–S19.

23. National Confidential Inquiry into Suicide and Homicide by People with Mental Illness. (2006) *Avoidable Deaths*. Centre for Suicide Prevention, Manchester.

24. Lewis, G. and Drife, J. (eds) (2004) *Why Mothers Die 2000-2002: Executive Summary and Key Findings* (The Sixth Report of the Confidential Enquiries into Maternal Deaths in the United Kingdom). RCOG Press, London.

25. Confidential Enquiries into Maternal and Child Health (CEMACH) (2007) *Saving Mothers' Lives: Reviewing Maternal Deaths to Make Motherhood Safer – 2003-2005*. CEMACH, London.

26. Frisher, M., Crome, I., Macleod, J. *et al.* (2007) *Predictive Factors for Illicit Drug Use among Young People: A Literature Review* (Home Office Online Report 05/07). Home Office, London.

27. Academy of Medical Sciences (2008) *Brain Science, Addiction and Drugs*. Academy of Medical Sciences, London.

28. Crome, I.B. and Ghodse, A.H. (2007) Drug misuse in medical patients, in Handbook of Liaison Psychiatry (eds G. Lloyd and E. Guthrie), Cambridge University Press, Cambridge, pp. 180–220.

29. Crome, I.B. and Bloor, R. (2008) Alcohol problems, in *Essential Psychiatry* (eds R. Murray, K.S. Kendler, P. McGuffin *et al.*), Cambridge University Press, Cambridge, pp. 198–229.

30. Crome, I.B., Rumball, D. and London, M. (2004) Health issues, in *Young People and Substance Misuse* (eds I.B. Crome, H. Ghodse, E. Gilvarry *et al.*). Gaskell, London, pp. 101–13.

31. Weaver, T., Madden, P., Charles, V. *et al.* (2003) Comorbidity of substance misuse and mental illness in community mental health and substance misuse services. *British Journal of Psychiatry*, **183**, 304–13.

32. Marsden, J., Gossop, M., Stewart, D. *et al.* (2000) Psychiatric symptoms among clients seeking treatment for drug dependence. *British Journal of Psychiatry*, **176**, 285–89.

33. Crome, I. and Chambers, P. (2009) The Relationship between Dual Diagnosis: Substance Misuse and Dealing with Mental Health Issues (SCIE Research Briefing 30). At http://www.scie.org.uk/publications/briefings/briefing30/index.asp (accessed 20 July 2009).

34. Burns, L., Mattick, R.P., Lim, K. *et al.* (2006) Methadone in pregnancy: treatment retention and neonatal outcomes. *Addiction*, **102**, 264–70.

35. Crome, I.B. and Bloor, R. (in press) Substance misuse and offending, in *Forensic Psychiatry*, 2nd edn (eds J. Gunn and P. Taylor), Hodder Arnold, London.

36. Stratton, K., Howe, C. and Battaglia, F.C. (eds) (1996) *Fetal Alcohol Syndrome: Diagnosis, Epidemiology, Prevention and Treatment*. National Academy Press, Washington DC.

37. Streissguth, A.P., Sampson, P.D., Olson, H.C. *et al.* (1994) Maternal drinking during pregnancy: attention and short-term memory in 14-year-old offspring – a longitudinal prospective study. *Alcoholism: Clinical and Experimental Research*, **18**, 202–18.

38. Day, N.L. and Richardson, G.A. (2004) An analysis of the effects of prenatal alcohol exposure on growth: a teratologic model. *American Journal of Medical Genetics Part C: Seminars in Medical Genetics*, **127C**, 28–34.

39. Royal College of Obstetricians and Gynaecologists (2006) Alcohol Consumption and the Outcomes of Pregnancy (RCOG Statement No. 5). At http://www.rcog.org.uk/files/rcog-corp/uploaded-files/RCOGStatement5AlcoholPregnancy2006.pdf (accessed 21 July 2009).

40. Department of Health (2007) *How Much is Too Much When You're Having a Baby?* Department of Health, London.

41. BMA Board of Science (2007) *Fetal Alcohol Spectrum Disorders: A Guide for Healthcare Professionals*. British Medical Association, London.

42. Mick, E., Biederman, J., Faraone, S. *et al.* (2002) Case-control study of attention-deficit hyperactivity disorder and maternal smoking, alcohol use and drug use during pregnancy. *Journal of the American Academy of Child and Adolescent Psychiatry*, **41**, 378–85.

43. Butler, N.R. and Goldstein, H. (1973) Smoking in pregnancy and subsequent child development. *British Medical Journal*, **4**, 573–75.

44. Goldschmidt, L., Richardson, G.A., Willford, J. *et al.* (2008) Prenatal marijuana exposure and intelligence test performance at age 6. *Journal of the American Academy of Child and Adolescent Psychiatry*, **47**, 254–63.

45. Barnes, W., Ismail, K.M.K. and Crome, I.B. (2008) Teenage pregnant substance misusers. *Midlands Medicine*, **25**, 113–18.

46. Bradley, K.A., Boyd-Wickizer, J., Powell, S.H. *et al.* (1998) Alcohol screening questionnaires in women: a critical review. *Journal of the American Medical Association*, **280**, 166–71.

47. Dawson, D.A., Grant, B.F., Stinson, F.S. *et al.* (2005) Effectiveness of the derived Alcohol Use Disorders Identification Test (AUDIT-C) in screening for alcohol use disorders and risk drinking in the US general population. *Alcoholism: Clinical and Experimental Research*, **29**, 844–54.

48. Chang, G., Wilkins-Haug, L., Berman, S. et al. (1998) Alcohol use and pregnancy: improving identification. *Obstetrics and Gynecology*, **91**, 892–98.
49. Bearer, C.F. (2001) Markers to detect drinking during pregnancy. *Alcohol Research and Health*, **25**, 210–18.
50. Raw, M., McNeill, A. and West, R. (1998) Smoking cessation guidelines for health professionals: a guide to effective smoking cessation interventions for the health care system. *Thorax*, **53**. Supplement 5.
51. Project MATCH Research Group (1998) Matching alcoholism treatments to client heterogeneity: treatment main effects and matching effects on drinking during treatment. *Journal of Studies on Alcohol*, **59**, 631–39.
52. Gossop, M., Marsden, J., Stewart, D. et al. (2003) The National Treatment Outcome Research Study (NTORS): 4–5 year follow-up results. *Addiction*, **98**, 291–303.
53. Tiet, Q.Q. and Mausbach, B. (2007) Treatments for patients with dual diagnosis: a review. *Alcoholism: Clinical and Experimental Research*, **31**, 513–36.
54. Molgaard, V., Kumpfer, K.L. and Spoth, R. (1994) *The Iowa Strengthening Families Program for Pre- and Early Teens*. Iowa State University, Ames IA.
55. Spoth, R., Redmond, C., Shin, C. et al. (2004) Brief family intervention effects on adolescent substance initiation: school-level growth curve analyses 6 years following baseline. *Journal of Consulting and Clinical Psychology*, **72**, 535–42.
56. Lejeune, C., Simmat-Durand, L., Gourarier, L. et al. (2006) Prospective multicenter observational study of 260 infants born to 259 opiate-dependent mothers on methadone or high-dose buprenorphine substitution. *Drug and Alcohol Dependence*, **82**, 250–57.
57. Weisdorf, T., Parran, T.V. Jr, Graham, A. et al. (1999) Comparison of pregnancy-specific interventions to a traditional treatment program for cocaine addicted pregnant women. *Journal of Substance Abuse Treatment*, **16**, 39–45.
58. Hankin, J., McCaul, M.E. and Heussner, J. (2000) Pregnant, alcohol abusing women. *Alcoholism: Clinical and Experimental Research*, **24**, 1276–86.
59. Manwell, L.B., Fleming, M.F., Mundt, M.P. et al. (2000) Treatment of problem alcohol use in women of childbearing age: results of a brief intervention trial. *Alcoholism: Clinical and Experimental Research*, **24**, 1517–24.
60. Chang, G., McNamara, T.K., Orav, E.J. et al. (2005) Brief interventions for prenatal alcohol use: a randomised trial. *Obstetrics and Gynecology*, **105**, 991–98.
61. Ingersoll, K.S., Ceperich, S.D., Nettleman, M.D. et al. (2005) Reducing alcohol-exposed pregnancy risk in college women: initial outcomes of a clinical trial of a motivational intervention. *Journal of Substance Abuse Treatment*, **29**, 173–80.
62. Higgins, S.T., Heil, S.H., Solomon, L.J. et al. (2004) A pilot study on voucher-based incentives to promote abstinence from cigarette smoking during pregnancy and postpartum. *Nicotine and Tobacco Research*, **6**, 1015–20.
63. Stanton, W.R., Lowe, J.B., Moffat, J. et al. (2004) Randomised trial of a smoking cessation intervention directed at men whose partners are pregnant. *Preventive Medicine*, **38**, 6–7.
64. Lingford-Hughes, A.R., Welch, S. and Nutt, D.J. (2004) Evidence-based guidelines for the pharmacological management of substance misuse, addiction and comorbidity: Recommendations from the British Association for Psychopharmacology. *Journal of Psychopharmacology*, **18**, 293–335.

65. Department of Health and the devolved administrations. (2007) *Drug Misuse and Dependence: Guidelines on Clinical Management 2007*. Department of Health, London.

66. Rayburn, W.F. and Bogenschutz, M.P. (2004) Pharmacotherapy for pregnant women with addictions. *American Journal of Obstetrics and Gynecology*, **191**, 1885–97.

67. Burns, L., Mattick, R.P. and Cooke, M. (2006) The use of record linkage to examine illicit drug use in pregnancy. *Addiction*, **101**, 873–82.

68. Fischer, G., Ortner, R., Rohrmeister, K. *et al.* (2006) Methadone versus buprenorphine in pregnant addicts: a double-blind, double-dummy comparison study. *Addiction*, **101**, 275–81.

69. Jones, H.E., Johnson, R.E., Jasinski, D.R. *et al.* (2005) Buprenorphine versus methadone in the treatment of pregnant opioid-dependent patients: effects on the neonatal abstinence syndrome. *Drug and Alcohol Dependence*, **79**, 1–10.

70. Lacroix, I., Berrebi, A., Chaumerliac, C. *et al.* (2004) Buprenorphine in pregnant opioid-dependent women: first results of a prospective study. *Addiction*, **99**, 209–14.

71. Martin, P.R., Arria, A.M., Fischer, G. *et al.* (2009) Psychopharmacologic management of opioids-dependent women during pregnancy. *American Journal on Addictions*, **18**, 148–56.

72. Tuten, M. and Jones, H.E. (2003) A partner's drug-using status impacts women's drug treatment outcome. *Drug and Alcohol Dependence* **70**, 327–330.

73. Jones, H.E., Haug, N., Silverman, K. *et al.* (2001) The effectiveness of incentives in enhancing treatment attendance and drug abstinence in methadone-maintained pregnant women. *Drug and Alcohol Dependence*, **61**, 297–306.

74. Nocon, J.J. (2006) Letter: Buprenorphine in pregnancy – the advantages. *Addiction*, **101**, 608–9.

75. Fiore, M.C., Bailey, W.C., Cohen, S.J. *et al.* (2000) *Treating Tobacco Use and Dependence* (Clinical Practice Guideline). Department of Health and Human Services, Rockville MD.

76. Benowitz, N.L. and Dempsey, D.A. (2004) Pharmacotherapy for smoking cessation during pregnancy. *Nicotine and Tobacco Research*, **6**, S189–S202.

77. NICE (2002) *Guidance on the Use of Nicotine Replacement Therapy (NRT) and Bupropion for Smoking Cessation*. NICE, London.

78. Coleman, T., Thornton, J., Britton, J. *et al.* (2007) Protocol for the Smoking, Nicotine and Pregnancy (SNAP) trial: double blind, placebo-randomised, controlled trial of nicotine replacement therapy in pregnancy. *BMC Health Services Research*, **7**, 2.

24

Foster parenthood

Yvon Gauthier

University of Montreal and Hôpital Sainte Justine, Montreal, Canada

24.1 Introduction

Foster parenthood is a rather recent phenomenon in the history of caring for abused children. We may remember that the problem of affective deprivation was brought to child psychiatry in the 1940s by René Spitz's research on children raised in institutions. His showing the severe developmental problems these children demonstrated in relation to the lack of the constant presence of a mother led to major changes in social policy in Western countries leading to earlier adoption of abandoned children.

Only in the 1960s did pediatricians and child psychiatrists realize that children not only could be abandoned but could also be victims of maltreatment in the hands of their own parents. Such observations made in pediatric emergency gradually led to child protection clinics in pediatric hospitals and later to child protection laws in several countries. Maltreated children can still be sent to institutions in some countries, but the appearance of foster homes can be seen as a result of such policy developments. Recent publications amply show the necessity of improving the foster care system even in developed countries, given the high risk of morbidity and mortality in maltreated children [1]. In this chapter, foster parenthood will be considered for children aged 0 to 3, since the situation with older foster children and adolescents is even more complex.

24.2 Foster children symptomatology

I still remember the day that pediatric colleagues came to me in the early 1990s to discuss their observations of young children placed in foster homes whom they followed in a special clinic which had been developed in our children's hospital in collaboration with protection services. They were worried about the frequent problems they were observing in these children – developmental delays in motor and cognitive spheres, particularly in language; sleeping

Parenthood and Mental Health: A Bridge between Infant and Adult Psychiatry   Sam Tyano, Miri Keren, Helen Herrman and John Cox
© 2010 John Wiley & Sons, Ltd

difficulties; behavior problems; difficulties in social relationships (withdrawal, indiscriminate sociability); frequent hospitalizations for physical ailments – and were wondering about their origin.

These colleagues were actually observing problems which have been described in several publications [2, 3]. We were in the following years frequently exposed to such problems in a clinic we set up to help protection workers deal with these children and their biological and foster families [4].

The question is: how can we understand such a symptomatology? In most countries, the placement of a child is the last resort in child protection, unless severe abuse is observed, in which case placement is immediately decided. Child workers usually spend much time evaluating the parents' parental potential, and putting into place measures to help them develop their abilities. Placement may be decided only after such measures do not appear to be efficient.

Once placement is decided however, the child who arrives in a foster home – unless placement is decided at birth or very early in the first year – may already be symptomatic, having suffered severe negligence or having been the object or witness of violence in his family: there already may exist developmental delays, dysregulation symptoms, even sadness at the loss of parental figures to whom an attachment has been made in spite of maltreatment. They already are difficult children who require from the foster parents an unusual amount of patience and understanding. Many of the children who arrive in a foster home may also have already been submitted to previous, even multiple, placements; those usually are the most difficult children to care for.

The symptomatology we then observe is the product of both the initial deprivation and/or abuse and of a dysfunctional protection system which can be summarized this way: a child is usually placed on a temporary basis, the plan is to send him back to biological parents as soon as possible. But parents do not improve as rapidly as expected, and the placement must continue. Two alternatives are then possible: a reunification is eventually made with the biological parents, but it does not work, parents have not really progressed, and a new placement has to be made, most often in a different foster family. This is where symptoms usually appear. This child cannot easily develop a new attachment, he does not know where he belongs, his symptoms can be a mixture of loss and of testing the new parents to see if he can really come to trust them.

Another possibility is also observed: the initial placement in a foster family has been long enough for a young child to develop a secure attachment to his foster parents. The court may then decide that the biological parents have progressed enough to get their child back. A progressive reunification is then attempted, leading to a strong reaction of the child who feels the loss of his foster parents who have become his 'psychological parents'. This child will often become a most difficult child, especially if the biological parents have not improved enough to be able to deal with him.

The optimal solution can also happily be observed: in face of a biological family that does not improve, the child is kept in the same foster family where he is already securely attached and a decision is made by the court toward permanency: placement to majority or adoption.

24.3 The use of attachment theory

Attachment theory is a most useful instrument to understand these children's needs and their symptomatic reactions to the decisions to which they are submitted. As he comes into this world, an infant is already a social being who needs human figures who are constantly present to answer his fundamental needs, physiological and relational. In the course of the first year this infant will come to feel that he can trust this (these) parental figure(s) who are sensitive to such needs, available especially when distress appears, and able to organize a daily and nightly routine around this developing human being: an attachment system is thus created between this child and his parents.

Whenever this system is severely hampered in its development because of parental dysfunction (severe negligence, physical and/or sexual abuse, conjugal violence, addiction to drugs, etc.), we will already observe behaviors which are manifestations of a disturbed attachment, resistant, avoidant or disorganized: constant search for proximity and comfort, tendency to withdraw into his own world, fear of the adult figure, etc. If a decision has to be made for this child to be placed in a foster home, the transition is usually difficult, because of the symptoms already present – only with a young infant can this transition be easy. The development of trust in the new parental figures will be possible, but often will take time and require special attention from them to the special needs of this disturbed child. If the process of placement has been repeated one or more times, the symptomatic responses already described will be even stronger and the development of trust even more hampered.

24.4 Foster children's special needs

Foster children present with special needs to the foster family. They have been neglected, affectively deprived, are often withdrawn and fearful, and show behaviors that suggest to the foster parents that they don't need care, whereas a special nurturing relationship has to be established to compensate for the deficient care they already have been submitted to. Foster families have to be aware of such realities. It is not by chance however that they are often the object of negative opinions, as if their only concern is not the child, but their own financial interest. Some of them actually fall into what has been described as the 'extended respite model' of foster care [5, 1], where the child is not affectively invested, his basic physiological needs are satisfied, but without the commitment that he deeply requires – and the system often actually tells these families not to let themselves be attached to the child.

In opposition to that type, the 'child-centered care' foster family is described in which we find psychological investment, a real commitment characterized by sensitive caregiving, a child valued as an individual and his needs prioritized. In such a model, we will observe as outcome a child who may improve in all developmental spheres: feeling safe in his family, he becomes securely attached, socially competent and emotionally well regulated. Such outcome is based on the plasticity of the young child's brain and evidently will also be function of the child's age at time of placement and of the severity of his initial symptoms.

Such a family is in the best interest of the child, but it should be realized that this foster family lives a complex dilemma: a woman is asked to invest in a child enough for him to develop a secure attachment, and to reciprocally develop her own attachment to a child without having any certitude of keeping this child, and then have to mourn this child if the biological family is successful in getting better. We often meet foster mothers who find it very difficult to invest a new foster child because of the painful memory of the previous lost child.

24.5 How to help foster parents to provide best care for the fostered child

Foster parents can be very unrealistic in their expectations of a rapid improvement of difficult children, as if only love is going to repair them, and they can feel overwhelmed by the complex behaviors they have to deal with. They have to be supported in their difficult tasks, and several programs have been developed to help them to better care for these children entrusted to them. For instance, in Louisiana, Heller's team [6] have found that these symptomatic children require comprehensive assessment and multidisciplinary intervention, while foster parents need the support of a clinical team. In this program, support takes the form of having foster parents record occurrences of problematic behavior in a diary, from which observations a behavioral program is designed which decreases the symptomatology and much helps to facilitate the relationship between foster child and caregiver. This team also suggests the development of a support and education group, foster parent/foster child playgroup, and interaction guidance following the McDonough technique.

Along the same lines, Mary Dozier and her group in Delaware have been very active in recent years. Inspired by Mary Main's work on the parent's attachment history through the Adult Attachment Interview and its influence on her child's quality of attachment to her, they examined the correspondence between foster mothers' state of mind and their foster children's attachment quality [7]. They then came to describe the specific problems foster parents have to meet, what they call 'critical needs'. These kids have often developed avoidant behavioral signals – 'I don't need you, I can do it on my own' – which lead nurturing caregivers to react in providing non-nurturing care. Foster parents also may not be comfortable in providing nurturance even though they want to foster difficult children; they often need help in providing a predictable interpersonal environment such that children develop better regulatory capabilities [8], and they particularly need to provide a non-threatening environment to children who often come from families where they have been threatened with abandonment if they did not behave [9].

Their work suggests that secure foster parents are the ones who can best care for these difficult children and their specific needs. Their own inner security seems to be an important variable in their ability to understand the complex signals sent by these very insecure kids. The study on infants placed with autonomous parents and at younger age shows higher and overall level of secure behavior, less avoidant behavior, more coherent attachment strategies compared with non-autonomous foster parents after two months of placement [10]. Following these findings, they developed a program – the Attachment and Biobehavioral Catch-up (ABC) – in which they train foster parents in targeting foster children's critical needs [11, 9]. In a randomized trial with 200 foster families, preliminary results show that foster children in this intervention, compared with the control intervention, had lower cortisol values, and caregivers reported fewer behavior problems for toddlers (18–36 months) than for infants (0–17 months) [12].

In Romania, Zeanah's team has developed an intervention for institutionalized children, comparing a group of still institutionalized children with a group of children placed in a foster home conceived as following the child-centered model, in which special attention is given to social workers and to foster families around the complex symptomatology presented by these kids in the transition to a foster home. In a random assignment of children to either foster care or to continued institutional care, they are reporting significant gains in the cognitive and language spheres for the children in foster care, as well as in attachment symptoms [13].

To summarize this gradual evolution in the care of young foster children, we can say that these difficult children need to be understood with the complex signals they send to their foster parents; they need to be tolerated at the same time that a structured environment will gradually give them a feeling of security. Foster parents on their part need to be better informed and trained to become more committed and efficient parents.

24.6 Kin vs. non-kin foster parents

In recent years a strong tendency has appeared towards placement in kin families rather than in unrelated foster homes, particularly in Britain and in the USA. Placement in a kin family has the definite advantage of sending a child to a person he already knows (grandmother, friend), thus favoring his sense of identity, culture and belonging, and thus decreasing his reaction to the separation from his parents. But social workers, even though they may have strong positive feelings toward kinship care, are usually concerned about a negative tradition of dysfunction within the family, the possibility of collusion and of alliances between relatives and parents or conflict between them, resulting in an increased feeling of risk to the child [14].

It remains essential here that the evaluation of the kin family system be made early in the decisional process so that a child is not transferred from a non-kin foster family to a kin family once an attachment system is already well advanced, thus creating a new loss in the child's life.

24.7 Visits to the biological parents

The question of visits to the biological parents during the early months of placement is often the subject of tension in the protection system. A young child on one hand needs the continuity of a parental figure to develop a secure attachment, and at the same time must continue to see his biological parents to keep their image in his mind, since the plan is for him to reintegrate his family. We often observe the anxious reaction of a child in such visits to his biological family, either because he is afraid of losing this new attachment figure or because the biological parents revive traumatic memories. It is suggested to include the foster mother in such visits so that the child is reassured that she is not going to leave him, but this is not always easy because of the tensions between the two mothers. We have heard foster mothers tell that they would not let the child leave on such a visit without a personal object of hers, as a way of telling him that he will necessarily come back to her. Such visits should be completely forbidden if the child has been traumatized by his biological parents.

24.8 Need for permanency

These observations in a field in which research is still in its early stages amply show how foster parenthood in the early years of a child is a necessary instrument in a situation of maltreatment, but fraught with significant tasks for foster parents and those working with them. The protection system has to deal with the biological parents' rights to be helped in developing or restoring their parental capacities and thus meeting their child's basic needs, make sure that foster parents keep their commitment to these difficult children, and at the same time keep in mind the child's need for permanency in the interest of his global development. Mary Dozier suggests 'that a system of temporary surrogate care simply does not make sense for young children' [15]. Quality of attachment is a most important variable in a child's development and continuity is essential for the development of a secure attachment. One can't repeatedly break the process of attachment within the biological family or a foster family without traumatic sequelae in the child's developmental process. Time in a child's life is very short and a decision toward permanency of affective ties should be made as rapidly as possible in his best interest.

24.9 References

1. Smyke, A.T. and Breidenstine, A.S. (2009) Foster care in early childhood, in *Handbook of Infant Mental Health*, 3rd edn (ed. C.H. Zeanah). Guilford Press, chapter 31, in press.
2. Leslie, L.K., Gordon, J.N., Ganger, W. and Gist, K. (2002) Developmental delay in young children in child welfare by initial placement type. *Infant Mental Health Journal*, **23** (5), 496–516.
3. Stock, C.D. and Fisher, P.A. (2006) Language delays among foster children: implications for policy and practice. *Child Welfare*, **85**, 445–61.
4. Gauthier, Y., Fortin, G. and Jeliu, G. (2004) Clinical application of attachment theory in permanency planning for children in foster care: the importance of continuity of care. *Infant Mental Health Journal*, **25**, 379–96.
5. Zeanah, C.H. (2005) Foster care – is it the solution or the problem for young children? Paper for *Congrès Attachement et Thérapeutique*, Paris.
6. Heller, S.S., Smyke, A.T. and Boris, N.W. (2002) Very young foster children and foster families: clinical challenges and interventions. *Infant Mental Health Journal*, **23**, 555–75.
7. Dozier, M., Stovall, K.C., Albus, K.E. and Bates, B. (2001) Attachment for infants in foster care: the role of caregiver state of mind. *Child Development*, **72**, 1467–77.
8. Dozier, M., Higley, E., Albus, K.E. and Nutter, A. (2002) Intervening with foster infants' caregivers: targeting three critical needs. *Infant Mental Health Journal*, **23**, 541–54.
9. Dozier, M., Lindhiem, O. and Ackerman, J.P. (2005) Attachment and biobehavioral catch-up: an intervention targeting empirically identified needs of foster infants, in *Enhancing Early attachments: Theory, Research, Intervention, and Policy* (eds Berlin L.J., Ziv Y., L. Amaya-Jackson and M.T. Greenberg), Guilford Press, New York, pp. 178–94.
10. Stovall-McClough, K.C. and Dozier, M. (2004) Forming attachments in foster care: infant attachment behaviors during the first 2 months of placement. *Development and Psychopathology*, **16**, 253–71.
11. Dozier, M. and Sepulveda, S. (2004) Foster mother state of mind and treatment use: different challenges for different people. *Infant Mental Health Journal*, **25**, 368–78.
12. Dozier, M., Peloso, E., Lindhiem, O. *et al.* (2006) Developing evidence-based interventions for foster children: an example of a randomized clinical trial with infants and toddlers. *Journal of Social Issues*, **62**, 767–85.
13. Smyke, A.T., Zeanah, C.H., Fox, N.A. and Nelson, C.A. (2008) A new model of foster care for young children. *Child and Adolescent Psychiatric Clinics of North America*, July 2009.
14. Peters, J. (2005) True ambivalence: child welfare workers' thoughts, feelings, and beliefs about kinship foster care. *Children and Youth Services Review*, **27**, 595–614.
15. Dozier, M. (2005) Challenges of foster care. *Attachment and Human Development*, **7**, 27–30.

25

Parenting the chronically ill infant

Barbara G. Melamed

Mercy College, New York, USA

You know, I don't think I'm ever going to accept the fact that my daughter has a life-long and serious illness. On most days, I have learned to come to terms with it, but I cannot accept it. [1]

25.1 Introduction

In recent years in high-income countries, medical technology has made it possible for children born with previously terminal illnesses such as cystic fibrosis or childhood cancer to enjoy increased longevity. Children born prematurely or having very low birth weight (VLBW), who would have died a decade ago, are beginning their lives in neonatal intensive care units (NICUs), often depriving them and their parents of the common bonding that facilitates both physical and social development. Therefore it is crucial to understand the psychological variables, adjustment and the family interactions both as an intervening variable between disability and adjustment and as potential for producing resilience or adverse consequences for the child and the family. In fact, the literature shows an increasing emphasis on family process approaches to understanding influences of chronic illness.[2]

The focus of this chapter is to evaluate which factors lead to vulnerability and which factors are protective of the infant's survival. Although many researchers have lumped chronic illnesses together, this chapter will focus on differences in adjustment in four different populations of children: asthma, congenital heart disease; cystic fibrosis and children of very low birth weight or preterm delivery.

Within these contexts the differences and similarities of the demands of these illnesses with regard to regimens, maintenance of relationships and parent and sibling relations are described. It is also necessary to examine the medical environment and the physicians' style of communication with the families to see the entire context of what dealing with the

Parenthood and Mental Health: A Bridge between Infant and Adult Psychiatry   Sam Tyano, Miri Keren, Helen Herrman and John Cox
© 2010 John Wiley & Sons, Ltd

disease requires. The actual severity and disease characteristics are only one factor in what adjustment to illness may mean. The caregiving for such infants involves communication with medical staff, shared parenting, job responsibilities, attention to other siblings ... a juggling act not easy to manage. At least one research or clinical study in connection with each disease has been described to encourage others on how to evaluate problems, interventions and hopefully prevention of adverse effects.

Extended life does not necessarily increase the quality of life for these children and their families. While recently acknowledging the need to measure quality of life, few measures exist in the area of infancy [2]. In fact, the quality of life as it influences marital quality, children's sibling relationships and adjustment is as important as the day-to-day management of illness symptoms.

First it is necessary to acknowledge [3, 4] that there are numerous problems that can exacerbate stress including:

1 Establishing relationships with medical personnel.

2 Coping with medical procedures associated with treatment.

3 Coping with symptoms associated with the condition.

4 Coping with hospitalization, the possible separation from parents, family members and delay of preschool environments.

5 Coping with new social pressures having a child chronically ill, or siblings who may never be like other children. Siblings may be embarrassed by their sick sibling, feel angry at attention they feel they are deprived of, or even guilty that they do not have the disease.

6 Coping with the limitations that can occur in a change in life style (e.g. diabetic children must change their diets, asthmatic children must exercise caution during physical activity.)

7 Coping with the added burden facing the entire family, including time, money and change in roles. In some cases families can be forced to relocate in order to get the medical care that the child requires.

Most parents during pregnancy say that their wish is not whether the child is boy or girl, but a healthy baby. What then is the reaction to finding out that your child is a preemie, may have Down's syndrome or need postnatal cardiac surgery? The parent may feel everything at once: discouragement, anger, love, guilt, despair and determination.

Even more distressing is finding out that your child suffers a chronic medical condition with all the uncertainties of survival and all the decision-making about how to support the necessary medical and growth needs, both social and physical, of such a child. Particularly first-time and single parents may cope with the news by shock, denial and guilt. They also face grief knowing that they have lost the dreams they have imagined for the life of their child. They tend not to know how to question decisions that are made in their behalf by the medical experts. Paternalism in physician behavior is still a widespread problem. Ethical and legal issues exist but are too extensive to deal with in this chapter.

Some general effects that have been found are that children from 6 months to 3 years separated from their parents due to hospitalizations have poorer attachment relationships. In children who enter life through NICUs during a time of high central nervous system vulnerability, immature regulation of blood–brain barrier, and rapid development of neuronal cytoarchitecture; medical procedures contribute to negative developmental outcomes, including attention, learning and memory problems which persist into childhood and adolescence. The challenge is even greater for involving parents. Fathers, who are often ignored, despite their risk of depression, need to keep the family together and provide financial support, and keep the hope alive that one day this child will be healthy and happy in the family home.

This chapter will focus on four common conditions: asthma, congenital heart disease, cystic fibrosis and very low birth weight infants. The specific issues raised for the family and health professionals with some recommendations for continued course of study and intervention are discussed.

25.2 Asthma

Mother with a child who has severe asthma:

> You can't even count on your own best friends. Even my mother is afraid. I've got to do some shopping and who wants to lug a screaming five-year-old boy through the lingerie department at Macy's. So, I call up Esther, my friend for ten years, and ask if Johnny (my son) can stay with her. Big pause on the phone.
>
> 'Uhh,' she says, 'What if something happens? You know, Lucille, I wouldn't know what to do. You better not leave him with me.'
>
> My mother? Same thing: What if, and What if, What if. I can't stand it. We haven't found a babysitter who would come and stay. We could get a nurse, but we can't afford it. [5].

In a range of high-income countries asthma is the most common disease of childhood. Despite significant advances in medical treatment, asthma morbidity and mortality rates have risen dramatically in the last two decades, especially in minority and socio-economically disadvantaged populations.

Description of the illness

Asthma is a lung disease characterized by airway obstruction, or narrowing that is reversible. Pathologically, it is characterized by a variety of features such as chronic inflammatory disease of the airways, with a granulocyticlympositic submucosal infiltration, epithelial cell desquamation and mucus gland hypertrophy and hyperplasia.

Prevalence

Asthma affects from 4% to 9% of children. As many as 50% of the cases are diagnosed before the child reaches age 2. The highest incidence seems to be from birth to age 4. It is the fastest growing problem in today's environment in several countries including the USA. The increase in outdoor air pollution, and the quality of the indoor environment as a result of exposure to maternal smoking and the high levels of dust mites appear to be relevant. One must also consider genetic factors, such as a positive family history, male sex, and low birth weight, and an increase in sensitization to inhaled allergens, such as their presence in house dust, cat fur and grass pollen.

Treatment

For a parent the management is geared towards relief of obstruction, restoration of oxygenation, and ventilation and prevention of complications. Each time a child has an asthmatic attack the parent fears death and, as the children begin to monitor their own regimens, misunderstanding of correct dosage and schedule, and omission of doses cause many children to be non-adherent. Over-protection by parents with infantilizing and isolating them from peers is common. Parents must work more closely with pediatric practitioners to understand the course of their child's symptoms and the need for action.

Research

In an exemplary prospective study [6], three variables were found useful for predicting asthma onset by age 3: elevated IgE levels measured when the children were 6 months of age, global ratings of parenting difficulties measured when the infants were 3 weeks old, and the higher number of respiratory infections in the first year of life. Maternal asthma and paternal asthma predicted asthma at ages 6 to 8 years when combined with these infancy variables. In a genetically at-risk group of children, psychosocial factors are related to asthma onset and persistence into childhood. The relationships between biological and psychosocial variables in the first year of life and subsequent school problems support formulation of asthma as beginning early in life. Mother's depression when the children were 6 years also contributed to problem behaviors. Parenting difficulties measured at 3 weeks were significantly correlated with 6-year measures of maternal depression. Mothers' ratings on the Child Behavior Problem Checklist showed they rated their children as being higher than population norms on internalizing scores. How much of this shy, withdrawn behavior is actually reinforced by the over-protective parent?

It might be possible to prevent secondary effects of asthma when intervention is directed at parenting difficulties. One study showed that family rituals and routines may protect children with asthma from anxiety-related symptoms [7]. Recommendations include reducing environmental pollutants and decreasing parental uncertainties through education and thoughtful interactions with health-care professionals. Repeated visits to seek emergency health care need to be used as a probe for how well the parent is defining and responding to the seriousness of symptoms.

25.3 Congenital heart disease

They didn't catch it at birth, but when he was about ready to come home from the hospital, he turned black and then that's when obviously there was something wrong. In the beginning, I pointed out to the nurse there several times that his color didn't look right. 'Oh, no, he just has to go to the bathroom or something.' Me and my wife would look and say 'something is wrong.' Then the day we were going to take him home, he turned black, and then that's when he was rushed over here. [8]

Description of the disease

Congenital heart disease (CHD) is one of the most frequent birth defects in children. Affecting approximately one in every 125 babies born around the world, congenital heart defects are the most common birth defect. In the USA twice as many children die each year from a CHD than all forms of pediatric cancers combined. The eight most common defects account for 80% of all congenital heart diseases, while the remaining 20% consist of many infrequent conditions or combinations of several defects. Ventricular septal defect is generally considered to be the most common type of malformation, accounting for about one third of all congenital heart defects.

Since many of these patients with the proper medical intervention lead relatively healthy lives it is important to evaluate the early response of the medical community and the reaction of the parents. Often the parent may learn in advance of delivery that their child may have a high risk of dying due to the abnormality of the heart. A baby's heart begins to develop shortly after conception. During development, structural defects can occur. These defects can involve the walls of the heart, the valves of the heart and the arteries and veins near the heart. Congenital heart defects can disrupt the normal flow of blood through the heart. The blood flow can slow down, go in the wrong direction or be completely blocked.

Advances in medical and surgical treatments over the past decades have led to more than 85% of these infants surviving to adulthood in high-income countries. Most interventions, however, have not been curative and about half of adults with congenital heart disease face the prospect of further surgery, arrhythmia, heart failure or premature death. The burden of pregnancy represents a new challenge in women with congenital heart disease. Annually, hundred of thousands of children worldwide died due to rheumatic fever and rheumatic heart diseases.

Treatment

Sometimes CHD improves with no treatment necessary. At other times the defect is too small to require any treatment. Most of the time CHD is serious and requires surgery and/ or medications. Medications include diuretics, which aid the baby in eliminating water and salts, and digoxin to strengthen the contraction of the heart. Some defects require surgical procedures and in some cases, multiple surgeries to help balance the circulation. Interventional cardiology now offers patients minimally invasive alternatives to surgery.

The treatment depends on the type and severity of the defect and a child's age, size and general health. Today, many children born with complex heart defects grow to adulthood and lead productive lives. Some defects need to be fixed as soon as the baby is born, others can wait. In the rare case of hypoplasias, heart transplant where available is the only solution.

In a questionnaire study [9] of how much information parents had it was found that only 50% knew about the disease as to its cause and hereditary roots. Although many knew about exercise appropriateness, fewer than 44% understood the medication functions and only 4% understood the side effects. Even the need for antibiotic treatment to prevent endocarditis was poorly understood. The parents' occupation and education were determinants of knowledge. The parents rate their children's quality of life (QOL) to be worse than the children themselves do. It may be affected by their expectations for the child and by the fact they have different definitions and understanding of a disease and its consequences for the future. In any case having to watch your child suffer through multiple surgeries and the fear and guilt associated with his or her vulnerability takes its toll on the entire family. Fathers especially experience conflicting feelings when they receive a diagnosis of their infant coping with severe congenital heart disease. They feel the joy of seeing the child born and becoming a father; the sadness and loss associated with the baby's illness; the challenge of becoming a father and becoming attached while dealing with the fears about the infant's vulnerability and potential death; and the need to try to maintain control and remain strong for others while hiding their intense emotions.

Research

Parents of the children with heart disease may experience higher stress levels than parents of children with other diseases, and may feel great stress in relation to such things as dilemmas of normality and social integration. Conflicting responses in the experiences of fathers of infants diagnosed with severe congenital heart disease frequently lead to depression [10]. On the other hand the parents' QOL may be more determined by spouses' satisfaction with each other or parental coping styles than by the child's handicap. QOL including energy, social impact, and physical and emotional factors may be related to financial stresses as well [11]. Studies show that children with CHD show more maladjustment and psychological problems from 2 years till 12 years [12].

Unrestricted parental presence in the NICU, parental involvement in infant caregiving, and open communication with parents are basic tenets of family-centered care [13]. By virtue of their continual presence and role in the NICU, nurses are in a unique position to support family-centered care. However, it was also shown that new nurses were more likely than other nurses in NICU to integrate the parent interaction that would seem necessary to provide for a healthy child within an informed family. In addition, there are often barriers to engaging fathers in NICU.

25.4 Cystic fibrosis

A father with a child with cystic fibrosis:

> There's a real problem in not losing friends. They're the people who end up under-standing and caring. I've lost a lot of acquaintances. For example, a family calls you up and wants to come visit. And you say you'd love to see them but, also ask if any of their kids have a cold. The parents answer, 'Oh sure you know, the ordinary sniffles.' Well ordinary sniffles could kill my kid. So I tell them they can't come over; they don't understand and get angry. [1]

Description of the illness

Cystic fibrosis (CF) is the most common life-shortening and autosomal recessive genetic disease of European and American Children. CF is lethal because of chronic broncho-pulmonary infections. In recent years prognosis of children with CF has improved. However, CF patients are multisynmptomatic, involving pulmonary and gastrointestinal dysfunctions.

Prevalence

Cystic fibrosis is an inherited chronic disease that affects the lungs and digestive system of about 30, 000 children and adults in the USA (70, 000 worldwide). A defective gene and its protein product cause the body to produce unusually thick, sticky mucous. From 1990 to

1992 the proportion of adults among CF patients in the USA increased to 33%, a fourfold increase from 1969. The median survival age was 29.4 in 1992.

The general consequences of malnutrition in CF may include growth failure, increased mortality, delayed puberty, decreased physical well-being and psychological disorders. Short stature and pubertal delay emphasize the differences between patients with CF and their peers, and may result in a greater impact on their quality of life than the longer term issues of compromised survival. Adjustment and self-esteem in patients with CF are less than peers, especially in girls. With intensive, coordinated care in a cystic fibrosis center, outcome and growth may improve independent of improved pulmonary function and normalize in most children with CF.

Growth itself is an important prognostic factor in survival of patients with CF. Analysis of data from 19, 000 patient records of the National Cystic Fibrosis Patient Registry showed that shorter patients are much more likely to die before taller patients. Short stature in CF may be a marker of more severe disease. The problem of worsening growth failure in children and adolescents with CF ironically is compounded by increased survival. As many patients live longer and their clinical symptoms become more severe, nutritional status may worsen, and growth remains impaired. It is important that linear growth be maximized through medical and nutritional intervention. Bone mineralization is decreased and rates of osteoporosis are significantly increased in patients with CF as they age; adults with late-stage CF are at high risk for fractures.

Treatment

The complicated regimen involves enzyme replacement and chest percussions to improve clearance of infected secretions. Its demands on the family are continuous. It also involves close attention to the child's physical condition (e.g. frequency of coughing, energy level, incidence of gastrointestinal complaints and weight). Physical therapy or postural drainage are required. Parents must also deal with their preschool children's distress in dealing with social demands, extreme thinness and the rigors of treatment regimen. Mealtime conflict is ubiquitous. Moreover parents must cope with the fact that their child has a limited life expectancy. Higher levels of parental distress, an avoidant coping style and low levels of family support put parents at risk for chronic, psychological dysfunction [14].

Research studies

The Diagnostic Depression Inventory found that parents with a child of CF less than 9 months of age at baseline had an elevated prospective risk of depression as did fathers. It is also important to consider the diagnostic phases.

A case study [15] of three children who were mildly malnourished demonstrated that a parent treatment program to reinforce better eating did influence important child health functions. The children's parents participated in a behavioral group-treatment program that focused on promoting and maintaining increased calorie consumption. Treatment included nutritional education, gradually increasing calorie goals, contingency management and relaxation training, and was evaluated in a multiple baseline design across four meals. Children's calorie intake increased across meals, and total calorie intake was 32% to 60% above baseline at post-treatment. Increased calorie consumption was maintained at the 96-week follow-up (two years post-treatment). The children's growth rates in weight and height were greater during the two years following treatment than the year prior to treatment. Increases in pace of eating and calories consumed per minute were also observed one year post-treatment. These findings replicated and extended earlier research supporting the efficacy of behavioral intervention in the treatment of malnutrition in children with CF. This type of research could easily be incorporated by clinicians' in their evaluation of individual patients.

It is necessary to monitor parental mood and explore preventive strategies early so the tasks do not overwhelm the family and lead to marital dysfunctions. Now that the genetic studies clearly show who is at risk, early intervention can begin prior to or at birth.

As a group, adults with CF do not demonstrate significant levels of depression, anxiety or other psychopathology. Psychological and psychosocial functioning in patients with CF are similar to that of healthy peers, at least until their disease becomes severe and their physical and social activities become increasingly limited. They may then have an increased risk for psychiatric problems, such as depression, and typically score poorly on physical functioning measures in QOL assessments. Coping styles have a large effect on QOL, and compliance is a complicated problem for many patients. Men may be at higher risk for depression and anxiety, and better lung function predicts less anxiety. Higher level of psychosocial support is a strong predictor of better psychological functioning. Major psychiatric illness may also occur in adults with cystic fibrosis, and both bipolar disorder and paranoia have been reported [16].

25.5 Very low birth weight infants

Description of the illness

Advances in neonatal intensive care have ensured the survival of 85% of VLBW infants and better care. These medically fragile infants remain at high risk for developmental delays, learning difficulties, and emotional and behavioral problems. They are at twice the risk of behavior problems and 2.5 times more likely to develop attention deficit hyperactivity disorder than a child at normal birth weight. These functional deficits persist in adolescence and early adulthood. VLBW children as young adults are more likely to exhibit chronic health problems and poorer academic achievement.

Prevalence

Extremely low birth weight (ELBW) is defined as a birth weight less than 1000 g (2 lb, 3 oz). Most ELBW infants are also the youngest of premature newborns, usually born at 27 weeks' gestational age or younger. Infants born at less than 1500 g are termed very low birth weight. Low birth weight (< 2500 g) was noted in 8.3% of all births in the USA in 2006, and very low birth weight was noted in 1.48% of all births; approximately 63, 137 such US births were reported in 2006.

Treatment

Studies on NICUs have often stressed the importance of support for the new parents. In one study [17], the similarity of maternal distress before discharge of their infants and then at 6 months (corrected age) to post-traumatic stress symptoms was apparent and related to maternal psychological well-being. Intervention to decrease maternal anxiety and improve developmental outcomes in VLBW children was conducted. NICU can be difficult for the infant and mothers. Investigators [18] have demonstrated that interactive maternal behaviors buffered the relationship between high pain-related stress exposure and poor focused attention in mothers who self-reported low concurrent stress.

Field [19] has demonstrated the positive effects of massage techniques. Mothers who were at high risk for preterm babies and were given pregnancy massages showed a reduction in stress, and reduced levels of cortisol, and an increase in the children's' birth weight. It should be possible to have the mothers and fathers participate in this stimulation. Using a breast pump cannot substitute for physical contact on the mother's body. The reluctance of neonatal specialists to allow touch in the risky babies has been tempered by the 47% weight gain of infants receiving this stimulation in the NICU. The babies were also discharged about six days earlier, saving much in the high cost of care of these infants.

The whole issue of how and when to discharge VLBW children is still controversial. While medical technological improvements would allow more at-home care, many parents are not ready or fear that their child might die if they do something wrong. In a study [20] where mothers of babies in NICUs had audiotapes of their conversations with a neonatologist, it was found that recall of information, attitude to and use of tapes, satisfaction with conversations did improve recall of information and psychological well-being. Again, if parents feel heard by their health-care provider they are more likely to be better deliverers of good care for their own offspring.

Intervention is targeted at parental sensitivity and maternal psychological distress as two important factors influencing development in VLBW children. Mothers who feel depressed have lower parental sensitivity and more intrusive parenting behavior in children's infancy and the infants show more internalizing behavior problems and poorer cognitive development at 24 months of age [21].

Research

A prospective study [22] looked at how characteristic of infants (i.e. birth weight and perinatal illness severity), mothers (anxiety level and level of education), and the social context (maternal received and perceived helpfulness of support) related to mother–child interaction at 3 and 6 months of age. Mothers who were better educated and less anxious at 3 months and reported higher perceived support were more sensitive and responsive to their infants in teaching interaction at 9 months.

A study [23] to evaluate coping in mothers whose 2-year-old children were born either at full term or at VLBW, found that stress was higher in the mothers of the VLBW babies because they understood the association between low birth weight and significantly higher than normal risk of mortality and various adverse outcomes. In caring for these children the families must deal with economic hardship, disruptions of work and household routines and the daily hassles of caring for a child with chronic illness, neurological deficits and developmental delays. About one third of mothers of VLBW children suffer from increased parenting distress and significant psychological stress, which may hinder the child's development.

Turning our attention to what helps these mother cope with stress, a study [24] on mothers of VLBW infants used a highly reliable measure of coping with 15 subscales which indicated acceptance, active, alcohol, disengagement, behavioral disengagement, denial, expression and venting of emotion, humor, mental disengagement, planning, positive reinterpretation and growth restraint, seeking social support for emotional reasons, seeking social support for instrumental reasons, suppression of competing activities and turning to religion. More use of avoidant and express emotions coping were significantly related to maternal depression and parenting strain. Religion coping was positively associated with maternal attachment to the infants and negatively associated with feeling that the child was demanding.

The Cues and Care Study protocol [25] provides a brief intervention designed to reduce anxiety and develop sensitive interaction skills. The strategy teaches empirically sound interventions and uses outcomes that are relevant. Cues involves teaching mothers to attend to their own physiological, cognitive and emotional cues that signal anxiety and worry and to use cognitive strategies to reduce stress. Those parents taught these strategies did far better than a control group of standard care. Mothers are also taught to understand infant cues and to respond sensitively to those cues. The Care group is a control for support and attention and educational information. Parents are not given sensitivity training.

The Cues intervention consists of six sessions identifying infant state cues and learning how to react sensitively with their infant. The sixth session is devoted to infant interaction during feeding. There is a telephone follow-up. The last session takes place in the mother's home two to four weeks after discharge. The mother is videotaped playing with her infant for 10 minutes. The intervener and mother then review the tapes to help the mother apply the skills learned in the intervention. Manuals are provided for the interveners. The videotapes are rated. The data is not yet published regarding the results of these interventions but it is likely that the sensitivity training makes a big difference.

A study of parent intervention using the Playing and Learning Strategies [21] showed strong changes in maternal affective-emotional and cognitive responsive behaviors and infants' development. Facilitation of maternal warmth occurred best with early intervention, while cognitive responsive behaviors were supported with the intervention in the toddler–preschool period.

25.6 Conclusions and future studies

Despite a limited sampling of the types of chronic medical disorders that children are born with, it is clear that maternal and paternal anxiety and depression produce further risks for these families. The factors that contribute to this are multidirectional. Certainly the degree of severity of the chronic illness influences parents' ability to meet the demands of the treatment and the developing child–family constellation. It is also necessary to consider the parents, sibling and marital dyad quality at the time of the occurrence of the event. If parents are already anxious or depressed, have had a previous negative birthing experience or have suffered from clinical illnesses, they are somewhat less resilient in facing the tasks that must be engaged in.

As to the children as they develop, the full range of developmental and childhood psychiatric disorders, including adjustment disorder, major depression, anxiety and delirium, are seen in children and adolescents with chronic illness. Psychiatric disorders are most likely to be present when the chronic physical disorder involves the brain. This argues for mental health assessment throughout the life of an individual who suffered from a childhood chronic medical illness. Some aspects of the treatment of life-threatening medical illness may be experienced as repeated trauma, which may not have an impact during or immediately after treatment, but rather appear as long-term effects on affect modulation and interpersonal relationships. There are treatment and intervention approaches that help. Matching individual factors rather than choosing interventions by disease is needed to maximize these effects. For instance, a poorly educated mother may need instruction on handling her child, particularly if she is an adolescent mother. Parenting self-efficacy is important to the resilience of the family in the face of coping with a sick child. Social support from family and health-care providers is a necessary ingredient. It is as important to give guidance and respite to parents as educational materials to help compliance and evaluation of changes needed. Follow-up in home visits by nurses who cared for the child in the hospital would certainly be a welcome addition. Certainly it would be important to show the cost-effectiveness of such treatment by such measures as fewer hospitalizations, more competent parenting and fewer medical complications.

In conclusion, a contextual family systems approach is needed to understand adaptation to chronic illness in children. This means that the health-care system must incorporate families in pediatric medicine. Many factors that influence the course of the disease are in part determined by genetic–environmental interactions. Chronic illness does not strike individuals; it strikes the whole living unit of the family. Every member is affected – the parents and brothers and sisters as well. Extended family relatives can provide respite. Parents want knowledge in three areas: the basic physiology of the disease; and the course and treatment of the illness or condition. This includes understanding of what to do to prevent problems. Family interventions need to be more replicable to evaluate individual differences in who benefits from which treatments. Involving fathers as participants and understanding their role in the care of a chronically ill child is of paramount importance.

25.7 References

1. Shayne, M. and Cerreto, M. (1981) Notes on Parent Group Meetings. Unpublished staff paper Vanderbilt Institute for Public Policy Studies. Tenn.
2. Levi, R. and Drotar, D. (2009) Critical issues and needs in health-related quality of life assessment of children and adolescents with chronic health conditions, in *Comprehensive Care for Children With Chronic Health Conditions* (ed. D. Drotar). Lawrence Earlbaum Associates, NJ.
3. Melamed, B.G. (2008) Parenting the ill child, in *Handbook of Parenting*, vol. **5** (ed. M. Bornstein). Lawrence Earlbaum Associates, NJ.
4. Melamed, B.G., Roth, B. and Fogel, J. (2000) Child health issues across the life span, in *The Handbook of Clinical Health Psychology* (eds A. Baum and T. Revenson) Guilford Press, New York.
5. Pediatric Health Care Division (1983) *Pediatric Ambulatory Care Division: Issues in Care of Children With Special Needs* (Videotape), Department of Pediatrics, Albert Einstein College of Medicine, New York.
6. Klinnert, M., Nelson, H.S., Price, M.R. *et al.* (2001) Onset and persistence of childhood asthma: predictors from infancy. *Pediatrics*, **108**, E69.

7. Markson, S. and Friese, B.H. (2000) Family rituals as a protective factor for children with asthma. *Pediatric Psychology*, **25**, 472–80.

8. Massie, R. and Massie, S. (1976) *Journey*. Knopf, New York, p. 12.

9. Cheuk, D., Wong, S., Chie, Y. *et al.* (2004) Parents' understanding of their child's CHD. *Heart*, **90**, 435–39.

10. Clark, S. and Miles, M. (1999) Conflicting responses: the experiences of fallacies of infants diagnosed with severe congenital heart disease. *Social Pediatric Nursing*, **4**, 7–14.

11. Turkel, S. and Pao, M. (2007) Late consequences of pediatric chronic illness. *Psychiatric Clinics of North America*, **30**, 819–35.

12. Arafa, M., Zaher, S., El-Dowarty, A. and Moneech, D. (2008) Quality of life among parents of children with heart disease. *Health Quality of Life Outcomes*, **6**, 91.

13. Miles, M., Funk, S.G., Kasper, M. (1991) The neonatal intensive care unit environment: sources of stress for parents. *AACN Clinical Issues Critical Care Nursing*, **2**, 346–54.

14. Drotar, D. (1997) Relating parent and family functioning to the psychological adjustment of children with chronic health conditions: what have we learned? What do we need to know? *Journal of Pediatric Psychology*, **22**, 149–65.

15. Stark, L.J., Stark, L., Knapp, A. *et al.* (2007). Increasing caloric consumption in children with cystic fibrosis: replication with a 2-year follow-up. *Journal of Applied Behavioral Analysis*, **26**, 435–50.

16. Glassco, C., Laucater, G., Smyth, P. and Hill, L. (2007) Parental depression following the early diagnosis of cystic fibrosis a matched prospective study. *Journal of Pediatrics*, **150**, 185–91.

17. Holditch-Davis, D., Bartlett, T., Blickman, A. and Miles, M.S. (2003) Posttraumatic stress symptoms in mothers of premature infants. *Journal of Obstetrical Gynecological Neonatal Nursing*, **32**, 161–71.

18. Lindsay, J., Roman, L., DeWys, M. *et al.* (1993) *Neonatal Network*, **12**, 37–44.

19. Field, T., Hernande, M. and Freedman, J. (2004) Stimulation program for preterm infants. *Social Policy Report*, **35**.

20. Koh, T., Buto, P., Coory, M. *et al.* (2007) Provision of taped conversations with neonatologists to others of babies in intensive care: randomized controlled trial. *British Medical Journal Publishing Group*, **334**, 28.

21. Landry, S., Smith, K., Swank, P. and Guttentag, C. (2008) A responsive parenting intervention: the optimal timing in early childhood for impacting maternal behaviors and child outcomes.

22. Tu, M., Grunau, R. *et al.* (2007) Maternal stress and behavior modulate relationships, between neonatal stress, attention and basal cortisol at 8 months in preterm infants. *Developmental Psychobiology*, **49**, 150–64.

23. Eisengart, S., Singer, L., Kirchner, H. *et al.* (2006) Factor structure of coping: two studies of others with high levels of life stress. *Psychological Assessment*, **18**, 278–88.

24. Feely, N., Gottlieb, L. and Zelkowitz, P. (2005) Infant, mother, and contextual predictors of mother-very low birthweight infant interaction at 9 months of age. *Journal of Developmental Behavioral Pediatrics*, **26**, 24–33.

25. Zelkowitz, P., Feely, N., Shrier, I. *et al.* (2008) The Cues and Care Trials: a randomized controlled trial of an intervention to reduce maternal anxiety and improve developmental outcomes in very low birthweight infants. *Biomed Central Pediatrics*, **8**, 38–48.

26

Parenting an infant born of rape

Frances Thomson Salo

University of Melbourne, Australia

(Kephisos) breaches the incest taboo and rapes his own daughter, thereby fathering Narcissus. [1]

26.1 Case vignette 1

A 15-year-old schoolgirl raped on her way home was devastated when she discovered she was pregnant, but felt that she should keep the infant. She felt that he was as much a victim as she was and she was not going to make him suffer. But she rejected him at birth because he resembled her attacker, said she could not look at him, did not want to hold him and asked for him to be taken away. However, she came to love him and said that it never ceased to amaze her that something so precious and wonderful had come from something so terrible and that she would not change him for the world.

26.2 Case vignette 2

The following case of intimate partner rape where the mother stayed with the father, whom she hated at times, is published in more detail [2]. Chantelle was born with severe respiratory distress syndrome. Her mother, Kerry, had received many diagnoses including borderline personality disorder. She revealed she had been born of a violent rape and had incorporated the fantasy of her father violating her mother and herself into her self-concept. As she looked into her infant's face, Kerry said that she saw a shameful, damaged image of herself reflected as bad, unwanted, abandoned and evil. This image of emptiness was what Chantelle may have seen reflected back to her through what she saw in her mother's face; she then avoided her mother's gaze. But both worked to overcome this and by the time Chantelle was 1 year old, her physical and social development seemed satisfactory.

26.3 Case vignette 3

A female patient in an in-patient psychiatric facility absconded and, repeating a pattern of experiencing intercourse as violent, became pregnant when raped by a very drunk, violent man. She had been sexually abused as a child and been a reluctant caretaker for her family. She was very fearful that her son would become like his father and sometimes felt that he was punishing her for the 'terrible things' that she had done. There was no contact with his father and she felt that caregiving had been imposed on her again. There were considerable negative attributions towards him, for example as a 1-week-old she described him as difficult and demanding. Her affect was incongruous, either depressed and mumbling, or giggling and manic. The mirroring he received contributed to a disorganized attachment by the time he was 1 year old: his mother, who found it hard to be empathic, increased his distress by laughing at him, so that he bit and hit out which increased her giggling.

26.4 Introduction

Despite acknowledgment for centuries about the frequency of rape, there is a paucity of data about parenting an infant conceived in rape. This important topic has been described by an experienced pediatrician as 'an unspoken subject'. A literature search in Pub Med, Ovid and the general infant mental health literature did not reveal many relevant references. Yet it is, for example, estimated that in recent conflict in Rwanda up to 10 000 infants were conceived in genocidal rape and in communities which are not at war, there are many thousands of undisclosed rape-related pregnancies a year. I surveyed over 80 professionals in the maternity services, the mental health services and the community,[1] and the help of all those who contributed directly or indirectly is gratefully acknowledged.[2] This chapter is written to outline some of the issues that caregivers face and in particular some maternal representations of the infant and the infant's attachment patterns and father representations.

While many victims of rape do not disclose the rape out of a sense of shame or fear of repercussions, many terminate the pregnancy before 20 weeks. A number arrange permanent care if they feel that the infant is innocent. Of those who keep the infant, a number are able to separate the nature of the conception from the child, while others are unable to be other than rejecting. While a particularly complex case may stand out in a clinician's memory, it is often not known how the mother parented her infant. Resources such as websites aim to publicize the effects of rape and help women access help for pregnancy but

---

[1] In Australia, Argentina, Germany, Japan, Pakistan, UK and USA and including academics, counsellors, hospital chaplains, midwives and nurses, pediatricians, physicians, protective workers, psychoanalysts, psychotherapists, psychiatrists, psychologists, social workers, speech therapists and teachers.

[2] In particular Campbell Paul, Amanda Jones, Judy Coram and Lisa Bolger.

until recently contained little about parenting infants conceived in rape. Three published case reports describe work with a mother who was conceived in rape who herself conceived a child in marital rape [2], and the psychotherapy of a 15-month-old infant and a 17-month-old infant of refugee mothers [3, 4].

26.5 Context

Different contexts of rape are considered as, along with psychosocial conditions and cultural background; these are likely to determine how well a mother comes to terms with the rape. The range of possible contexts makes it difficult to cover all the likely consequences. The severity of the effects will depend on the woman's experience, her internal and external supports and subsequent life events. What little is known currently applies more to clinical populations; much less is known about mothers who make a more successful adaptation to their infant's existence. The following subdivisions indicate the range of contexts rather than constituting a classification. In complex cases there can be a considerable number of compounding factors for women who already suffer a number of disabilities. Clinical and research evidence suggests a probable link between child sexual abuse and a woman being re-victimized in rape.

Within the family

Intimate partner violence

Intimate partner violence is universal but little is known about it [5]. It may be regarded as part of some subcultures. If the mother does not want an infant but feels that she had to conceive one for a partner, she could feel raped. Adolescent girls may continue a pregnancy under duress from the father or their family; health professionals tend to support adolescent girls who are experiencing non-voluntary sex, rather than rigorously enforcing statutory rape law.

Incest

Some professionals advocate replacing the term 'incest' with 'rape' because use of power in family relationships is abusive. Some young mothers may want the pregnancy to continue so that the rape is revealed. In other cases where incest is suspected and the infants are globally developmentally delayed, the women often conceal paternity, provide 'names' of putative fathers and rarely consent to DNA tests.

In the community

'Date rape'

The incidence of non-voluntary sexual experiences in adolescence which lead to pregnancy is greater than previously thought. Women who become pregnant through 'date rape' may not know who the father is, if they have been drugged.

Rape of sex workers by client or employer

While sex workers have a low rate of continued pregnancy, underage girls are particularly vulnerable to rape during prostitution or enslavement.

Rape while homeless

Homeless women are raped more than housed women and mothers who taking care of young children represent two of the most rapidly growing subgroups of this population [6].

Rape during impaired consciousness

The influence of drugs or alcohol and the experience of serious mental illness are likely to affect a woman's capacity to protect herself (including during in-patient psychiatric admissions). Substance-using women often experience a considerable degree of violence throughout their lives and some counselors suggest that the women expect to have forced sex; they often say that the infant is 'unplanned'.

Rape in a cult

Little is known, although exploitation of the transference seems implicated.

Breakdown of civil order

This includes rape during war or imprisonment with (gang) rape, and rape as ethnic cleansing or torture [7]. Sexual violence against women and girls has been described as the 'war within the war' with them as the invisible victims. Rapes by official personnel such as the UN peacekeepers have been documented including in post-disaster contexts such as a tsunami.

In exile, refugee camps or during resettlement

About 80% of refugee women are estimated by the United Nation's High Commissioner for Refugees to have been raped; children as young as 10 are bearing infants [8]. The women often face isolation, feelings of loss and survivor guilt in addition to the trauma of rape.

26.6 Outcomes of pregnancy

Termination

Many women, particularly when they have been raped as a weapon of war, feel unable to care for the infants and try to abort or abandon them, often refusing to look at them. Some clinicians report a high level of abortion in cultures with considerable violence towards women (although if the pregnancy is not terminated, the mother may be relatively accepting of the infant).

Continuation of the pregnancy

Clinicians working with women who present to support services for sexually assaulted women find that their first thoughts are about the infant, whether positive or negative. Often women do not feel that anything good can come from their body, which is felt to be bad. Some women may, despite facing several difficulties such as supporting substance use by sex work, decide to do what is best for the infant and arrange good antenatal care, including meeting the foster parents. If they keep the infant, they have often found that the infant can become a driving force for a better life.

26.7 Perinatal period

Clinical experience suggests that birth can be difficult, re-traumatizing women, triggering flashbacks and dissociation. The mothers may push the infants away and find it difficult to bond. They may find aspects of breastfeeding difficult especially if suckling reminds them of the rape or if they feel they cannot control those watching them feed. Other women feel breastfeeding helps them view their body more positively and to bond with their infant.

Some mothers feel uncomfortable or distressed touching their infant, particularly during bathing and nappy changes. Some may find that caring for an infant of one gender is more difficult than the other: when a son gets an erection they cannot look at or touch his penis and are unsure how to diaper him; others find cleaning their daughter's genitals stressful. The difficulties with loving touch may continue so that kissing and demonstrativeness are affected.

26.8 Maternal representation of the infant

Most of the psychological, social and cultural effects of rape have repercussions for the mother-infant dyad including fear and anger and perhaps particularly shame, which contributes to the subject being covered up to protect mother and child. Guilt and self-blame felt may lead them to feel that they should acquiesce with the pregnancy. Their fantasies and difficulties during pregnancy and birth are likely to have a highly significant effect on their identifications with their infants. They have to care for an infant while recovering from the trauma of being assaulted. They are likely to be suffering post-traumatic stress, and without help this may become chronic. They report a continuum of oscillating states from rejecting to accepting the infant.

When infants are conceived in rape many mothers wish that they or their infants would die. Looking at the infant can be very painful, reminding the mother of the perpetrator and of herself as victim [2, 4]. She may have very negative projections about her infant, who can be seen as punishing and evil. The mother may defend against shame by responding to her infant with anger, rejecting the infant and trying to pass on the pain. She may have difficulty resolving her responses. She may be very depressed and traumatized. She may want to hurt and humiliate her infant the way that she felt treated, and cannot bear to hear his or her crying out of fear and have to respond to this, let alone the ordinary baby needs which may feel like the demands of an adult man. Fear and feelings of lack of control in pregnancy, birth and early parenting may connect in the mother's mind to an earlier experience of rape, even if the infant is not conceived in rape.

If mothers do not disclose around the birth they are likely to close up about the subject, unless they overtly reject the child. They may only later define the experience as rape. If they can talk about it, their self-blame and sense of violation can lessen, increasing the possibility of re-finding internal and external loving figures. If there is a perception within the culture the woman lives in that rape is not so violent an act or she feels that she contributed to it, this may lessen her ambivalence. If she is in a relatively satisfactory relationship, she may be able to compartmentalize the rape.

Mothers with a religious faith and family support are more likely to accept the infant. Some mothers feel that they do not want to victimize their innocent child. They feel that to not terminate is a way to heal the inner infant and make a new start. Some feel that if they can get through the pregnancy they will have conquered the rape and reclaimed lost self-esteem and that giving birth is a generous and courageous act. While many women steadfastly maintain that to sever emotional ties they do not wish to see the newborn infant, some find that they are won over immediately. Some feel convinced they made the right decision, that it was love at sight and surprisingly easy to love the infant. Others feel that the infant brought peace and healing to their lives. One substance-using mother who made good foster care arrangements wanted to hold her daughter once at birth and, when she saw her, cancelled the fostering arrangements. A Bosnian single mother, who had been raped by soldiers, said that her son was her whole life and that he would be a good man. A mother has to work through seeing the infant as the damaged part of herself to being able to feel that she is the infant's mother, that she has chosen to love and protect her infant who is a new person rather than a representative of hate, a raping penis.

26.9 Maternal attachment

If the infant is experienced as an alien object invading her body there may be a transgenerational transmission of trauma. The following are important factors: the mother's mental state at the time of the rape (whether endured for survival for herself or her children and the intactness of her mind under the effect of pain, terror or disintegration), what she felt was in the perpetrator's mind and whether she felt the rape was denied or condoned e.g. in a breakdown of civil order. A boy's approach to his mother may act as a trauma trigger so that she may startle or freeze. Girls may also trigger such responses if the mother is obsessed by the need to protect her child's vulnerability. Harmless acts that resonate with the trauma, e.g. a mother's tears, may dysregulate feelings and activate insecure or disorganized attachment behaviors [4, 9, 11]. A denial of the impact of the rape can lead to mothers avoiding intimacy in the relationship with their infant; they encourage early independence. Some mothers transmit difficulties with self-esteem, assertion and joyful sexuality. The effects of the mother's difficulties are discussed further under '26.11 Infant attachment'.

Cultural differences are important: when having children is highly valued, many mothers seem to do well and to be able to put aside the nature of the infant's conception. Some are more idealizing of the infant and try psychically to obliterate the nature of the conception and compensate with the quality of their mothering. Some women parent very well, e.g. becoming clean of drugs and finding housing, supported by relatives and other services. Many mothers are resilient, becoming protective on behalf of their infants. One mother who had horrific experiences (she saw her husband murdered, endured gang rapes during months of imprisonment while pregnant and infected with HIV), was nevertheless able to overcome this. Some resilient infants also help ease their mothers' pain and suffering, and are able to re-connect quickly if their mother becomes sensitively available.

Mothers may be concerned for the safety of their infant, particularly in times of armed conflict. They often prefer to have a girl who will resemble them more than the rapist; more girls are kept than boys. Conception in intimate partner rape is usually hidden for the sake of the children whom the mother tries to protect by staying with their father.

26.10   Infant attachment

If as a result of the rape mothers have a fear of attachment and feel rejecting of the infant, a wide range of psychological difficulties are likely [10]. If the pain, shame and the fear arising from the violence and the powerlessness remain unresolved for the mother, this is likely to predispose the infant to having a disorganized attachment style with its expectation of catastrophe [11]. This attachment style would be over-represented in comparison with the norm. If infants conceived in rape arouse fear in their mothers, they grow up unable to understand this, and lack a representation of a mother to turn to for help. They may then lose awareness of wanting a response from her and feel that they have to protect themselves. To achieve coherence infants may develop irrational fears or become aggressive, projecting their own fear while trying to make sense of their mother's fear of them. They use freezing or hypervigilance to cope with feeling frightened and unwanted. If they have identified with their mothers' projections of them as violent, violence may be a way of getting their mother to experience their feelings of terror and rage when they feel abandoned.

26.11   Representations of the father and disclosure to the infant

The possibility of someone filling the father role is important. The myth of Narcissus, conceived in rape, who drowns while gazing at his reflection, points to the difficulty of a boy growing up in a mother–son dyadic relationship who, without a father, is vulnerable to a lack of separation between mother and child [1]. Children try to construct a representation of the father, to complete the representation of their own self. How a mother tells her child about their conception depends on whether she has been able to maintain an internal good father representation alongside the biological father representation. Mothers whose infants present with difficulties and who say that the father is not around face the clinician with whether or not to explore this with the mother.

Mothers often fear that giving their infants information about their father will damage them. Often the conception is not discussed so as not to 'hurt' the child, although they may be concerned about whether it would be worse if the secret were revealed. While telling the child may never arise when the infant is born of intimate partner violence, in other situations it may be of major concern for those involved. Questions about when and how to tell a child feature prominently on websites about parenting infants conceived in rape. Some mothers plan to tell the infant using a 'short truth', e.g. 'Your biological father and I were together (for a short time) and it didn't work out.' Others describe a 'soft truth', e.g. a mother told her son that his father and she were friends but he wanted her more than she wanted him and he thought they should make a baby; further details were added later as appropriate. Others suggest telling the infant that their father made a mistake and hurt the mother (emotionally), while stressing to the infant that they are the most important part of their life.

A number of women from African countries report acceptance of the infant who was conceived of rape, such as a Rwandan mother who said that she would tell her son about his conception and add that God is not angry with either of them, that it happened because of war, and that God loves them [12]. In therapeutic groups for mothers and infants who have experienced family violence, the mothers seek help about explaining this to the infant while often wishing to deny that questions will arise in the child's mind before adolescence.

In online debates, parents discuss whether to provide their child with the name and location of the father and allow telephone communication. One mother, who was very loving towards her son, initially tried to get the father involved because she did not want her son to resent her for not knowing him. She did not plan to tell him the details of his conception as she did not want him to think that he was unwanted, but would support him if he wanted to find his father when he was older. Some adoptive parents who wish for or have an open adoption are aware that biological and adoptive mothers need to agree on what they say to the infant. If the rape was carried out with extreme severity, some adoptive parents are determined to protect the adoptees from knowing the father or his family, to the extent of changing the child's name, and dread being asked about him.

The older infant with an absent father has fantasies and questions about him. The infant son of an adolescent asylum-seeking mother was at birth given the surname meaning 'God's child'. His mother could only care for him if she imagined she had conceived him with God, as his father was a brutal military guard and she needed this defense for a long time. But after his second year, he began to ask where his father was (Jones, personal communication, 21 June 2009). Mothers have to balance the information the infants ask for about their father's whereabouts and what they can cope with [12]. Is it enough to say he is 'far away'? If infants are told that the father who does not live with them was bad, they might worry that if they are 'bad' they could also be removed. When a mother cannot allow a space for the infant's questions about the father, curiosity may be inhibited. Some mothers, however, encourage the child's reflective function by saying they do not understand why he did what he did. When 2½-year-old Sara's mother said that her daughter's aggression reminded her of her father's violence, Sara stopped playing and said to her mother, 'No, no mama, no dadda, (pointing towards herself) Sara' [3].

26.12 Adoptive and foster parenting

Little is known about the situation for an infant in permanent care or adopted. Children construct representations about their biological parents while there is considerable variation about the information adoptive parents are given about whether the infant was conceived in rape or incest, and how open the adoption is (see previous section). A Bosnian woman conveyed her claiming of her adoptive son. She was terminally ill and in great conflict about whether to tell him that his Muslim mother had been raped by a Serbian soldier, and had abandoned him. His adoptive mother did not think he should try to find his biological mother as he was loved by the adoptive parents, his mother especially. Adoptive parents may give a sanitized story to their adopted children but some have not liked discovering the distortion. Adoptees sometimes trace their biological mother, occasionally to thank her for her courage in continuing the pregnancy.

26.13 Siblings

There is a potential for splitting of maternal ambivalence towards siblings depending on their conception. One mother responded very differently to her two children, her first having been conceived in rape in a refugee camp. When she was settled in another country, she re-partnered, had another infant and rejected the older child who became emotionally disturbed.

26.14 Being parented in ongoing difficulty

If mother and infant continue to live in a situation of ongoing violence, this increases the likelihood of the infant being aggressive. For mothers to feel attached and attuned to their infants is very difficult if they are in a situation where they are being tortured while they are pregnant and lactating. In situations of armed conflict when women are raped by members of the opposing side, mothers may be rejected with their children labeled as children of the attackers. Mothers may protect the fact of the children's conception from everyone including husbands out of fear of the children being regarded as 'filth' or 'children of hate' [10].

Cases in the child protection system of infants conceived in rape are heavily weighted with violence, drug and alcohol use and transience; the rape is usually by a 'stepfather' rather than the father. Sometimes the mother continues to be raped in the home in the presence of an older toddler; one mother was threatened with a gun and raped by the father of the toddler who witnessed the rape.

26.15 Support and therapeutic intervention for the family

Reports in the literature of cases treated by individual or group psychotherapy are infrequent. Clinicians report that patients either leave therapy early or that aspects other than the rape were more challenging. While a crucial role for health professionals is to help lessen the powerful projections onto the infant, women may present with infants with a range of common infant mental health pediatric problems and be unable to divulge their rape.

The following infant mental health intervention shows how enduring the effects of rape can be despite the mother appearing to have accepted it. Elle, a 20-year-old mother in a refugee camp, had a very ambivalent relationship with her second child, 1½-year-old Dee, who was failing to thrive. She had been in the hospital nutrition ward for six weeks for a ruptured bowel and food refusal. She lay quietly on the bed emaciated, miserable and completely disinterested, with her arm covering her face. When the clinician talked gently to her about how fed up and sad she looked, Dee held her gaze expressionless. Elle brightly related that Dee had been a happy infant who had breastfed fed well and only refused food when recently weaned and, still brightly, told a story of loss and trauma. As a 14-year-old Elle had been forcibly held down by the friends of a 35-year-old man who raped her and she became pregnant with her first child, now 6 years old, but he abandoned them when she became pregnant with Dee. The clinician reflected that she might be feeling very angry.

At the next visit Elle and Dee's mood had changed. Elle was sadder, admitting that she thought Dee would die. Dee was more irritable as Elle struggled to console her, handling her roughly on the bed; only when placed on her back did she quieten. When the clinician produced a small soft toy dog Dee screamed and attacked it. The clinician attuned to her anger by smacking the dog, saying 'naughty dog'. Dee made a rapid recovery and was discharged. Once Elle had been able to talk about the rape, and both expressed anger, Dee improved immediately. (Elle's only strategy had been to lay Dee on her back in a sacrificial way; once she lay resignedly with Dee on top of her for over an hour, reminiscent of Dolto's conceptualization of infants born of violence while their mothers lay down as if dead [15].)

26.16 The infant's view of their life

There are occasional autobiographies or survivor accounts on the Internet. Some wonder whether they have inherited evil genes, and will develop psychological problems. A series of interviews with children conceived in rape in a war situation revealed that the mother–child relationships were traumatic as they reminded the mothers of the perpetrator [14]. Some children who have been hated by their caregivers have found it helpful to know the reason, rather than it remain a secret. A 17-month-old boy, whose mother had been coerced by her partner into conceiving him, was chained to a tractor and beaten after he urinated. He was treated with extreme cruelty by biological and foster parents. On learning this as a 16-year-old from a clinician, he thanked her, volunteering that it was better to know what had happened. Such resilient children seem to develop a capacity to be reflective.

26.17 Conclusions

The chapter, with four illustrative case vignettes, has outlined some issues that caregivers face as well as likely infant attachment patterns, father representation and development of a positive self-representation. Mothers who keep the infant experience a continuum of states of mind from acceptance to rejection. In terms of implications for practice and policy it is important for support services for women who have been raped, and for hospital staff, police and mental health services to be linked to make it easier for women and their infants to feel safe enough to receive effective intervention. More therapeutic services are needed and further systematic studies are indicated.

26.18 References

1. Teising, M. (2007) Narcissistic mortification of ageing men. *International Journal of Psychoanalysis*, **88**, 1329–44.
2. Paul, C. (2008) Working with a sick infant born of a rape. *The Signal*, **16**, 1–5.
3. Bekos, D. (2007) *Sara: psychotherapy with a mother-infant dyad with a background of violence*, in *The Infant as Subject: New Directions in Infant-Parent Therapy from the Royal*

Children's Hospital, Melbourne, 2nd edn (eds F.Thomson Salo and C. Paul). Stonnington Press, Melbourne, Australia, pp. 202–12.

4. Jones, A. (2008) Raped in utero. *The Signal*, **16**, 5–9.
5. McFarlane, J. (2007) Pregnancy following partner rape: what we know and what we need to know. *Trauma, Violence and Abuse*, **8**, 127–34.
6. Goodman, L. (September 2006) *No Safe Place: Sexual Assault in the Lives of Homeless Women*. VAWnet, a project of the National Resource Center on Domestic Violence/ Pennsylvania Coalition Against Domestic Violence, Harrisburg, PA. Retrieved 16 April 2009, from http://www.vawnet.org.
7. Carpenter, R.C. (2007) *Born of War: Protecting Children of Sexual Violence Survivors in Conflict Zones*. Kumarian Press, Bloomfield, CT.
8. Eckert, R. and Hofling, J. (2008) *Breaking the silence: Women and Girls at Risk and Children of Rape.* http://www.crr.unsw.edu.au/documents/ARRA%20Children%20of%20Rape.pdf. Accessed 30 May 2009.
9. Main, M. and Hesse, E. (1990) Parents' unresolved traumatic experiences are related to infant disorganized attachment status: Is frightened and/or frightening parental behavior the linking mechanism? in *Attachment in the Preschool Years: Theory, Research and Intervention* (eds M. Greenberg, D. Cicchetti and E.M. Cummings). University of Chicago Press, Chicago, pp. 161–82.
10. Papineni, P. (2003) Children of bad memories. *Lancet*, **362**, 825–26.
11. Hopkins, J. (2008) Discussion. *The Signal*, **16**, 9.
12. Wax, E. (2004) Loving the children born of hate: insight. *The Age*, **3.4.2004**, 6.
13. Thomson Salo, F. (2007) Relating to the infant as subject in the context of family violence, in *The Infant as Subject: New Directions in Infant-Parent Therapy from the Royal Children's Hospital, Melbourne*, 2nd edn (eds F. Thomson Salo and C. Paul). Stonnington Press, Melbourne, Australia, pp. 182–98.
14. Nikolic-Ristanovic, V. (ed.) (2000) *Women, Violence and War: Wartime Victimisation of Refugees in the Balkans*. Central European University Press, Budapest.
15. Keren, M. (2008) Editor's perspective: Infants born of rape, raped infants … the need to have them in mind. *The Signal*, **16**, 19.

27

Parenting an infant with a disability

Sheila Hollins,[1] Stella Woodward[2] and Kathryn Hollins[3]

[1]St George's University of London, UK
[2]Medical student, Cardiff University Medical School, UK
[3]Chelsea and Westminster Hospital, London, UK

27.1 Introduction

Discovering that your newborn baby is not the hoped-for healthy baby, but has significant physical or mental impairments, is a significant source of physical, emotional and spiritual distress for parents as well as siblings and the child's wider family. Parents face the painful process of understanding and adapting to the diagnosis and its implications for their future. Becoming a 'good enough' parent may require significant changes of life routine and role to provide the care the child requires. Ensuring good mental and physical health of such a child's parents is important, and providing parents with support, information and psychological or psychotherapeutic interventions, when needed, will enable them to care more effectively for their growing disabled child and the whole family.

Some of the problems and challenges faced by parents will be similar regardless of the cause of the child's impairment. This chapter will explore the various ways in which stressors affect parental mental health.

27.2 Parental expectations

Reconciling expectations of having a normal child with the reality of giving birth to a baby with a disability is an ongoing process, throughout which may not be easy for the couple to agree about. Often, something akin to a bereavement reaction will accompany the birth or diagnosis of an infant with a disability as parents grieve the loss of the 'dreamed of' child and perhaps of their personal freedom. This sense of loss may remain over time and become more tangible at particular moments, for example, when the child fails to reach expected milestones or engage with the usual rites of passage.

Parenthood and Mental Health: A Bridge between Infant and Adult Psychiatry   Sam Tyano, Miri Keren, Helen Herrman and John Cox
© 2010 John Wiley & Sons, Ltd

Diagnosis is often the point at which parents begin the process of adaptation to their child's disability and is also the point at which access to services and support networks relevant to the child's condition may begin. Early access to support services can have a beneficial effect on parental well-being as they identify goals towards which they can work in partnership with relevant professionals.

27.3 Antenatal diagnosis

In the UK, routine antenatal investigations can identify women carrying a baby at increased risk of having a disability. For example, screening for Down's syndrome, usually using the triple or combined test, is now routinely offered to expectant mothers. Women with a 'screen positive' result (a chance of having a baby with Down's of more than 1 in 250) are offered a definitive test to confirm or refute the diagnosis, usually fetal karyotyping using amniocentesis or chorionic villus sampling [1].

A diagnosis of significant abnormalities will then present parents with an important decision, as they must quickly decide whether to continue with or terminate the pregnancy. Some studies have shown that the information given to parents about their child's disability is often presented in a negative manner assuming that parents will wish to terminate the pregnancy [2]. Staff attitudes towards disability in the context of antenatal screening have important implications for the decisions parents make.

Choosing to have a termination for fetal abnormalities can be a complex and painful decision. For many couples it can be the right decision to take for their own personal reasons. Some couples are able to come to terms with this and move on with their lives despite their sadness about this longed-for child. Others are traumatized by the experience, which may affect further parenting. These parents can benefit from specialist psychotherapeutic treatment to help process their experience of loss.

27.4 Case vignette 1

An Australian couple decided to terminate their first pregnancy at a very late stage due to the sudden discovery of severe abnormalities in their unborn baby. They had to make this decision within days. A year later they presented to a specialist perinatal psychotherapy service, as the woman was still in an extremely distressed and depressed state. It seemed as if the loss had occurred the day before, so acute was her grief. The couple's relationship was strained and she was unable to work. It emerged that she felt she had killed her unborn baby. This unresolved grief was having profound implications in preventing the couple think about having another child The woman undertook psychotherapeutic treatment to help address her grieving, traumatized state.

27.5 Case vignette 2

A South American couple decided not to terminate their first pregnancy even though the unborn baby had a severe neurological condition and chances of survival were poor. They had a few weeks to prepare for her birth. The baby girl died two days after birth but the couple felt grateful to have become her parents even for this brief period. After burying their daughter they were able to begin processing their grief with psychotherapeutic treatment, hopeful that they would be able to go on to have more children in the future.

As shown in the above examples, for those parents who choose to continue with an affected pregnancy, knowledge of the child's disability before he or she is born can affect their reactions to the diagnosis in different ways. For some, it allows time to prepare for and come to terms with the prospect of having a disabled child, making it easier to cope once the child is born. For others, receiving unwelcome news during pregnancy and facing a difficult decision about whether to proceed with the pregnancy, which may not have been easy for the couple to agree about, can result in disruption of bonding during pregnancy between mother and unborn baby and/or significant maternal anxiety. Chronic anxiety in pregnancy is known to have adverse consequences for a baby's healthy development. The high cortisol level in the mother is believed to affect the development of the physiological stress response in the child. It has been associated with disturbed antenatal attachment and disturbed infant behavior and temperament, as well as behavioral and emotional problems in children [3].

27.6 Postnatal diagnosis

If pregnancy has gone well with no problems picked up on routine screening or scans, the birth of an infant with severe disabilities is a devastating shock. The new parents are faced with sudden grief, disbelief and overwhelming disappointment at the loss of their dreamed-of child. They may also be dealing with confusion and anger about whether there has been hospital negligence in not identifying the problems earlier.

27.7 Case vignette 3

One new mother from North Africa had an emergency Caesarean for maternal health reasons, only to discover that her baby had severe abnormalities. On the first day she sat in the middle of her bed, stock-still, unable to move physically or emotionally in the midst of her pain and shock. The next moment she would be weeping with upset and anger, not understanding how this could have happened without warning. Helping her cope with this experience, and to grieve for the baby she had hoped for, enabled her to begin to love and accept her baby. In order to establish bonding and breastfeeding, these first few days are important for the mother–infant relationship.

How the news of the impairment is broken to parents will be influential. Sensitive and constructive disclosure may help parents to adjust to the reality of the ways in which this baby will be different from most other babies. Ensuring parents are well informed from the time of diagnosis seems to enhance long-term coping mechanisms. Research suggests that maternal satisfaction at method of disclosure significantly affects maternal adaptation [4].

Several examples are given by Hollins [5] of parents' recollections of how the news of their baby's condition was given to them.

27.8 Case vignette 4

One mother recalled how the midwife and the doctor had seemed reluctant to give them any information except the bare minimum. She thought they knew that her daughter had something seriously wrong with her, and indeed there were signs that all was not well in her appearance. As time went by she experienced a similar reluctance from other professionals. But she says that she and her husband really needed a guide whom they could trust to be open and honest so that they could get on with their parenting role, knowing the worst from the beginning rather than having to face repeated disclosures. Looking back she realized that it was possible that the staff could not have known the extent of her multiple impairments. However she felt that it had been down to her and her husband to know what questions to ask. Why hadn't they helped them to find out rather than leaving them to make sense of it on their own?

27.9 Diagnostic uncertainty

The importance of diagnosis to mental health outcomes goes beyond when and how it is delivered. Diagnostic uncertainty can be a major psychological stressor that contributes to the long-term emotional burden of having a child with a disability. Mothers of children with an intellectual disability of unknown origin show psycho-emotional disadvantages compared to mothers of children with Down's syndrome, where the diagnosis is usually obvious [6]. In fact, a definite diagnosis of Down's syndrome has been associated with emotional outcomes similar to those of parents with non-disabled children. This may relate to the nature of the diagnosis. Down's syndrome carries a good prognosis, standards of care are well established, many support groups exist and it is well known to members of the general public – all factors that may increase acceptance of the disability both by parents and by the wider community. However, the good outcome seen in parents of children with Down's syndrome may also reflect the psychological benefit of a definite diagnosis.

27.10 Parental responses

How parents respond to their child's disability will be affected by previous experience, personal psychological factors and social circumstances. One influence will be their prior experience or knowledge of disability. They may have had no experience of disability at all. Some will have had a disabled sibling or other family member while others may have had a previous child with a disability. A positive experience of coping with disability in their family will enhance parental ability to cope and will ease the process of adjustment. A negative experience, however, may result in maladaptive responses, which can affect the development of a secure attachment and have long-term implications for the relationship between parents and their child. A particular disability may be more devastating than others depending on personal circumstances, such as deafness in a musical family, or a severe physical disability in a family who live in inaccessible housing.

Perhaps more importantly it is a time in which parents' own psychological states will help determine the personal resources they bring to parenthood. The personal meaning for a particular mother or father in giving birth to an infant with a disability will play a central role in their parenting ability. This means that some parents will struggle to adjust to what others may see as quite minor challenges and others will appear to cope with unthinkable adversity.

Early help-seeking may result in better outcomes: Sloper *et al.* [7] found that turning to informal sources for emotional support at the time of diagnosis was related to high satisfaction at the time of the study and that the use of informal support at times of crisis also had a protective effect. In terms of social circumstances, working parents were found to show lower levels of negative affect and better psychological well-being, suggesting that taking a break from caregiving and engaging in other tasks may protect parents from acute stress [8].

However what also needs to be considered is whether parents are able to make the changes necessary to parent a child with more complex needs. This may mean working less outside the home, and being able to provide appropriate education, treatments and appliances/aids. Having support from their extended family and community and from local services will be key in making this possible.

27.11　Parent–infant relationship development

Being able to parent an infant with a disability can be affected by factors such as the severity of the condition and feeding and communication problems [7]. An infant with severe developmental delay due to physical and/or intellectual impairments will have more demanding needs, for example he or she may not sleep as well as other infants. However such problems can be exacerbated by a mother's own difficulties.

27.12　Case vignette 5

One new mother described her infant as crying all the time and hardly sleeping. At times she admitted hating him for not letting her feel competent as a mother. In these moments she could find herself feeling desperate and shouting at him angrily. At just a few months old, this baby began avoiding his mother's gaze, which made her feel even more useless.

The resulting exhaustion and sense of failure in not being able to settle or comfort her infant made this new mother feel useless and frustrated. His poor sleep and crying were in part related to his condition, but her high level of anxiety and fury also seemed to be affecting his ability to be soothed. His avoidance of her gaze suggested that he was overwhelmed by her anger and distress and this in turn disrupted the development of a loving relationship. What emerged in parent–infant psychotherapy was how critical this mother was of her own successes and failures in life and how emotionally deprived her own childhood had been. This helped her understand why she found it so hard to contain her baby's distress and respond to his extreme neediness. Through understanding her own emotional needs better, she became more able to provide for his needs and he became a calmer, more communicative baby.

　　Parents of infants with developmental delay may also find their child difficult to 'read', resulting in problems with interpreting their needs, and therefore being less able to provide sensitive and responsive caregiving. An association has been demonstrated between infant disability and insecure or disorganized parent–infant attachment [9].

　　A recent study looked at mother–infant interactions in high-risk infant siblings of children with autism [10]. It found that these infants were less attentive to their mother, had less positive vocalizations and were more neutral in affect. It also showed their mothers had less sensitive responsiveness to their infants. This team are exploring what interventions may help reduce the chances of autism developing, for example by helping parents to continue interacting positively with their infants, even if they are not receiving the level of feedback and reinforcement they would naturally expect. This will be pertinent to relationships with other infants with disabilities, who may not be able to interact with their parents in the way their normal siblings can. Interventions that support parents in the task of good communication with their child will assist the child's long-term emotional and cognitive development.

27.13　Case vignette 6

An English couple were surprised by how quiet and unresponsive their infant was when they talked and sang to him. Eventually, profound deafness was diagnosed. The whole family decided to learn British Sign Language, so that their son would be able to develop his linguistic and cognitive skills from infancy onwards and participate as much as possible in family life.

This couple were able to come to terms with the specific needs of their son, and the commitment that they needed to make in order to improve his emotional and cognitive development. Parents who find it too hard or painful to acknowledge the huge changes that need to be made can be affecting their child's future outcome and may need considerable practical support or psychotherapeutic treatment in order to make this happen.

The extent to which parents are able to adjust to their child's disability can also have implications for the development of a secure attachment. Parents with unresolved feelings towards their child's diagnosis may display reduced sensitivity and emotional attunement to their child, resulting in insecure parent–child attachments. Conversely, parents whose grief or disappointment has resolved may form more secure attachments.

Parents can become over-protective of their disabled child, which restricts the abilities of the child to make friends, gain independence and become part of the wider society. This pattern can begin in infancy with parents being unable to let other people help care for their child, feeling that no one else will be able to manage well enough. It is important to support parents in allowing others to help, as this will also benefit the child as he or she grows and develops.

27.14 Depression in parents of children with a disability

An association between parenting a disabled child and maternal depression has been found in a number of studies over the past 25 years, with risk factors for parental depression being identified. Mothers are more likely than fathers to report depressive symptoms. The experience of being pregnant with a child with severe abnormalities can result in considerable feelings of guilt in women, with feelings of shame and failure in not producing a healthy child. These feelings of guilt can be even more acute in women who recognize that their child's disabilities are the result of their own health problems or behavior during pregnancy. For example, women who drink excessively in pregnancy can cause fetal alcohol syndrome in their infant, which includes both physical and intellectual impairments. Women with anorexia nervosa are more likely to give birth to premature and underweight babies.

This higher risk of depression may also reflect the fact that mothers take on a larger portion of the care and work that a disabled child requires. They are more likely to give up employment and may be unable to pursue their own interests. Their psychological well-being may be more related to their level of fulfillment as a mother, making them more vulnerable to depression when difficulties arise. It is possible that fathers may show their distress in ways other than depression [11], but it is also possible that we under-diagnose new fathers with depression, expecting depression to be found only in mothers.

While the strength of the association between maternal depression and parenting a disabled child is disputed, it nevertheless requires the attention of health professionals, as poor maternal mental health is known to adversely affect child behavior and development. For children with disabilities, whose development and well-being are already compromised, parenting practices that further impair their development can place them at significant disadvantage (12, 13).

Certain characteristics of the child are also related to maternal depression. A diagnosis of autism and significant behavioral problems are highly associated with depressive symptoms, suggesting that challenging behavior is more difficult to cope with than physical or intellectual impairments on their own [14]. High maternal stress levels, poor coping styles and poor physical health are also associated with depressive symptoms. Disabled children and their families are more likely to experience poorer health associated with their socio-economic conditions. Good family support and social cohesion are key determinants of psychological well-being reflecting the importance of good support to maternal mental health.

27.15 Responses of family, friends and wider society

The response of family and friends to the birth of an infant with a disability can have a large impact on parental experience and well-being. Parents may feel that friends and family fail to understand their situation and seem uncomfortable in dealing with their disabled child. This can result in isolation from potential sources of support and can reinforce the difference between their situation and that of other families.

In many countries, the place of the disabled child in society has altered dramatically over recent decades although in the past the shame associated with having a disabled child often resulted in the institutionalization of the child. Bringing about an end to institutional care remains a crucial goal, which is well advanced in Western countries but has not achieved the same political imperative in many others. National strategies ensuring the availability of community-based services for disabled children and their families are still a distant aspiration in many low- and middle-income countries, despite the scandals in some Eastern European countries in recent years. The WHO have recently launched a major program in several low- and middle-income countries that will include attention to the needs of disabled children and their families and is concerned with identifying disabled children, supporting their families and developing community-based rehabilitation.

27.16 Economic and social implications

The practical effects of having a disabled child can take their toll. In many families, having a disabled child necessitates one parent, usually the mother, leaving the workforce to look after the child, thus limiting the family income. Also, work mobility and the ability to accept promotions that require relocation may be lost as families feel unable to leave behind the professional and community support networks they have fought for and developed over time. Sometimes the child's additional health needs require repeated hospital visits and admissions, often in an emergency, for example, a child with severe epilepsy. Families can therefore find themselves in a state of relative poverty. Leaving the workforce also has implications for psychosocial well-being; it may precipitate a strong sense of loss and social isolation which, coupled with a diminished social network, can impair parents' ability to cope with stress. If the child has physical impairments requiring lifting by carers, parents may develop back problems themselves. Unless social care agencies are able to provide short breaks to allow parents to recharge their batteries, the burden of caring can become too much.

Woodgate *et al.* interviewed parents of children with autism to gain insight into their experiences and needs [15]. An overriding theme was that parents felt 'in a world of their own' to the point that their role as parent of an autistic child defined their experience of life was the essence of their experience. In response to this, parents struggled to preserve a sense of self and to maintain some routine in their lives. A sense of isolation was felt to result from society's lack of understanding of their child's disability, however parents may also isolate themselves from social contact for fear of awkward encounters [16].

27.17 Positive implications

Although parenting a disabled child may be experienced as stressful and can be associated with negative mental health outcomes, there is also evidence that it can have a positive impact on parental mental health, creating opportunities for personal and social development that would not have otherwise arisen [17].

Parents of disabled children learn to speak out; they become the child's advocate and find themselves taking on new and fulfilling roles such as group leaders, teachers and writers. Many parents are aware of becoming more compassionate, less self-focused and of developing greater personal strength. Parents find that their marriages are strengthened and their friendship networks expanded, with relationships operating at a deeper level. Parents may experience a change in their outlook on life that renders them more resilient; for example, by trying to make the most of and appreciate each day [17]. Parental perception of the child having a positive impact in their life can moderate the relationship between the challenge posed by the child's behavior and parental stress. Thus, the positive effects of parenting a disabled child in turn promote good parental mental health [18].

27.18 Supporting parents

The twenty-first century has seen significant changes in the attitudes of governments, health professionals and indeed of society towards disability. New aims have emerged, the most important being to provide practical, emotional, professional and financial support for families of children with disabilities, to reduce stigma and to include children in communities.

To effectively cater for the needs of parents, their own perceptions of the support they require must be sought. Beresford *et al.* have investigated the outcomes parents of disabled children desire for themselves and their child [19]. As found by Woodgate *et al.*, (ref 15) parents described a loss of personal identity, with the role of carer dominating how they felt about themselves and how others see them. Therefore work, interests and personal relationships, which play a key role in an individual's sense of identity, were identified by parents as vital to their wellbeing, as was being able to sustain family life. Many parents felt that aspects of their personal identity had been lost, with the role of carer dominating how they felt about themselves and how others see them. Since work, interests and personal relationships play a key role in their sense of identity, maintaining these aspects of life as well as sustaining family life is all of importance to parental well-being.

MacDonald *et al.* found that in infancy, informal support was readily accessed. Family and friends were comfortable with helping as care needs were generally in line with 'normal' infant care [20]. After starting school however, the child's differences became more obvious, and these researchers reported caregiving becoming increasingly onerous as family and friends became less involved. Parents experienced fatigue, depression, boredom, isolation and an inability to work outside the home. They also found it more difficult to allocate time to their other children. This is also illustrated in the stories of six families quoted by Hollins [5].

Parent groups and workshops can strengthen solidarity among parents, and provide a robust source of emotional support. In the UK as soon as the diagnosis is made, parents must be informed of relevant voluntary organizations, which may be able to provide them with relevant information and contacts, or be put in touch with parent support groups for families parenting children with similar impairments. For example a pregnant woman who is known to be carrying a baby with Down's syndrome can be offered an introduction to the Down's Syndrome Association.

Parents require professional support, both practical and emotional, to enhance their coping skills and to avoid 'burnout'. Adequate financial support for families is vital as the additional costs of parenting a disabled child can be considerable, particularly if a parent gives up work to become a full-time carer. Adequate social worker or health visitor input can offer emotional support and facilitate access to practical help and services. Respite care in familiar surroundings, both on a planned basis and in response to acute 'crises', gives the family a break as well as giving the child the opportunity to develop other relationships.

Child and adolescent mental health services (CAMHS) are an important source of help and treatment for families with a child with a disability. This can address the experiences of being disabled as well as secondary depression or emotional and behavioral problems. CAMHS may be needed at different stages during infancy, childhood and adolescence, for the child with the disability, for siblings and for parents. This may involve behavioral methods or cognitive-behavioral treatments, family therapy or individual child psychotherapy.

27.19 Conclusion

In this chapter we have reviewed recent research about the mental health of parents following the diagnosis of an intellectual, physical or sensory impairment in their infant and during the early childhood years. While parents who have a disabled child will face additional challenges, the majority will still enjoy the rewards of parenthood. The early period following diagnosis appears to be the most challenging for parents with respect to their own adjustment and well-being. Sensitive multidisciplinary assessment of the child's needs at an early stage is vital if parents are to gain and sustain access to the support they require. They need help to anticipate their infant's needs and how they may differ from those of other children in the years ahead. The needs of the baby and those of the family evolve continually over time; therefore regular reassessment is required, to ensure that service provision remains appropriate and optimal. Parents recognize that they need to be physically and emotionally healthy in order to properly look after their child. Many parents describe accessing and dealing with services as stressful and distressing and have identified having to use inadequate or inappropriate services as a source of anxiety. Clearly, it is important that parents feel confident about the services they are using and know that professionals are working in partnership with them.

27.20 References

1. Morris, J.K. (2009) The National Down Syndrome Cytogenetic Register 2007/8 Annual Report. Barts and the London School of Medicine and Dentistry. Queen Mary University of London.
2. Partington, K.J. (2002) Maternal responses to the diagnosis of learning disabilities in children: a qualitative study using a focus group approach. *Journal of Intellectual Disabilities*, **6**, 163.

3. O'Connor, T., Heron, J., Glover, V. *et al.* (2007) Antenatal maternal stress and long-term effects on child neurodevelopment: how and why? *Journal of Child Psychology and Psychiatry*, **48**, 245–61.

4. Dagenais, L., Hall, N., Majnemer, A. *et al.* (2006) Communicating a diagnosis of cerebral palsy: caregiver satisfaction and stress. *Paediatric Neurology*, **35**, 408–14.

5. Hollins, S. and Hollins, M. (2005) *You and Your Child: Making Sense of Learning Disabilities*. Karnac Books, London.

6. Lenhard, W., Breitenbach, E., Ebert, H. *et al.* (2005) Psychological benefit of diagnostic certainty for mothers of children with disabilities: lessons from Down syndrome. *American Journal of Medical Genetetics A*, **133**A (2), 170–75.

7. Sloper, P. and Turner, S. (1993) Risk and resilience factors in the adaptation of parents of children with severe physical disability. *Journal of Child Psychology and Psychiatry*, **34**, 167–88.

8. Ha, J.W., Hong, J., Seltzer, M.M. and Greenberg, J.S. (2008) Age and gender differences in the well being of midlife and aging parents with children with mental health or developmental problems: report of a national study. *Journal of Health and Social Behaviour*, **49**, 301–16.

9. Howe, D. (2006) Disabled children, maltreatment and attachment. *British Journal of Social Work*, **36**, 743–60.

10. Wan, M.W., Green, Elsabbagh, M. and Johnson, M. (2008) Mother-infant interactions in high-risk infant siblings of children with autism. *International Meeting for Autism Research London*. http://imfar.confex.com/imfar/2008/webprogram/Paper1788.html (viewed 14 September 2009).

11. Olsson, M.B. and Hwang, C.P. (2001) Depression in mothers and fathers of children with intellectual disability. *Journal of Intellectual Disability Research*, **45**, 353–43.

12. Bailey, D.B., Golden, R.N., Roberts, J. and Ford, A. (2007) Maternal depression and developmental disability: research critique. *Mental Retardation and Developmental Disabilities Research Reviews*, **13**, 321–29.

13. Feldman, M., Mconald, L., Serbin, L. *et al.* (2007) Predictors of depressive symptoms in primary caregivers of young children with or at risk for developmental delay. *Journal of Intellectual Disability Research*, **51**, 606–19.

14. Bromley, J., Hare, D.J., Davison, K. and Emerson, E. (2004) Mothers supporting children with autistic spectrum disorders: social support, mental health status and satisfaction with services. *Autism*, **8**, 409–23.

15. Woodgate, R. (2008) Living in a world of our own: the experience of parents who have a child with autism. *Qualitative Health Research*, **18**, 1075–10.

16. Gray, D. (1994) Coping with autism: stress and strategies. *Sociology of Health and Illness*, **16**, 275–300.

17. Scorgie, K. and Sobsey, D. (2000) Transformational outcomes associated with parenting children who have disabilities. *Mental Retardation*, **38**, 195–206.

18. Blacher, J. and Baker, B.L. (2007) Positive impact of intellectual disability on families. *American Journal of Mental Retardation*, **112**, 330–48.

19. Beresford, B., Rabiee, P. and Sloper, P. (2007) Outcomes for parents with disabled children. *Research Works* 2007-03, Social Policy Research Unit, University of York, York.

20. MacDonald, H. and Callery, P. (2007) Parenting children requiring complex care: a journey through time. *Child Care, Health and Development*, **34**, 207–13.

28
Being a parent with a disability

Adil Akram and Sheila Hollins

St George's University of London, UK

28.1   Being a disabled parent

Being a parent is a richly varied social role that is highly valued as a cornerstone of society. Parenting has public and private facets and can be one of the most enriching and fulfilling experiences a person can have. Being disabled, be it from a physical or a mental cause, can often conversely lead to social exclusion, discrimination and a negative attitude from services. Despite this, it should be remembered that living with a long-term impairment might also for many be an enriching and fulfilling life experience. In 2001 the World Health Organization (WHO) disability and rehabilitation team declared that:

> States must introduce comprehensive mandatory anti-discrimination laws to secure the systematic removal of environmental and cultural barriers to disabled peoples' meaningful participation at all levels and in all areas – economic, political and social – of mainstream community life. [1]

To be a parent is in essence to be at the heart of community life. In this chapter, we touch on parents with physical or intellectual impairments, or parents having a mental illness. It is important to state at the outset that although we may speak of 'being a disabled parent', that the disability itself frequently arises from the social and environmental barriers and restrictions that people with impairments face in their communities. It follows that the degree of someone's disability may then differ across each country and community, to the extent that people in some nations may not even identify themselves as being 'disabled', even if they have some form of recognized impairment.

Parenthood and Mental Health: A Bridge between Infant and Adult Psychiatry   Sam Tyano, Miri Keren, Helen Herrman and John Cox
© 2010 John Wiley & Sons, Ltd

In the USA over 8 million families include at least one parent with a long-term illness or impairment [2]. Worldwide there are millions of parents raising children and living with a disability. They comprise a widely heterogeneous group and their parenting needs may vary depending on the nature of their specific impairments, the support they receive and the societal barriers they face over time. But there is a dearth of literature on parenting with a disability, despite the increasing numbers of these parents and the development of supportive networks online to allow disabled parents to share their experiences. The majority of studies that have looked at parenting and disability come from high-income nations such as the USA, Australia, Canada and the UK. Our discussion of the literature is mainly from a UK perspective as one model of a nation which, over the past 20 years, has been developing social policy and awareness around disability and parenting. Useful practice points and important issues arising from the literature in these areas is discussed and highlighted.

28.2 The UK context

In the UK there are 14.1 million parents. About 12% of these parents identified themselves as disabled [3], or up to about 2.1 million people [4]. The largest UK study on parenting and disability to date is by Olsen and Clarke [5]. They interviewed disabled parents from 67 families. Their impairments were categorized as physical, mental, 'physical and mental' and 'physical and sensory'. Of note, their study did not include parents of African or Caribbean ethnicity and only 10 disabled fathers took part. This highlights some of the major gaps that still exist in the research into this area.

The authors of this important study comment on this and describe the 'invisibility' of disabled parents in the literature [5]. Previously researchers have specifically excluded parents with disabilities from potentially positive and empowering studies about education and support of parents in the parenting role. In this way, research focus itself has served to further isolate and marginalize disabled parents into studies that focus solely on what 'deficits' may exist in their parenting. They had also previously been excluded from UK policies and initiatives to promote social inclusion, parenting and family welfare, virtually up to the end of the twentieth century. In some cases parents may be parenting while experiencing both physical *and* mental illness or other impairment. The effects of each may also differentially impinge on parenting over time as symptoms change.

A UK taskforce on supporting disabled adults as parents heard from disabled parents that 'negative attitudes towards disabled parents and unequal access to support' [6] was the main obstacle or difficulty they faced in being able to effectively exercise their role as a parent, rather than any inability arising from a physical impairment, intellectual disability or mental illness.

28.3 Parents with physical disability

The Olsen and Clarke [5] study highlights the 'pathologising' perspective from which physical disability and parenting is viewed in the literature. The essence of parenting is the relationship between parent and child. Yet studies have tended to focus on searching for deficiencies or inadequacy of parenting and looking for direct causal associations, often negating other important social factors such as home environment and social support.

The term 'physical disability' includes a wide range of diverse physical health problems and their subsequent impairments, such as cancer, rheumatoid arthritis, multiple sclerosis, cerebral palsy, spinal cord injury, musculoskeletal injury or neuromuscular diseases like motor neurone disease. Parents may have sensory impairments such as blindness or deafness. Parents with physical impairments may then experience disability and exclusion through a lack of assistance with practical tasks, poor access to facilities for family social activities or even their child's school, poor transportation and poverty [7]. The poverty trap faced by parents with physical impairments is especially harsh due to the fact they are more likely to need financial welfare benefits compared to other parents, having additional costs to overcome their disabling environment, e.g. for home adaptations, adequate transport and social family activities [7].

Parenting assessments by statutory services often get reduced or operationalized into a series of tasks which may translate into easy-to-measure research outcomes or 'tick box' checklists for professionals to assess. This reductionist 'task-based parenting' approach serves to further exclude and undermine disabled parents, who may be unable to meet some of these mainly practical criteria without support or adaptations. Being a parent encompasses much more than task-based activity, including providing emotional support, guidance and love – arguably among the most important aspects – and also the most difficult to assess, measure and research.

A UK taskforce identified major obstacles to supporting disabled adults as parents [6], which are summarized in Box 28.1. These barriers result in poor and inadequate service provision and increase the risk of family breakdown and of disabled parents losing children into care [6].

Box 28.1   The barriers to supporting disabled adults as parents in the UK [6]

- A lack of consultation or involvement of disabled parents in developing policies to support their role as parents

- Disabling attitudes such as: 'impairment . . . in itself, and inevitably, leads to child deprivation, potential harm or abuse' or 'disabled parents are considered in need of "care" rather than in need of assistance' [6]

- Poor access to information to help support a disabled parent in the parenting role

- Poor quality information that does not address their concerns and fears

- Health-care and social workers lacking in knowledge, expertise or confidence in supporting disabled parents in their parenting role

- Confusion about disabled peoples' rights to community care

- Labeling disabled parents' children as 'in need' to get assistance

- Differential national access in the UK to direct payments for supporting disabled parents

- A lack of promoting and enhancing parenting by disabled adults, instead viewing assessments through the prism of 'incapacity'

- A lack of joint working between children's and adults' services.

28.4 Parents with intellectual disability

Parents with intellectual disability tend to face more social barriers and discriminatory attitudes than other groups of disabled parents. The number of parents with intellectual disability in the UK is unknown, which makes service provision and resource planning difficult [3, 8]. Of the limited research that has been done, it is clear that many parents with intellectual disability are rendered further disabled by poverty, reliance on services that presume parental incompetence, and professionals that do not have adequate training in supporting their needs in the family unit [3, 5, 8, 9].

There is particular difficulty around accessing support for parents identified as having 'mild to moderate' intellectual disability [3]. This group of parents may not meet threshold criteria for community support provided for adults with intellectual disability. The dual role of social workers is also an issue due to conflicting responsibilities of supporting the family unit with one hand and intervening if things deteriorate with the other. This may serve to promote a fatalistic attitude of the disabled parent being unable to cope. Social services may then only respond to crises when children have been identified as 'at risk' with the emphasis shifted to a child protection 'judgemental' perspective. This is a missed opportunity to provide adequate support early and 'think family' and 'think parent' [8, 9]. Most research in this area has not looked at how to support the parent in their family role [3].

This professional perspective is disempowering to disabled parents and can result in children being taken into care. Disabled parents with intellectual disability or mental illness are most vulnerable to this outcome and most likely not to have had a needs assessment from adult services, as is their right in the UK [6]. This is just one example of 'system abuse' – where people's difficulties are exacerbated by the very services designed to support and protect them [10]. Types of system abuse have been analyzed using case studies of parents with intellectual disability and have been described by Booth and Booth [10], but all parents with disability have been shown to be at greater risk of experiencing these [3, 5, 6, 9, 11]. These are outlined in Box 28.2.

Box 28.2   Types of 'system abuse' experienced by parents with intellectual disability [10]

- Unintended negative outcomes from services intervening
- Misadministration
- Buck-passing between professionals and agencies
- Setting unrealistic or impossible standards
- Double standards
- Exclusion from decision-making
- Poor communication
- Poor access to professionals
- Lack of continuity in services provided

Another important UK qualitative study of parents with intellectual disability by Booth and Booth [11] used the research methodology of exploring parents' 'life stories' by in-depth interviewing. This gave rich levels of detail as to the under-examined lives of parents bringing up children and living with an intellectual disability. Twenty families took part in this study and fourteen of these families had experienced one or more children placed into care. Most of these parents had experienced the trauma of losing a child into care, permanently [8, 11].

At first glance, the findings suggest that parents with intellectual disabilities are seemingly doomed to failure. However, in many cases, 'parents were not given the opportunity to demonstrate their capacity to look after the child' [11]. In one case a parent was presumed incompetent due to low intelligence. This highlights one common misassumption prevalent among professionals – that people with intellectual disability are simply unable to learn new skills – which is patently untrue. Compare this to the wide perception of new parents needing time to learn the skills to look after a baby and all the statutory support that is typically provided to ensure this happens (antenatal classes, GP check-ups, midwifery services, health visiting). This is in addition to the extended family support and skills passed on from grandparents and other relatives that most new parents enjoy and can access. Parents with intellectual disability often have no sound experiences of being parented themselves to draw on, may have a reduced or absent family network, may be excluded from antenatal classes and thus have reduced opportunities to develop parenting skills over time [3, 5, 8, 11].

The personal stories described by Booth and Booth [11] form a valuable resource for highlighting the challenges and obstacles faced by this vulnerable and relatively 'hidden' group in society. The researchers strove to obtain and understand the experiences of these parents directly, compiling data from hours of taped interviews, phone calls, meetings, photographs and social outings. For example, to recount the story of one subject, 'Rosie Spencer', required frequent contact over 18 months and over 100 hours of time getting to know her [11]. This level of intensive working and analysis is arguably what health and social care professionals should be striving for to support their clients with intellectual disabilities and children. This can lead to assessing relative strengths as well as problems that parents with intellectual disability may experience [8, 11].

What appears clear is that the majority of problems that parents with intellectual disability encounter are in fact the same types of problems as all parents may face – social problems with inadequate housing, poor access to transport, financial difficulties and poor social support networks. What also is evident is the additional burden of social isolation, discrimination, negative attitudes from services and lack of parenting skills from personal childhood experiences [3, 5, 8, 12].

Generally the research on parents with intellectual disability has focused on mothers, with fathers relatively ignored [3]. Studies in this area have limitations in their methodology, for example small sample sizes, lack of control groups or explanations about data collection. This may affect the validity and reliability of results. There is a dearth of studies looking at parenting with intellectual disability across the life cycle as the child grows up and how the parenting roles and responsibilities change over time [3].

Key messages from the UK experience include the need for statutory services to first and foremost recognize the parenting rights and responsibilities of parents with intellectual disability, to develop and deliver parenting skills training packages that are home-based and to promote self-determination in decision-making around parental issues [3].

28.5 Parents with mental illness

Historically people with severe and enduring mental illness (SMI) were largely institutionalized and removed from society and the chance to engage in wider social roles. Efforts were made to deny or prevent the opportunity to become parents by controlling their fertility, including enforced sterilizations or abortions for women. Traditional neuroleptic medications also had significant sexual side effects affecting fertility [13].

Over the past 30 years things have changed in the UK and other high-income countries as care of people with mental illness has gradually moved out of the asylum into the community, with new opportunities to take on meaningful social roles in work and family arenas. Studies from Norway and the USA have also suggested that the fertility of women with severe mental illness has increased with deinstitutionalization [13, 14]. Reproductive rates among women with SMI such as schizophrenia were similar to healthy controls in US studies [13]. In addition, second- and third-generation neuroleptic medications have less effect on fertility. These factors have contributed to the increasing number of parents who live with severe and enduring mental illness such as bipolar affective disorder and schizophrenia.

There has been little research into the needs of women with SMI who may wish to become, or in many cases already are, parents. Studies have tended to focus on the potential risks of negative outcomes for the children of mothers with SMI and the deficits in the mothers' parenting skills [15]. Hardly any studies have been published on SMI and the impact on fatherhood [16].

Limited data from other countries indicates that the sexual health of women with SMI is much more at risk than for women in the general population. They appear to have higher rates of unprotected sex, coerced sex, unwanted pregnancies, terminations, children taken into care and sexually transmitted infections [12]. Women with SMI may also have more lifetime sexual partners and be at greater risk of violence in pregnancy but less likely to receive antenatal care than controls [12].

There is little data about the attitudes of mental healthcare professionals towards supporting patients in their role as a parent. One review by Miller [13] argues that reproductive health services should be offered in conjunction with mental health services, as the logistics of attending separate clinics may be a barrier preventing women with SMI from seeking advice about family planning. Locating the perinatal psychiatry services in the same location as the obstetric and gynecology services would also allow pregnant women with SMI access to psychiatry care in the same vicinity as where they attend for routine antenatal checks and ultrasound scans [17]. This would also help reduce stigma and barriers to accessing appropriate care in a timely, convenient way.

In the UK maternity services often do not make adequate provision for the complex situation of pregnancy and severe mental illness or of pregnant women who have experienced major trauma. There is variable access to perinatal psychiatry services to support such women through pregnancy and the postnatal period, nor to support them in parenting their new infant.

28.6   A recovery perspective on disabled parents with mental illness

The traditional research perspective in this area has focused on deficits in parenting, based on the views of children being at risk from maltreatment, abuse and mental illness themselves [5]. Supporting people with mental illness in their role as parents has been largely ignored both clinically by healthcare professionals and by researchers. This is despite the parenting role potentially having an important 'normalizing' therapeutic social role to play from a 'recovery' perspective of well-being.

The recovery model has now been widely accepted across many high-income nations as the favored approach to delivery of mental health services. Important central elements of a recovery perspective include instilling hope, providing a secure base, supporting a sense of self empowerment, social inclusion, developing personal coping strategies and a sense of meaning [18]. This approach can also easily translate to a framework for the rights to and services from social and healthcare services that disabled parents with mental illness should be offered and expect. There is now increasing recognition in the UK that mental health policies should explicitly acknowledge the needs of parents with mental illness [6].

28.7   The social model of disability

This model, described by Oliver [19], proposes that the extent of any disability that results from an impairment is a function of environmental factors. These are external social barriers and include things like negative attitudes, poor access, inadequate facilities and provision of services. By definition, Oliver's model strongly argues that disability is not located within the person with impairment, but exists around them in society. The general findings from studies of disabled parents certainly support this view and more studies incorporating a social perspective of disability could elucidate the social barriers to parenting with a long-term physical or sensory impairment or illness [5, 11].

28.8   Cultural representations of parents with disabilities

Depictions of disabled parents in popular culture through film and television largely serve to perpetuate entrenched societal attitudes that disabled parents are inadequate parents. They almost without exception portray negative role models and usually show family discord or breakdown as a result of the disability, rather than of other significant disadvantages that disabled parents may face, such as poverty, poor access to support, social deprivation and having to overcome discrimination.

Despite this, films such as 'I am Sam' (US) [20] attempt to dramatically explore the fictional experiences of disabled parents (in this case with intellectual disability). These dramatic interpretations may serve to raise some wider awareness about the struggles disabled parents face behind closed doors. However, the vast majority of films from both high and low-income nations depicting disabled parents only reinforce the negative stigmatizing stereotype described above of parents unable to adequately raise their children and who ultimately always lose their children into care.

28.9 UK policy perspectives

Over the past 20 years the UK has developed and published a range of policies for social and health-care services meant to apply to all members of society. More recently at the outset of the twenty-first century, policies have specifically been introduced to support and recognize the needs of disabled people. These are outlined in Box 28.3. In general these policies and guidelines all promote values of equality of access to statutory support for and recognition of disabled peoples' right to engage in parenting roles. Despite this, studies still show a failure of systems and professionals in meeting these values [3, 5, 6, 8, 9, 11].

Box 28.3   UK policies to support the rights of disabled parents [3]

- The Disability Discrimination Act (1995, 2005)

- The Community Care Act (1996)

- Human Rights Act (1998)

- Department of Health (2000) Framework for the Assessment of Children in Need and their Families

- Health and Social Care Act (2001)

- Department of Health (2003) Fair Access to Care Services

- Prime Minister's Strategy Unit (2005) Improving the Life Chances of Disabled People.

28.10 Solutions to support disabled adults as parents

There has been an increase in the peer support available worldwide through online forums and organizations which are accessible through the Internet, e.g. Parents with Disabilities Online [2], Disabled Parents Network [21]. The rise of these groups has increased the availability of useful information by and for disabled parents, allowing a pooling together of experiences and resources, as well as being a source of support. Positive stories of parenting while managing a physical or intellectual disability or mental illness help to counter negative public and professional attitudes or assumptions head-on with enlightening snapshots of real family life. These online groups demonstrate how disabled parents are sharing practical advice about parenting (e.g. shopping, pregnancy, wheelchair adaptations to carry children) and overcoming barriers by sharing their expertise with others. At least in the UK, disabled parents themselves are now, more than ever before, in a position to challenge societal discrimination and demand their right to an equal opportunity to raise their children and provide care with the same statutory obligations for support from services that non-disabled parents are entitled to [5].

Development of innovative services and new professional roles can help bridge the gaps between different professions expertise. For example, the development of a specialist mental health midwife role recognizes that women with severe mental illness can and do choose to have babies and will require appropriate support during pregnancy and after delivery as do other women [17].

Parents with intellectual disability can benefit from educational programs to develop parenting and other life skills. These may be most effective if delivered in the home environment, provided that this is stable [3]. Recognizing that adults with intellectual disability may take longer to learn skills or concepts, but that learning is possible is vital. Effective forms of teaching may include practical 'hands on' experiential learning, using reinforcement, visual aids and repetition [3].

Case working and service provision for disabled parents can be done from different *enabling* or *impeding* professional perspectives. In the literature on parents with intellectual disability, Mount and Zwernik [10, 22] differentiate between a 'deficiency orientation' and a 'capacity perspective'. A 'deficiency orientation' focuses on personal limitations and deficits. A 'capacity perspective' focuses on personal strengths and abilities. Booth and Booth [11] in their biographical study describe one case through these opposing perspectives. They argue that a deficiency orientation results in an assumption of incompetence, apportioning blame for difficulties on parents themselves rather than external factors.

Support can come in different guises that can serve to enhance or impede independent parenting. Tucker and Johnson [23] have defined these 'competence-promoting' or 'competence-inhibiting' types of support, also discussed in the cases studied by Booth and Booth [11, 23]. These are shown in Table 28.1

Table 28.1   Types of support for parenting [11, 23]

Competence-promoting support

- Parents feel in control

- Advocacy offered

- Involved in making decisions about what support they need

- Feeds back the usefulness of the support offered

- Acknowledges relative parenting strengths

- Attempts to build skills within the family unit

- Practical assistance with finances, benefits, appropriate furniture

- Perspective aimed at promoting self-reliance in community.

Competence-inhibiting support

- Professionals prejudge parental incompetence

- Assume outside intervention required

Table 28.1   (*Continued*)

- Does not encourage development of parenting skills

- Professionals provide assistance as they judge or see fit

- Lack of acknowledgement of parenting strengths

- Isolating perspective from wider social networks.

Environmental pressures on the parents can influence these models of support offered by social services. In one case of parents with intellectual disability, these were identified as including debt, discrimination, social isolation, lack of means of communication or transport, deprived neighborhood, and lack of exposure to parenting or life skills due to separate upbringing of disabled people from the mainstream [8, 11]. The difference between the controlling and enabling aspects of support offered by the professionals directly involved may make the vital difference between keeping or losing the child into care.

Confusion about whether support should come under adult or child services often leads to professionals lacking confidence in offering support to disabled parents or knowing what form effective support may take [3, 6, 7, 8, 9]. Studies have found that insufficient joint working exists between agencies such as health, housing and education to support disabled parents, with confusing legislation [3, 6, 8, 9]. However, it was also found that the best solutions came from disabled parents themselves, often finding creative, simple and small-scale ways to meet their needs. These are summarized in Box 28.4. An important message from the studies conducted was for policy-makers to 'think parent' and not equate 'disabled parent' with 'child in need' [3, 5, 8, 9, 10, 11]. This highlights the cultural shift required in 'placing support for disabled parents within a broader strategic commitment to the principles of independent living across social care, housing, health and employment.' [9].

Box 28.4   Supporting disabled adults as parents [8, 9]

- Make information accessible on an equal basis to all parents as required, e.g. school reports in Braille or on tape

- Recognize individual needs differ, even between parents with the same impairment, i.e. 'one size does not fit all'

- Supporting family life in ways that help disabled parents exercise control and choice, e.g. through individual budgets

- Giving adequate training to professionals in disability issues

- Making support more flexible, timely and responsive to the changing needs of disabled parents as their children grow up

- Providing support that is also in keeping with the parents' and families' cultural background, e.g. around language, food customs and interaction

- Setting up peer support groups to share ideas and experience, e.g. online

---

Discussion with disabled parents and professionals conducted by Olsen and Tyrer [9] led to a set of principles of good practice for supporting disabled parents, set out in Box 28.5.

Box 28.5   The nine principles of good practice with disabled parents

1 Focus on rights and entitlements of disabled parents

2 Focus on how barriers to fulfillment of the parenting role can be tackled

3 Be needs led and recognize the needs of disabled parents vary greatly

4 Promote parental choice and control

5 Involve working in partnership across teams and agencies, and with parents themselves

6 Work from a sound knowledge base of practice, policy, legislation and research

7 Involve management commitment and strategic direction

8 Underpin rather than undermine parents in fulfilling their parental role

9 Be non-discriminatory to disabled people as parents.

(Adapted from Olsen and Tyrer, 2004 [9])

28.11 Involving disabled parents in research

In the last 20 years there has been a small but gradually increasing research interest in the experiences of disabled parents. The studies discussed in this chapter are located within a social model of disability and sought to examine the interface between societal barriers and individual impairment in causing and exacerbating disability. They acknowledge that employing both quantitative and qualitative research methods bring about the most useful insights into the lives of parents with disability.

Qualitative biographical methodologies such as life stories and in-depth interviewing have allowed participants to tell their stories: '. . . it is essential for the researcher first of all to listen to those who know' [11]. A biographical approach avoids the pitfalls many researchers and professionals make of over-simplifying the family relationships being assessed, comparing parents with intellectual disability against inappropriate standards, ignoring parental achievements and assuming inadequate care solely results from poor parenting [3, 5, 8, 11].

UK-based knowledge reviews and research briefings from the Social Care Institute for Excellence (SCIE) have identified a need for more research into disability and parenting [3, 7, 24]. There is a need for more research into the changing nature of parenting with a disability across the lifecycle, as parents become grandparents and continue caregiving as part of the wider family. The studies that have been done so far have generally been limited by small sample sizes, lack of replication and focusing on the experiences of mainly disabled parents from Caucasian populations living in high-income countries. There is a need for the development of innovative services and promotion of inter-agency working to support disabled parents. Just as pressing is the need for research into the effectiveness of these models to combat the social constructs of disability and exclusion. There is also a startling lack of accurate data about the numbers of disabled fathers and their experiences and parents with intellectual disability and their needs, not just in the UK but also worldwide.

28.12 Conclusion

There are a large number of disabled parents around the world. They comprise a diverse group of people who number in the millions, but have been largely ignored in the parenting literature. Studies conducted in high-income countries suggest they often have difficulty accessing services, and services have often not suitably been meeting their diverse parenting needs. In large part however, their needs are likely to be the same as non-disabled parents in today's society, namely the opportunity to access support and advice about their parenting role, suitable childcare and nursery facilities, receiving health care and social care according to individual need. More research is urgently needed to examine the experiences of disabled parents in middle- and low-income countries and look at developing social care and health policies and models of service delivery in these diverse populations.

The combination of disability and additional social factors such as ethnicity (cultural and language barriers), poverty, social exclusion, social deprivation and poor housing also need to be further explored. The limited research that does exist has been done almost exclusively in high-income countries. From these studies on parents with impairment of any form, what is clear is that environmental external barriers that exist in society have a major impact on an individual's ability to parent, as argued by the social model of disability. Essentially living with an impairment and being a parent need not mean being *disabled as a parent*. Unfortunately, the significant additional barriers in society faced by these parents have often resulted in doing just that. It is hoped that with increasing awareness of the issues at stake, more research and strong advocacy by disabled parents themselves setting the agenda using new technologies to share support and promote good practice, that the twenty-first century will finally herald the wider social acceptance of parenting with a disability.

28.13   References

1. World Health Organization (WHO) Disability and Rehabilitation team (2001) Rethinking care from the perspective of disabled people. Conference report and recommendations. http://whqlibdoc.who.int/hq/2001/a78624.pdf.
2. http://www.disabledparents.net.
3. Social Care Institute for Excellence (SCIE) (2005) Research briefing 14: Helping parents with learning disabilities in their role as parents. Policy Press, London.
4. Stickland, H. (2003) *Disabled Parents and Employment*. Department of Work and Pensions, London.

5. Olsen, R. and Clarke, H. (2003) *Parenting and Disability. Disabled Parents' Experiences of Raising Children.* The Policy Press, Bristol.
6. Morris, J. (2003) *The Right Support: Report of the Task Force on Supporting Disabled Adults in their Parenting Role.* Joseph Rowntree Foundation, York.
7. Social Care Institute for Excellence (SCIE) (2005) Research briefing 13: Helping parents with a physical or sensory impairment in their role as parents. Policy Press, London.
8. Booth, T. (2003) Parents with intellectual disabilities (article). http://www.intellectualdis-ability.info/lifestages/ds_parent.htm.
9. Olsen, R. and Tyrers, H. (2004) Think parent: supporting disabled adults as parents. The National Family and Parenting Institute, London. Also online summary 'Findings Nov 2004' Joseph Rowntree Foundation. http://www.jrf.org.uk/sites/files/jrf/n34.pdf.
10. Booth, T. and Booth, W. (1998) *Growing up with Parents Who Have Learning Difficulties.* Routledge, London.
11. Booth, T. and Booth, W. (1994) *Parenting under Pressure: Mothers and Fathers with Learning Difficulties.* Open University Press, Buckingham.
12. Andron, L. and Tymchuck, A. (1987) Parents who are mentally retarded, in *Mental Handicap and Sexuality: Issues and Perspectives* (ed. A. Craft), D.J. Costello, Tunbridge Wells.
13. Miller, L.J. (1997) Sexuality, reproduction, and family planning in women with schizophrenia *Schizophrenia Bulletin,* **23** (4), 623–35.
14. Odegard, O. (1980) Fertility of psychiatric first admissions in Norway 1936–75 *Acta Psychiatrica Scandinavia,* **62**, 212–20.
15. Mowbray, C.T., Lewandowski, L. Bybee, D. and Oyserman, D. (2004) Children of mothers diagnosed with serious mental illness: patterns and predictors of service use. *Mental Health Services Research,* **6** (3), 167–83.
16. Styron, T.H., Pruett, M.K., McMahon, T.J. and Davidson, L. (2002) Fathers with serious mental illness: a neglected group. *Psychiatric Rehabilitation Journal,* **25** (3), 215–22.
17. Akram, A. (2009) Good practice – The specialist midwife in mental health. *Disability, Pregnancy and Parenting International Journal,* **66**, Summer.
18. Care Services Improvement Partnership (CSIP), Royal College of Psychiatrists, Social Care Institute for Excellence (SCIE) (2007) A common purpose: Recovery in future mental health services. Joint position paper 08. London.
19. Oliver, M. (1990) *The Politics of Disablement.* Macmillan, Basingstoke.
20. Nelson, J. (2002) *'I am Sam'* (US) New Line Cinema.
21. www.disabledparentsnetwork.org.uk. Disabled Parents Network, 81 Melton Road, West Bridgford, Nottingham, NG2 8EN, UK. Tel: 0044 300 3300 639.
22. Mount, B. and Zwernik, K. (1988) It's Never Too Early, It's Never Too Late: A Booklet about Personal Futures Planning. Metropolitan Council, St Paul, MN, USA.
23. Tucker, M. and Johnson, O. (1989) Competence promoting vs. competence inhibiting social support for mentally retarded mothers. *Human Organisation,* **48** (2), 95–107.
24. Social Care Institute for Excellence (SCIE) (2006) Knowledge review 11: Supporting disabled parents and parents with additional support needs. Policy Press, London.

29

Parenthood: the impact of immigration

Olivier Taïeb,[1] Thierry Baubet,[1] Dalila Rezzoug[1] and Marie Rose Moro[1,2]

[1]Avicenne Hospital, APHP, Paris 13 University, Seine-Saint Denis, France
[2]Cochin Hospital, APHP, Paris Descartes University, France

29.1 Introduction

Culture and parenthood, in the meaning shared by psychoanalysts, psychologists, psychiatrists and pediatricians, and also philosophers, teachers, social workers and policy-makers, is the challenge of the twenty-first century [1]. It is tempting to suggest that the most important issue is for each individual to find their own style of parenthood, to transfer or pass on the bond, the tenderness, the protection of self and others or – in a word – life. Oddly enough, the English *parenthood* has only in recent years appeared other languages (French, Spanish or Italian) as a neologism (such as *parentalité* in French). It is as if we have only recently realized that we have in our hands something precious, and that parents all over the world possess it. We have seen that some parents, those that are vulnerable or that find themselves in difficult or even inhuman situations, are so preoccupied with finding strategies to survive – in all senses of the word, mentally or materially – that they find it difficult or impossible to pass on anything but the precariousness of their surrounding world. This is why it is important to study migratory situations, since for the parents these situations lead to changes and in some cases to breakdowns that make the establishment of parent–infant relationships more complex. And indeed, today, migrations are part of modern societies, which are multiform and multicultural, and migration should be a focus of our clinical concerns. This is all the more true because once this variable is taken into account, the risk is converted into creative potential, both for the children and their families and for caregivers, as will be seen hereafter from a French experience in infant care set up in Avicenne Hospital and Jean Verdier Hospital in the Paris multicultural suburbs [2, 3, 4, 5, 6, 7].

29.2 The ingredients of parenthood

You are not born a parent, you become one. Parenthood is constructed from complex ingredients. Certain of these are community ingredients, and belong to the society as a whole; they change over time, they can be historical, legal, social and cultural. Others are more personal and private; they may be conscious or unconscious, they belong to each parent as separate persons and future parents, to the couple, and to the family history of each parent. What is played out here is the part that is passed on and the part that remains hidden, childhood traumas, and the way each individual has patched them up.

There is also another set of factors belonging to the child, who changes those who gave him birth into parents. Certain infants are more gifted than others, some are born into an environment that makes things easier; others, because of the circumstances of their birth (prematurity, neonatal distress, physical or mental handicap), have numerous obstacles to overcome, and must develop numerous, often costly strategies to enter into a relationship with the distressed parent. Since the work by Cramer, Lebovici, Stern and many others, we know that the infant is an active partner in the parent–infant interaction, and thereby in the construction of parenthood [8, 9]. The infant contributes to the emergence of the maternal and paternal identities of the adults around him that are handling him, feeding him, and giving him pleasure, within a process of exchange of actions and affects that are a central part of the first moments of life [10].

There are very many ways of being a father and being a mother, as has been shown by a large volume of work by sociologists and anthropologists (for instance [11, 12, 13, 14, 15]). The difficulty for professionals resides in the need to leave room for these potentials to emerge, and to refrain from any form of judgement on the 'best way' to be a father or a mother. It is a difficult task, because any professional will tend to think he or she knows better than the parents how they should behave with their child, what his needs are and what his expectations are. Social and cultural elements contribute to the construction of parental functioning [16, 17, 18]. Cultural elements have a preventive function and enable anticipation of how to become a parent, if need be giving meaning to the daily ups and downs of parent–child relations, and preventing distress from setting in.

Early on, cultural elements mingle and become profoundly entangled with individual, family and social elements [19, 20, 21, 22]. Pregnancy, on account of its initiatory nature, recalls our mythical, cultural and fantasized belonging. How can we protect ourselves in exile? How can we have fine and healthy children? In some places the pregnancy must be concealed, in others certain fish should not be eaten, or certain tubers that soften when cooked; in others again the husband should not eat certain sorts of meat while his wife is pregnant, or dreams must be kept and interpreted and the demands made complied with, because in dreams it is the child who is speaking [13]. In exile these elements belonging to the private sphere can find themselves in contradiction with new, outside, medical, cultural and social manners of thinking.

Then comes the moment of childbirth. Here again there are many ways of giving birth, receiving the child, presenting him to the world and thinking about his otherness and sometimes his distress. There are also all sorts of 'trivial' things that are reactivated in situations of crisis, reawakening representations that may have remained dormant, or that were thought to have been outlived.

In the name of a sort of empty universality and simplistic ethics, we professionals do not integrate these complex manners of thinking in the design of prevention and care provision, nor in our theorizing. The issues we approach rarely enter the cultural dimension of parenthood, and above all we do not view these ways of thinking and doing things as being of use in establishing an alliance, understanding, anticipating and providing care. We no doubt feel that technique is unclothed, that it has no cultural impact, and that it is enough to observe a protocol for the action to be correctly implemented.

Yet several clinical experiences [2, 7] show that once these different representations are shared, efficiency is patent. From a theoretical viewpoint they renew our manners of thinking, lead us to 'de-center' and complexify our models and to set aside our over-hasty judgement. Apprehending this otherness is to enable these women to experience the different stages of their pregnancies and parenthood in a non-traumatic manner, and to become familiar with other ways of thinking and other techniques. Migration does entail the need to change. But ignoring otherness is not only to miss the creative side of the encounter, but also to run the risk that these women will never find their place in our prevention and health systems, and it also restricts them to solitude of thought and living. To engage in thought we need to build together, exchange ideas, confront perceptions with those of other people. If this is not possible, then thought rests on itself and its own mechanisms. Non-confrontation of this sort can also lead to rigidity and withdrawal. It is exchanges with others that enable us to change.

Psychic transparency, cultural transparency

Besides these social and cultural dimensions, paternal and maternal function can be upset by manifestations of individual mental functioning, or by earlier suffering that has not found relief, appearing often in a sudden and violent manner at the time when the line of descent is being enacted: for instance the various forms of post-partum depression, and even psychoses, leading on to loss of meaning. The vulnerability of the mother – whoever she is – in this period is well known and has been theorized, in particular via the concept of 'psychic transparency' (*transparence psychique*). By transparency what is meant is that, in the perinatal period, the mental functioning of the mother is easier to read and perceive than it usually is [23, 24]. Indeed, the alterations occurring during pregnancy are accompanied by a more ready, more explicit expression of desires, conflicts and impulses. In addition, childhood conflict is relived, reactivated in particular by Oedipal revival. Later, functioning once again becomes opaque. This psychic transparency is less recognized in fathers, who also experience upheavals relating to the reliving of their own conflicts, to the re-enacting of their own status as a son, and to the shift from being a son to being a father. The perinatal period thus enables regression and expression that are quite specific to it.

Exile merely potentializes this psychic transparency, which expresses itself in the two parents in different ways in the mental and cultural spheres. In the mental sphere it is expressed by the reliving of conflicts and the expression of emotions. It is expressed in the cultural sphere by way of the same process but here applied to cultural representations, and ways of doing and saying things that are specific to each culture. All these cultural elements, which we thought belonged to the preceding generation, are reactivated, and suddenly become valuable and alive. Thus it is appropriate to suggest the concept of cultural transparency to apprehend and represent what the parents are experiencing. Their relationship with their culture and their own parents is altered.

Early prevention of setbacks in parenthood

In this reality in which different levels interact one with another, the psychological dimension has a specific position in terms of prevention and care. Prevention, indeed, starts with the pregnancy. It is important to provide help for mothers experiencing difficulties in thinking of the baby to be born, in investing in it, and in welcoming it despite their solitude – which is social and, even more so, existential. Sharing a culture makes it possible to anticipate what will happen, to think about it, and to establish protection. The culture is a base on which to build a place for the child to be born. The setbacks in this construction of the parent–infant bond find cores of meaning within the experience of the social group; but these meanings are far more difficult to apprehend in a migrant situation. In this case the only fixed elements are the body and the individual mental make-up, since everything else has become shifting and precarious. Women living in their communities but excluded from their own societies, equally isolated, also find themselves alone in the task of humanizing the child, a task common to all births. The child is a stranger that the mother must learn to know and recognize.

In the perinatal period, adjustments are needed between mother and infant, and also between husband and wife. Dysfunction is possible, sometimes inevitable, but it is often short-lived if early intervention is possible. To intervene early, demands need to be recognized in their somatic or functional 'translations' – these demands are often difficult to express because individuals do not know to whom they should be addressed, or how this should be done. It is therefore important to learn to recognize the distress and doubts of migrant women through small things (somatic complaints, complaints concerning the child, requests for social assistance). Most important of all, they should be allowed to say things, in their own language if necessary, through other women in their community.

Early prevention is positioned from the start of life in prevention centers, maternity wards, pediatric departments, infant welfare centers and GP consultations. This perinatal prevention work is essential because the period is crucial for the child's development; it is also the time when the child's place in the family is constructed.

Prevention is an important issue, but care is another. The day-to-day difficulties of migrant or socially underprivileged families and their children are leading us to alter our psychological care provision techniques and our theories so as to adapt them to increasingly complex clinical situations [25]. This in turn leads us to alter our own frameworks so as to adequately cater for these children and their parents, and to refer them on to specialized consultations if necessary, within a network enabling links and to-and-fro movements between prevention and care facilities: this complementary functioning is essential. The aim is to enable the parent to move from the inside to the outside that he or she is afraid of, and to be what Michel Serres [21] called the 'weaver', working to seam together two worlds set apart by a sudden catastrophe.

The tree of life

Each of us, according to Serge Lebovici, carries a trans-generational mandate: it can be said that our 'tree of life' sends its roots down into the earth that has soaked up the blood from the wounds caused by the childhood conflicts of our parents [8, 9, 26]. Yet our roots, he says, can enable the tree of life to develop and blossom, if they are not so far buried in the soil that they are inaccessible. Generally – and happily so – filiation, with its neurotic conflicts, does not prevent the processes of cultural affiliation. The child's tree of life, that is to say the mandate he is given via trans-generational transmission, thus brings his grand-parents' generation into his psychic life through the childhood conflicts of his parents, whether pre-conscious or repressed [8, 9].

More contemporary conflicts, and in particular migratory trauma for instance, can also take their place in this tree of life, and such events of course give new meaning, in the aftermath, to childhood conflict and traumas. This is the case for migratory traumas. When the weight of transmission is too great and translation too direct, this becomes for the child a 'pathology of destiny' [26]. This is when there are 'ghosts in the nursery' [27]. These are visitors that re-emerge from the parents' forgotten past, visitors that were 'not invited to the christening'. In favorable circumstances the ghosts are driven away from the nursery and return underground. But in some unfavorable circumstances these representations of the past in the present take over the field, settle there, and seriously affect the mother–infant relationship. The therapeutic challenge resides here: with the mother and those around her, starting from the child as an interactive partner, to create and co-create the conditions needed to identify the ghosts, and rather than chasing them away to negotiate with them and in a sense to humanize them. Once again, the task is to make something human even out of trauma, whatever its nature; here the breakdown arising from exile.

29.3 Pregnancy and childbirth in exile

Traditionally, childbirth is an initiatory moment during which the mother-to-be is neces-sarily supported by other women from the group: accompaniment, preparation for the different events, interpretation of dreams and so forth [3, 28]. Migration leads to several breaks in this supportive process that constructs meaning. First there is the loss of the accompaniment by the group, by the family, by cultural and social support, and an inability to give a culturally acceptable meaning to dysfunction, such as the mother's sadness, feelings of inability, or inharmonious mother–infant relations.

In addition, migrating women are confronted with medical methods that do not allow for traditional protective strategies. For these women, Western medical practice can be violent, indecent, traumatic and even 'pornographic' (a word used by several patients). We became acutely aware of the scale of the violation experienced by the pregnant migrant women from the start of our work with them. The women referred to here are migrants from the rural areas of North Africa, sub-Saharan Africa, or Sri Lanka. For city-dwellers, these effects are also present, but probably in less explicit manner.

Medina's story: every day is a lifetime

I[1] received Medina, a Soniké woman from Mali, who had been referred to me for post-partum depression, apparently accompanied by elements of delirium, but this later was shown to be the cultural expression of a traumatic experience, following trans-cultural evaluation. There was no delirium, only trauma, even if its expression was unusual. Medina is a fine, tall woman with a deeply sad look in her eyes. At our first encounter she was wearing a bright yellow *boubou* and a cloth of the same color covering her hair. On her serious face there were ritual scarifications: a vertical line on the chin, two horizontal lines on the cheek-bones, and a small vertical mark on the forehead. She spoke Soniké in a monotonous voice. From time to time a few tears ran down her cheeks. She took no notice and went on talking about her complete incomprehension of what had happened to her while her son Mamadu was still in her womb. On that day she had Mamadu on her back, he was 2 months old and her first child. The child was very small, was not feeding well, was crying a lot and moaning painfully. She was not able to breastfeed him, he sucked the breast very feebly, and in addition Medina was convinced she had no milk, or at any rate that her milk was not nourishing enough for the child. Medina had been in France for one year, where she had come to rejoin her husband in the country for the previous eight years.

There are several moments that can take the form of genuine mental and cultural violations for these women from rural areas. But before any analysis is made, it is important to emphasize that what is violent is the fact that actions are performed without preparation. These technical acts are closely linked to the Western cultural context. For those who do not share it, these acts, by their implicit content, become veritable inductors of mental violation. The women can neither imagine nor anticipate them. The conclusion to be drawn is not that such acts should not be performed, which would be quite unacceptable both in terms of ethics and in terms of public health. To refrain from practising these acts would amount to excluding the women further from our health-care system, and contribute to socially marginalizing them. On the contrary, the task is to ensure that these acts are efficacious and fulfill their purpose. To adapt our care and prevention strategies we need to apprehend this otherness so that, instead of being an obstacle to interaction, it can become the opportunity for a new encounter.

Reporting the pregnancy

Traditionally, pregnancy should be hidden as long as possible, or at least it should be spoken of as little as possible so as not to arouse envy among sterile women, or women who have not had a boy, women who have had too few children and women who are outsiders. This explains the fear that Medina experienced when she went to see the social worker for her to complete the required pregnancy certificate forms. She felt threatened and unprotected. Anything could happen to her, she could even be 'bewitched' and lose the child she was carrying. This fear was with her throughout her pregnancy, and even when the child was born she was still terrified: the child was not protected, he could at any time return to the world of the ancestors, that is to say he could die.

---

[1] Marie Rose Moro

The ultrasound scan

In hospital things continued along the same lines for Medina. They took 'photos' that showed what she had in her womb, that showed 'what God was still keeping hidden' she said. For her, the scan was almost pornographic. All the more so because the medical team had shown her the images almost without comment, since she understood very little French. These images without words, and without accompaniment, were all the more violent. The practitioner performing the scan did not understand her refusing to look, talked to her, no doubt encouraged her to look, not to worry . . . She closed her eyes to avoid seeing. He interpreted this refusal to look at the images as a difficulty in investing herself in the child. In contrast, for other migrant women in the habit of asking for divinatory acts during pregnancy, such as the Mina or Awa women from Togo or Benin, the scan is sometimes associated with these practices, in which case it is felt to be familiar. Every situation is unique.

Childbirth

Then Medina gave birth, on her own, without an interpreter, with the virtually compulsory presence of her husband, who was brought into the labor room because things were not going well. A Caesarean was envisaged, which the husband, terrified, refused. Finally they waited a little, and Medina was calmed by bringing in another Soniké woman who had just given birth in the same ward. Then, she said, the child consented to come out 'on his own'. We now know the importance of allowing for the physiological labor wherever possible; that is to say so long as the lives of the mother and child are not at risk.

For Medina there was the recurrent idea that the child she had borne and that came into the world in these conditions was not protected; he was in danger, and so was she. In this case it was the category 'lack of protection of mother and child', and also its cultural consequence, vulnerability towards an 'attack by witchcraft', that was the right category for us to envisage, as was confirmed in subsequent work with Medina.

Medina did indeed begin to feel calmer following certain cultural acts that contributed to shoring up the breach, the inadequate protection: the couple asked their families in Mali to perform protection rites for their son Mamadu, so that the child was brought into the generational chain and the wider family. At the same time, we explored the mother's sadness with her, and her lost support, by bringing to life cultural representations that had lost their meaning because of exile and family conflict; in other words the cultural prop was partly reconstructed in the therapeutic group. She had left Mali without her father's consent, and therefore her first child was unprotected. This work of co-construction of cultural meaning was the first step, that of the construction of a framework.

In the second stage, the many losses that Medina had suffered were approached. Her mother had died when she was born and she had been brought up by her father's other wife. In addition she was distressed and sad in her life of exile, separated from her sisters, one of whom died before she could seen her again. Supported by the group [6] and the framework offered, Medina went on to elaborate her sadness, she found meaning for everything that had happened during her all-too-lonely pregnancy, and she constructed a secure relationship with her son Mamadu. The protection of the maternal grandfather requested and obtained by Medina then took effect.

In the preventive sphere, it can be seen from this story, and many others like it, that there is a need to enable pregnant women to have a culturally acceptable representation of what is done to them. They can then build an individual strategy enabling them to shift from one world to another without having to relinquish their own representations – thus constructing a genuine *métissage* or cultural hybridization.

In intra-cultural situations, through pregnancy and childbirth a woman positions herself in the line of mothers and grandmothers, thus finding efficient support (whether family, medical or friendly). In a trans-cultural situation the women will no longer find the outside support required to shore up their internal disarray, leading to a 'potentialisation of the mechanisms of confusion through exile' [2].

Other attitudes observed among mothers need to be understood to be linked to the trauma of certain exiles, and the way in which this reactivates previous conflict. There is first of all the apparent 'opting out' of certain mothers: it is as if they are saying that the abilities are with someone else, with the foreigners. They then go on to over-hasty acculturation: everything that comes from me is bad, and everything good comes from outside. Or, conversely, there is the development of cultural rigidity: the women tend to return to practices that may be outlived in their original families, and there is, more importantly, a loss of their adaptive flexibility to any culture, and more rigidity in behavior; there are above all thoughts that are secondary to a trauma that cannot be expanded upon.

Pregnancy and childbirth in a situation of migration reactivates the loss of a framework. When events are not accompanied by the group, their traumatic nature is enhanced. Thus it is for childbirth, the time of a breach in the maternal shell, both mental and physical, which is often a factor that reactivates the sufferings of exile.

Thus it can be seen that caring for migrant women and their infants is a quite specific task: if there is a pathology of exile, the pathology cannot be positioned on the level of content, since it is invariant and universal; however its nature can be sought in the functioning of the 'containers', and the internal and external frameworks.

29.4 The infant, a cultural being

The infant develops within a cultural shell that pre-exists his birth. What is the nature of the infant? Where is he from? These questions on his ontology have been with human beings through time and under all latitudes. The questions seek to apprehend the otherness of the infant by establishing him within ontological representations that are specific to each cultural group. The infant is above all a stranger who will have to be identified [2].

These questions, and their answers, pervade the whole of family discourse. Overall, they are an attempt to determine whether the infant is a 'virgin' being, or whether he has arrived already possessing his own abilities. In North Africa it is sometimes said that the infant is an angel until his first chuckles – so long as he has not opened his mouth, they say, he is pure, and if he dies he will go straight to heaven. In India in some families it is sometimes said that the infant is a trans-migrant, loaded with baggage containing tendencies and experiences from his previous life [22]. In certain West African countries it is said that the infant is not human; he is a stranger from another world, a visiting stranger, who may leave again without notice if the world of humans does not please him. Thus it is the infant that decides his own death, and this strange ability is all the more significant of his otherness. In so-called traditional societies where infant mortality is still high, this ontological representation is an attempt to give an acceptable meaning to this unacceptable event. In other places, it is thought that the infant will only really achieve human status when he has reached the age of talking and walking: after two years of life, the risk of mortality decreases markedly. In Mongolia in certain regions it is only with the first haircut – between the ages of two and five – that the child shifts from an intermediate being to a human being [29].

In western Europe between the two world wars popular representations saw an infant carrying no trace of any sort, a dough or clay that was to be shaped; educational prerogative belonged to the parents, who were supposed to shape the infant in their own image. Later academic theory, with pedo-psychiatrists like Lebovici, Cramer or Brazelton, set out very different representations: the infant then came to be thought to arrive in the world with a baggage of abilities that the adults had the task of bringing out [8]. If this theory had such success, it is because popular representation had already noted, beyond prevalent discourse, the specific abilities of the very young infant.

The 'enculturation' of the infant as defined by Margaret Mead in 1928 and 1930 is enacted through the body, care and mothering, and also through education, speech and the implicit components of discourse [14, 15]. Enculturation is the incarnation of culture in each one of us. Culture embeds itself in perceptions and sensations as the child develops. In Niger, in order to be considered handsome, Peul infants should have a thin nose; among the Touaregs, the mother will pull and pinch the child's nose, a symbol of honor. In West Africa, Bambara women massage their infants energetically so that later they will have 'sure feet in the bush' and become brave hunters [11]. Thus each of these mothers implicitly passes on a fundamental value belonging to the group to her child. This enculturation is part of what Devereux has referred to as the cultural 'envelope' or shell, a shell that clothes each one of us and forms a sort of second skin [30].

Enculturation of the human child becomes a more delicate matter when it occurs in a cultural environment that is not that in which the mother and those around her have grown up. The mother, undergoing the multiplicity of the worlds around her, is more prone to states of confusion, and even perplexity, and this will make her function of 'object-presenting' to the baby more difficult [10]. The mother will in this case transfer her own perception of the world, a kaleidoscope perception, sometime pervaded with anxiety. Her classic function of guarding the infant from over-excitation is compromised; she has difficulty presenting the world 'in small doses' so that the child is constantly at risk from encountering the world in a traumatic manner.

However certain interactive patterns, even if altered by migration, retain coherence and are performed and passed on with sufficient serenity to enable good-quality mothering. This is true for instance of massages performed on the infants. Enculturation transits via specific interaction modes – the voice, the ways of looking and touching, kinetic stimulations. These patterns are variously implemented according to the cultural group into which the infant is born. Thus mothers in sub-Saharan Africa and Asia do not talk much to their babies and avoid visual interaction: the voice and the eyes can be filled with evil intentions. There are various practices aiming to counter the effects of the evil eye or the evil tongue. It is easy to understand that in this cultural context the voice and the eyes are not the main channels for interaction. Our 'quite natural' way of smiling and talking to babies is thus often seen as threatening by mothers from other cultures.

Naming the infant is the first step in humanization. In sub-Saharan Africa, to affiliate a child to the community and to his mother, the main task is to separate the child from the 'other world' from which he is supposed to have come: the superhuman and supernatural world of the ancestors and the genies. Generally, when the infant is seven days old, the ritual of naming the child is performed, and this will consist in identifying which ancestor (or which genie) is returning in the child. The infant is indeed a messenger moving from one universe to another, and to correctly identify the ancestor is to apprehend the message the child brings. It is when the ancestor has been correctly identified that the infant can embark on a process of humanization. There is then a breaking-off between the superhuman world and the human world. This breaking off is the *sine qua non* condition for the infant to be able to develop harmoniously and finally settle among humans.

In this mode of humanizing the infant, the primary separation is seen first of all as occurring between the ancestor and the infant. This separation enables the child to settle into the primary relationship with the maternal figure. In this logic, the infant is not at first in a symbiotic relationship with his mother. The child does not belong to the mother. If there is symbiosis, it is with the 'other world', the world of the ancestors. So long as this symbiosis is sustained the child cannot become human, and may present serious somatic or mental dysfunction, described by different etiological theories, such as that of the child-ancestor or a *djinna* baby [7, 18]. Through the naming ritual and primary separation can be seen a whole theory of the humanization of the infant: so long as those receiving the child have not settled their accounts with their ancestors and forerunners, the child runs the risk of paying dearly. Psychoanalysis confirms this, in particular in studies on trans-generational issues. The naming rituals as practised in sub-Saharan Africa are an attempt to guard against subsequent serious disorder by forcing each member of the community to see him- or herself as part of a chain of generations, in a trans-generational interaction that is cleared of major conflicts that could hinder the child's development.

29.5 Conclusions: parents in exile

The consequences to be drawn for day-to-day work with parents and future parents in a situation of immigration are considerable [6, 16, 31, 32, 33, 34, 35]. The task, for psychologists and psychiatrists, midwives and child nurses, obstetricians and nurses, social workers and child education specialists, is to attempt quite simply to do their job better by way of an adaptation to these families from elsewhere [36]. This work, sometimes seen as fraught with difficulty, once one becomes involved, proves rewarding and fascinating. To be affected and 'transported' by these parents and their infants is necessary to allow them to draw on their own resources. Better understanding, better care, better provision for migrants and their children are the challenges for early prevention and clinical care in today's society.

29.6 References

1. Bornstein, M.H. (ed.) (2002) *Handbook of Parenting*. Erlbaum, Mahwah, NJ.
2. Moro, M.R., Nathan, T., Rabain-Jamin, J. *et al.* (1989) Le bébé dans son univers culturel, in *Psychopathologie du bébé* (eds S. Lebovici and F. Weil-Halpern), PUF, Paris, pp. 683–750.
3. Moro, M.R. (1994) *Parents en exil. Psychopathologie et migrations*. PUF, Paris.
4. Moro, M.R. (2000) *Psychopathologie transculturelle des enfants et des adolescents*. Dunod, Paris.
5. Moro, M.R. and Ferradji, T. (2000) Nourritures d'enfance. *L'autre, Cliniques, Cultures et Sociétés*, **1**, 1.

6. Moro, M.R. (2003) Parents and infants in changing cultural context: immigration, trauma and risk. *Infant Mental Health Journal*, **24**, 240–64.

7. Nathan, T. and Moro, M.R. (1989) Enfants de djinné. Evaluation ethnopsychanalytique des interactions précoces, in *Evaluation des interactions précoces* (eds S. Lebovici, P. Mazet and J.P. Visier), Eschel, Paris, 307–40.

8. Lebovici, S. (1983) *Le nourrisson, la mère et le psychanalyste*. Le Centurion, Paris.

9. Lebovici, S. (1993) On intergenerational transmission: from filiation to affiliation. *Infant Mental Health Journal*, **14**, 260–72.

10. Winnicott, W. (1979) *L'enfant et sa famille*. Payot, Paris.

11. Delaisi De Parseval, G. and Lallemand, S. (1980) *L'art d'accommoder les bébés, 100 ans de recettes françaises de puériculture*. Le Seuil, Paris.

12. Devereux, G. (1968) L'image de l'enfant dans deux tribus: Mohave et Sedang. *Revue de Neuropsychiatrie infantile et d'hygiène mentale de l'enfant*, **4**, 25–35.

13. Lallemand, S., Journet, O., Ewombe-Moundo, E. *et al.* (1991) *Grossesse et petite enfance en Afrique noire et à Madagascar*. L'Harmattan, Paris.

14. Mead, M. (1963) *Mœurs et sexualité en Océanie*. Plon, Paris.

15. Mead, M. (1973) *Une éducation en Nouvelle-Guinée*. Payot, Paris.

16. Moro, M.R. (2007) *Aimer ses enfants ici et ailleurs. Histoires transculturelles*. Odile Jacob, Paris.

17. Nathan, T. (1986) *La folie des autres. Traité d'ethnopsychiatrie clinique*. Dunod, Paris.

18. Réal, I. and Moro, M.R. (1998) De L'art d'humaniser les bébés. Clinique transculturelle des processus de socialisation précoce. *Champ Psychosomatique*, **15**, 91–108.

19. Rabain-Jamin, J. (1989) La famille africaine, in *Psychopathologie du bébé* (eds S. Lebovici and F. Weil-Halpern.), PUF, Paris, pp. 722–27.

20. Rabain-Jamain, J. and Wornham, W.L. (1990) Transformation des conduites de maternage et des pratiques de soin chez les femmes migrantes d'Afrique de L'Ouest. *La Psychiatrie de L'Enfant*, **33**, 287–319.

21. Serres, M. (1977) Discours et parcours, in *L'identité* (ed. C. Lévi-Strauss), PUF, Paris, pp. 25–39.

22. Stork, H. (1988) *Enfances indiennes. Etude de psychologie transculturelle et comparée du jeune enfant*. Le Centurion, Paris.

23. Bydlowski, M. (1991) La transparence psychique de la grossesse. *Études freudiennes*, **32**, 2–9.

24. Bydlowski, M. (1997) *La dette de vie, itinéraire psychanalytique de la maternité*. PUF, Paris.

25. Tamminen, T. (2006) How does culture promote the early development of identity? *Infant Mental Health Journal*, **27**, 603–5.

26. Coblence, F. (1996) *Serge Lebovici*. PUF, Paris.

27. Fraiberg, S. (1999) *Fantômes dans la chambre d'enfants*, Presses Universitaires de France, Paris.

28. Seeman, M.V. (2008) Cross-cultural evaluation of maternal competence in a culturally diverse society. *American Journal of Psychiatry*, **165**, 565–68.

29. Fontanel, B. and D'Harcourt, C. (1998) *Bébés du monde*. La Martinière, Paris.

30. Devereux, G. (1970) *Essais d'ethnopsychiatrie générale*. Gallimard, Paris.

31. Koniak-Griffin, D., Logsdon, M.C., Hines-Martin, V. and Turner, C.C. (2006) Contemporary mothering in a diverse society. *Journal of Obstetrical, Gynecology and Neonatalogy Nursing*, **35**, 671–78.

32. Kotchick, B.A. (2002) Putting parenting in perspective: a discussion of the contextual factors that shape parenting practices. *Journal of Child and Family Studies*, **11**, 255–69.

33. Bornstein, M.H. and Cote, L.R. (2004) Mothers' parenting cognitions on cultures of origin, acculturating cultures, and cultures of destination. *Child Development*, **75**, 221–35.

34. Moro, M.R. and Serre, G. (2002) Désirs d'enfant. *L'autre, Cliniques, Cultures et Sociétés*, **3**, 2.

35. Cauce, A.M. (2008) Parenting, culture, and context: reflections on excavating culture. *Applied Developmental Science*, **12**, 227–29.

36. Moro, M.R., Neuman, D. and Réal, I. (2008) *Maternités en exil. Mettre des bébés au monde et les faire grandir en situation transculturelle*. La pensée sauvage, Grenoble.

30

Parenting and poverty: a complex interaction

Mark Tomlinson

Stellenbosch University, South Africa

30.1 Introduction

In 2005, 1.4 billion people in low- and middle-income (LAMI) countries were living in extreme poverty – on less than $1.25 a day [1]. Of the 559 million children under 5 years old in LAMI countries, 219 million can be considered to be disadvantaged (stunted or living in absolute poverty) which equates to 39% of all under-5 children in LAMI countries [2]. Parenting is a complex and difficult task even when conditions are optimal. In the context of poverty, parenting is likely to be compromised. Parenting and poverty are complex areas of contestation in their own right, with divergent views of the causal role of parenting in child outcome [3], and considerable debate about definitions of poverty and its measurement.

In this chapter, consideration will be given to the complex interplay between parenting and poverty and whether poverty is directly and causally related to poor infant and child outcome or whether there is a distal effect magnifying vulnerabilities and adding to stress that in turn affects outcome, the effect of which is mediated by other factors. This will be done by way of an examination of concepts such as absolute and relative poverty and the concept of upstream and downstream effects. I will outline some of the complexities of conceptualizing the relationship between parenting and poverty using a systems model that takes account of both individual (micro) and institutional and structural (macro) factors.

Parenthood and Mental Health: A Bridge between Infant and Adult Psychiatry   Sam Tyano, Miri Keren, Helen Herrman and John Cox
© 2010 John Wiley & Sons, Ltd

Finally, I will focus on two areas central to the early life of infants – maternal depression and malnutrition/non-organic failure to thrive – in order to elucidate the complex interplay between poverty and parenting.

30.2 Poverty

In the 60 years since the end of World War II, the world beyond North America and Western Europe has seen breathtaking improvements in health care and living conditions [4]. There have been improvements in life expectancy, the eradication of smallpox, lower infant mortality rates, better access to safe water, the availability of health-care services, and improving levels of literacy in LAMI countries. This improvement is misleading however, in that due to population growth the actual number of people living in poverty has hardly changed. The worst 'performer' has been Sub-Saharan Africa where almost 50% of the population lives in extreme poverty [5].

Absolute versus relative poverty

The most widely used definition of poverty makes a distinction between absolute poverty and relative poverty. Absolute poverty is defined as the severe deprivation of human needs such as food, safe water and basic shelter [6], the form of poverty characteristic of many LAMI countries. It often includes a lack of education and access to services. Relative poverty, on the other hand, refers to income in relation to the average of that particular country. Relative poverty is no less detrimental and it has been shown that morbidity is more closely related to relative income within countries than to differences in absolute income, while countries that have lower levels of relative deprivation tend to have lower national mortality rates [7]. The concept of relative poverty or of 'relative deprivation' is crucial in any discussion of parenting because it is likely that the effect of relative poverty on parenting occurs via psychosocial mechanisms [8].

30.3 Upstream and downstream factors

Parenting occurs in and is particularly sensitive to perturbations in the psychosocial context. Link and Phelan argue that behavioral or proximate risk factors are simply the mechanism through which the more fundamental societal and contextual factors operate [9]. This interaction can be conceptualized using the concepts of upstream and downstream determinants. Upstream determinants are defined as features of the environment, such as socio-economic status or levels of discrimination in a society [10]. Downstream determinants on the other hand are physical health, parenting and disease. One of the tasks is to determine how upstream determinants or specific social environments 'get under the skin' and affect downstream variables such as parenting and infant outcome [10]. Halpern has described this as trying to understand how poverty (which appears to be such a global variable) comes to influence specific processes in the lives of infants and children [11]. Research that looks at poverty and the specific processes in people's lives has often found that the role of poverty is smaller than more immediate factors (partner violence) in, for example, the development of mental disorders. This is a common mistake that assumes that upstream variables are less important because of their smaller effect sizes [12]. This is misleading in that upstream factors (for example poverty) exert their influence by way of the downstream factors (parenting).

30.4 Parenting and its determinants

Bronfenbrenner's ecological model of human development offers a systems perspective that describes the factors that influence the interaction between parents and their children [13]. Bronfenbrenner's model is a hierarchical one with four levels. These four levels of factors are:

1 Socio-cultural (macro system)

2 Community (exo system)

3 Family (micro system) and

4 Individual (ontogenic).

The model outlines how social, community, family and individual factors contribute to developmental outcome. With specific regard to parenting, the premise of the ecological model is that the effect of parenting is embedded in a myriad of social factors that may affect child development [14], and the model is useful in that it considers the ecological niche in which infants and children live. An important premise of this model is that there is a potentially inexorable co-variation of risk factors in the environment of any child [14]. The seminal work of Sameroff illustrates how consideration of a single risk factor in the etiology of infant and child outcome is problematic [15]. Sameroff and colleagues developed a multiple risk score based on 10 environmental variables. Risk variables included maternal mental illness, education (maternal), family size, family support and stressful life events. They found that the severity and chronicity of the mental disturbance combined with persistent poor environmental conditions such as poverty and family instability [15] were more important than the specific psychiatric diagnosis of the mother.

In such a systems understanding it is important to consider how poverty not only affects parenting, but parenting may also have an effect on poverty, creating 'cycles of disadvantage' [16]. So for example, a poor diet and smoking during pregnancy is associated with low birth weight. Low birth weight infants require heightened levels of parental care and medical resources. Parents in poverty are less able to provide the heightened care necessary and may have little or no access to adequate medical interventions as a result of weak health systems. As a consequence the infants have an increased likelihood of developing later developmental and cognitive deficits which place increased demands on parents. Children, when performing poorly at school, are likely to drop out. When this occurs in a poor environment characterized by high crime levels and gangsterism the child is more likely to join a gang (if a boy) or fall pregnant (if a girl), which in turn creates additional stress in a parenting system that is by this time severely compromised. This has implications for the parenting of that child but also other siblings. Adolescent girls in this context are more likely to take substances and eat poorly, which is likely to result in the second generation infant having a low birth weight, thus completing the cycle of disadvantage.

30.5 Parenting and poverty

In the light of Bronfenbrenner's model it is important to distinguish between the immediate and direct consequences of poverty on infant and child development (which will in turn effect parenting given the vulnerable infant), and the more indirect effects such as those mediated by depression and parenting practices. Various stress models describe the family as an interconnected, interdependent system in which different factors play a role in determining stressful experiences that in turn influence parenting and infant and child development. These factors include the individual psychological characteristics of parents, the couple characteristics, antecedent factors from each parent's family of origin, child characteristics and environmental characteristics [17]. Belsky has described three sources of influence on parental functioning: parental factors and the personal psychological resources of the mother (father); child characteristics such as temperament and gender; and finally contextual sources of stress and support [18].

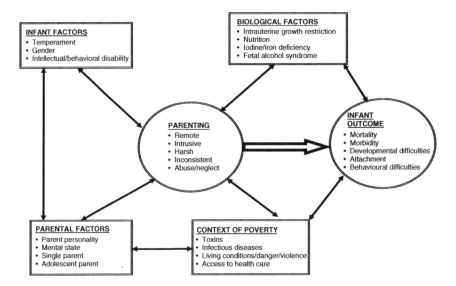

Figure 30.1 Poverty and parenting: complex interactions within an ecological niche

Figure 30.1 illustrates some of these interactions and attempts to account for the complexity of the relationship between poverty and parenting within an ecological niche. Poor living conditions (context) and a violent community will affect the choices parents make in order to protect their children. This might for instance result in harsh and intrusive parenting. In this scenario, poverty exerts its influence on infant and child outcome in a distal way via parenting practices. Poverty may also contribute to familial stress and maternal depression which in turn affects parenting, and by extension child outcome. Biological factors such as nutrition and intrauterine growth restriction may affect outcome in a proximal way (increased mortality and morbidity), but also in a distal way by increasing the vulnerability of the infant to an already stressed and adverse environment. Factors such as fetal alcohol syndrome may result in mental impairment which may result in heightened levels of abuse and neglect. Parenting is rendered more difficult with a child who has fetal alcohol syndrome, but it is the mental impairment that compromises parenting practices rather than the direct effects of poverty. Halpern has described a negative triad of a constitutionally vulnerable infant, and a vulnerable parent in an unsupportive community context [11].

Biological factors

Poor maternal nutrition and infections during pregnancy (common in many LAMI countries) are linked to intrauterine growth restriction [19]. Low birth weight is associated with lower cognitive scores at age 2 and 3 years, greater inhibition, less vocal and less happy children [19], while in China low birth weight has been associated with a greater risk of behavioral problems in adolescence [20]. Alcohol use during pregnancy is a major problem in many LAMI countries, and children with fetal alcohol syndrome are less likely to complete school and also have a variety of concentration and behavioral difficulties [21]. All of these factors (and there are many others) are related to poverty and in turn to various aspects of infant and child functioning. The infants and children with these behavioral problems are more difficult to parent and place additional strain on what is often already a sub-optimal parental system, and increase the likelihood that the parenting practices that develop in response will be negative further compromising development.

Context of poverty

Parents living in poverty face a broad range of issues other than material deprivation that may affect their ability to effectively parent. These include low levels of education, lack of access to jobs and services, social isolation, mental and physical ill health and domestic violence [22]. These factors may act independently to influence childrearing outcome, but they are also likely to interact with one another and complicate outcomes. The correlates of poverty, such as unemployment, low income and poor housing, are associated with higher rates of child maltreatment, particularly physical violence and child neglect [23]. Family conflict is associated with higher rates of child maltreatment, hostile parenting and behavioral problems [24]. Low-income parents are likely to be less nurturing, use more inconsistent, erratic and harsh discipline and are more likely to inadequately supervise their children [25]. Poverty and poor education are strong predictors of poor infant and child safety. The breakdown of the family and lone parenting is strongly associated with parenting difficulties and adverse outcomes for children, due to reduced family resources as well as psychological distress [26].

Large families also tend to be more stressful as parents have to manage a combination of increased demands and limited material and resources to meet these demands. High-risk contexts for child maltreatment are areas that are physically degraded and run-down, where relationships between neighbors are less positive, and those that lead to more stressful day-to-day interactions for families [27], resulting in parents who are depleted and unable to muster the necessary energy to parent [11]. Ghate and Hazel have argued that while many parents do well (even those living in poverty) parenting in environments characterized by poverty is more 'risky' than parenting elsewhere, and that the poorer the environment the more difficult parenting becomes [26].

Infant factors

A limitation of early work on parent–child interaction was the emphasis placed on the role of the parent in determining the nature of the interaction. It is increasingly understood that effects in parent–child relationships are in fact bi-directional [14]. Difficult temperament in infancy may undermine parental functioning [18]. Kochanska [28] has shown how depending on whether the child is temperamentally fearful or more aggressive (fearless) the optimal parental response is in fact gentle control (for the fearful child) or firmer control (for the fearless child) in order to achieve the same emotional regulation. When partner and extended family support is optimal and financial concerns do not predominate, the chances of the parental system being able to respond to a temperamentally 'difficult' (or fearless) infant or child are increased. An adolescent poor single mother with no support is unlikely to be able to muster the psychological or emotional resources to appropriately parent such a 'difficult' infant.

Parent factors

According to Hoff, Laursen and Tradif [29] parents with lower socio-economic status are more likely than parents with a higher socio-economic status to adopt an authoritarian parenting style. Authoritarian parents are demanding and directive towards their children, and less likely to be responsive [30]. Katz and colleagues argue that parenting styles should be separated from parenting goals and parenting practices [22]. According to this argument two sets of parents who use similar parenting practices in different contexts may have different child developmental outcomes depending on the parenting style. They also hypothesize that the difference in parenting style among poor parents may not necessarily be the result of deficit role modeling or inadequate socialization, but rather responses to their environment. Attempts at increased monitoring in order to protect the child from dangerous environments or from associating with an 'inappropriate peer group' may result in the escalation of the harsh and coercive aspects of caregiving [22]. Halpern has also described how if a mother had been hurt as a child she might struggle to identify with her young child's need for protection and in trying to avoid her own painful memories might in fact begin to avoid the infant [11]. Propper and colleagues have shown how the impact of income on development is in fact small [31] and that it is rather the mother's health together with early life events that play a more important role in infant and child development.

30.6 Maternal depression

One aspect of parental functioning in the context of poverty that has attracted significant research attention is that of maternal depression. Brown and Harris [32] have elaborated the link between poverty and maternal depression and argue that there are two main factors implicated in the etiology of maternal depression: provoking events, such as stressful occurrences (retrenchment), and vulnerability factors, which are personal factors that increase the odds of developing depression when there is a stressful event. With regard to parenting, depression is important in that it interferes with the ability to adequately parent. This has particular resonance with regard to infants, as they are born primed for interaction with others, and are particularly vulnerable to perturbations in interaction with their caregivers.

Wilson [33] found that parents living in poverty were less happy and less involved in their children's lives than parents who experienced fewer stressors. Highly depressed, poor mothers also hit and yelled at their children more frequently and relied less on reasoning when disciplining them than their non-depressed counterparts [34]. Negative mood may negatively bias a parent's reactions and credit for their children's behavior, and may cause parents to selectively attend only to negative child behaviors [35], causing parents to become more controlling, punishing or avoidant of child interaction [36].

In a study of the emotional well-being and behavior of adolescents, Conger and colleagues [24] found that behavior was negatively affected, mainly due to disruptions in parenting during economic hardship rather than from direct effects from the hardship itself. Parents who moved into poverty became distressed and depressed and experienced marital deterioration. This in turn leads to disruptions in their parenting practices. However, parents with a robust marriage and social support were less likely to become depressed. Poverty increases familial stress which may lead to depression [37], which in turn is associated with harsher and/or more inconsistent parenting. In this cycle, it is the depression (proximal) in the context of poverty (distal) that affects parenting and outcome [26].

30.7 Poverty, parenting, depression and infant attachment

A study conducted in a peri-urban settlement in South Africa, in conditions of extreme social adversity and very high rates of post-partum depression, illustrates the complexities of the relationship between parenting and poverty. In this study the prevalence rate of post-partum depression was 34.7% [38]. Post-partum depression was also associated with impaired mother–infant interaction. Cooper and colleagues have argued that maternal depression and the endemic high levels of social adversity both have a significant adverse impact on maternal sensitivity. However, the same team found that despite this adverse context 61.9% of the infants were securely attached at 18 months [39].

Tomlinson and colleagues have argued that one of the reasons for the high rates of secure attachment in a context of extreme poverty was the protective contribution of social and cultural organization that characterized the community. Despite the extreme levels of adversity and the legacy of the apartheid system that systematically attempted to destroy family structures and community cohesion, there still exists a humanity and compassion for neighbors and the wider community. In African parlance this notion of community spirit and compassion for others is known as *Ubuntu*. Infants and young children are seen as belonging, to some extent, to the community, and responsibility for their safety and well-being is seen as a collective responsibility. In addition, the combination of extremely close dwellings and small houses facilitates a great deal of social interaction in the narrow portions of space in front of houses or in the street. This high-density living, and the communal nature of the culture, combined with the survival imperatives of living in extreme poverty (many mothers depend at times on the assistance of friends and neighbors to, quite literally, feed their children) may mean that some of the more negative social consequences of poverty that are often present in more developed societies do not arise.

There is also the possibility that the poverty experienced by many of the women is attributed to the effects of decades of apartheid rule in South Africa [39]. Babarin and Richter [40] make the point that much of the evidence of the relationship of income poverty, material disadvantage and child development has been gathered from poor living conditions in countries with high standards of living. They argue that the meanings ascribed to poverty and the allied negative or positive status ascribed to it may be very different across contexts [40]. The psychological consequences of poverty may be very different when the experience of poverty is a common and widely shared one, when it is attributed to external sources rather than internal sources, and when it is treated with empathy rather than moral censure [40]. In rich countries, being poor is often seen as evidence of 'failure' while in poorer countries the ubiquity of poverty may carry less of a moral judgement. Parents who feel that they have 'failed' are likely to find sensitive parenting a challenge.

With regard to the role of poverty in infant attachment outcome, it was the features of the mother–infant relationship, post-partum depression, and the mother's experience of partner support that were the strongest predictors of infant attachment outcome [39], rather than poverty. This in no way omits the role of poverty and adversity in contributing to increased levels of post-partum depression or the lack of partner support (poverty is instrumental in the genesis of both). Rather, these findings suggest that the simple measurement of socio-economic adversity is not, in itself, sufficient for a full understanding of the factors involved in understanding parenting, poverty and infant and child developmental trajectory.

Similarly, caution must be exercised in ascribing a causal role to parenting factors when in fact there are a number of other unmeasured confounders (such as inherited factors) or even unrecognized factors that we are not able to measure using available instruments. With regard to poverty and parenting, the reality is that it is likely that the relationship between poverty and parenting is a synergistic one.

30.8 Malnutrition and non-organic failure to thrive

Another area that aptly illustrates the complexities of the relationship between poverty and parenting is that of non-organic failure to thrive. In a recent *Lancet* series, it was estimated that stunting, severe wasting and intrauterine growth restriction were responsible for 2.2 million deaths for children under 5 years of age [41]. Poverty and poor nutritional intake are significant causes of high levels of poor infant and child physical growth. In young children, underweight and stunting have found to be associated with apathy, less positive affect, lower levels of play and insecure attachment [19]. Traditionally, malnutrition and poor infant physical development have been seen as a function of food intake and by extension fundamentally a pure issue of poverty. In certain instances however, the picture is in fact more complex. Other factors such as socio-cultural practices and maternal mental health also need to be considered in how they may impact upon infant and child physical development. For instance, it is well recognized that abuse or neglect may have an adverse influence on infant physical growth [42].

Research conducted into infants who fail to thrive has typically examined the role of factors such as abuse or neglect in the infant's failure to gain weight. When this impairment is as a result of non-organic factors it is known as non-organic failure to thrive (NOFT). The proximate etiology of NOFT is insufficient nutrition [43] but there is often a complex interaction of factors [42]. Given that infant feeding is such an interactive process, one of the hypotheses is that anything that interferes with, for example, the ability of the mother to be sensitive and responsive to cues from her infant during feeding, may then play a role in under-nourishment NOFT and be implicated in later growth difficulties. This may include depression, worries about debt and financial problems or domestic violence. All of these factors may be more prevalent in poor areas.

A number of studies have investigated the association between malnutrition and mother–infant interaction. Associations have been reported between malnutrition and low levels of home stimulation, low sensitivity and responsiveness [44], and disturbed attachments [45]. Under-nourished infants were also less competent in manipulation of toys during play and were more passive when in contact with their mothers. Richter and Griesel [46] have argued that the conditions associated with malnutrition are the same conditions that are likely to give rise to depression and thus compromise interaction with an infant.

Is it the case that under-nutrition causes impairment in the mother–infant interaction, in that underweight infants may be impaired in their ability to elicit and engage in positive social interactions [45]? Alternatively, does maternal insensitivity and lack of responsiveness lead to faltering weight? Most likely the interaction would again be a transactional one [47], where the impairment in the infant's ability to elicit positive social interactions (due to under-nutrition) occurs in tandem with the mother's difficulties in sensitive and responsive caregiving, resulting in maladaptive interactions between the pair. This is a further example of the bi-directionality of the interactions between parents and their children but on this occasion occurring in an adverse environment.

30.9 Conclusions

Many infants and children do remarkably well, even in the context of poverty. Many infants and children however do not. It is undoubtedly the case that one of the reasons for this is poverty. Poverty magnifies vulnerabilities and stigmatizes people as failures [11], contributing both directly and indirectly to poor parenting and poor child outcome. The relationship between parenting and poverty is a complex one, and due caution must be exercised in drawing causal or inferential links between the two, or from one or both to simple notions of infant and child outcome as there is a potentially inexorable co-variation of risk factors [14]. There is no clear-cut or causal link between poverty and parenting as individual vulnerabilities and strengths as well as the severity and chronicity of the poverty will determine how people with respond to the stress of poverty. Finally, poverty must be understood not just in terms of absence of resources but as part of a complex of social, interpersonal and psychological factors which impact on individuals, groups and entire societies. As such it exerts a 'distal' rather than a 'proximal' effect on parenting and infant and child outcome.

30.10 References

1. United Nations (2009) *The Millennium Development Goals Report.* United Nations, New York.
2. Grantham-McGregor, S., Cheung, Y.B., Cueto, S. *et al.* (2007) Developmental potential in the first 5 years for children in developing countries. *Lancet,* **369**, 60–70.
3. Harris, J.R. (1999) *The Nurture Assumption: Why Children Turn Out the Way They Do.* Free Press, Illinois.

4. Desjarlais, R., Eisenberg, L., Good, B. *et al.* (1995) *World Mental Health: Problems and Priorities in Low-Income Countries.* Oxford University Press, New York.

5. United Nations Population Fund (2008). *State of the World Population: Reaching Common Ground: Culture, Gender and Human Rights.* New York: United Nations.

6. United Nations (1995) *World Summit of Social Development, Copenhagen.* United Nations, New York.

7. Wilkinson, R.G. (1997). Socioeconomic determinants of health: health inequalities: relative or absolute material standards? *British Medical Journal,* **314,** 591.

8. Hiliemeier, M.M., Lynch, J., Harpe, S. *et al.* (2003) Relative or absolute standards for child poverty: a state-level analysis of infant and child mortality. *American Journal of Public Health,* **93,** 652–657.

9. Link, B.G. and Phelan, J. (1995) Social conditions as fundamental causes of disease. *Journal of Health and Social Behavior,* **35,** 80–94.

10. Gehlert, S., Sohmer, D., Sacks, T. *et al.* (2008) Targeting health disparities: a model linking upstream determinants to downstream interventions: knowing about the interaction of societal factors and disease can enable targeted interventions to reduce health disparities. *Health Affairs,* **27,** 339–349.

11. Halpern, R. (1993) Poverty and infant development, in *Handbook of Infant Mental Health* (ed. C.H. Zeanah), Guilford Press, New York, pp.73–86.

12. Corrigall, J., Lund, C., Patel, V. *et al.* (2008) Poverty and mental illness: fact or fiction? A commentary on Das, Do, Friedman, McKenzie & Scott (65:3, 2007, 467e480). *Social Science and Medicine,* **66,** 2061–2063.

13. Bronfenbrenner, U. (1979) *The Ecology of Human Development: Experiments by Nature and Design.* Harvard University Press, Cambridge.

14. O'Connor, T.G. and Scott, B.C. (2007) *Parenting and Outcomes for Children.* Joseph Rowntree Foundation, London.

15. Sameroff, A.J. and Seifer, R. (1983) Familial risk and child competence. *Child Development,* **54,** 1254–68.

16. Rutter, M. and Madge, N. (1976) *Cycles of Disadvantage: a Review of Research.* Heinemann, London.

17. Cowan, C.P., Cowan, P.A., Homing, G. *et al.* (1985) Transition to parenthood: his, hers, and theirs. *Journal of Family Issues,* **6,** 451–81.

18. Belsky, J. (1984) The determinants of parenting: a process model. *Child Development,* **55,** 83–96.

19. Walker, S.P., Wachs, T.D., Gardner, J.M. *et al.* (2007) Child development: risk factors for adverse outcomes in developing countries. *Lancet,* **369,** 145–57.

20. Liu, X., Sun, Z., Neiderhiser, J.M. *et al.* (2001) Low birth weight, developmental milestones, and behavioral problems in Chinese children and adolescents. *Psychiatric Research,* **101,** 115–29.

21. Viljoen, D, Gossage, J.P., Brooke, L. *et al.* (2005) Fetal alcohol syndrome epidemiology in a South African community: a second study of a very high prevalence area. *Journal of Studies on Alcohol,* **66,** 593–604.

22. Katz, I., Corlyon, J., Placa, VL. *et al.* (2007) *The Relationship between Parenting and poverty.* Joseph Rowntree Foundation, London.

23. Dietz, T.L. (2000) Disciplining children: characteristics associated with the use of corporal punishment. *Child Abuse and Neglect,* **24,** 1529–42.

24. Conger, R.D., Conger, K.J., Elder, G. *et al.* (1993) Family economic stress and adjustment of early adolescent girls. *Development Psychology*, **29**, 206–19.
25. Elder, G., van Nguyen, T. and Caspi, A. (1985) Linking family hardship to children's lives. *Child Development*, **56**, 361–75.
26. Ghate, D. and Hazel, N. (2002) *Parenting in Poor Environments: Stress, Support and Coping.* Jessica Kingsley Publishers, London.
27. Garbarino, J. and Kostelny, K. (1992) Child maltreatment as a community problem. *Child Abuse and Neglect*, **16**, 455–64.
28. Kochanska, G. (1997) Multiple pathways to conscience for children with different temperaments: from toddlerhood to age 5. *Developmental Psychology*, **33**, 228–40.
29. Hoff, E., Laursen, B. and Tardif, T. (2002) Socioeconomic status and parenting, in *Handbook of Parenting*, vol. **2** (ed. M. Bornstein), Lawrence Erlbaum Associates, London.
30. Baumrind, D. (1991) The influence of parenting style on adolescent competence and substance use. *Journal of Early Adolescence*, **11**, 56–95.
31. Propper, C., Burgess, S. and Rigg, J. (2004) *The Impact of Income on Child Health: Evidence from a Birth Cohort Study.* CASE Paper 85. CASE, London School of Economics, London.
32. Brown, G.W. and Harris T. (1978) *Social Origins of Depression: A Study of Psychiatric Disorder in Women.* Free Press, New York.
33. Wilson, H. (1974) Parenting in poverty. *British Journal of Social Work*, **4**, 241–54.
34. Longfellow, C., Zelkowitz, P. and Saunders, E. (1982) The quality of mother-child relationships, in *Lives in Stress: Women and Depression* (ed. D. Belle), Sage, Beverley Hills, CA, pp. 163–76.
35. Jouriles, E.N., Murphy, C.M. and O'Leary, D.O. (1989) Effects of maternal mood on mother-son interaction patterns. *Journal of Abnormal Child Psychology*, **17**, 513–25.
36. Crnic, K. and Acevedo, M. (1995) Everyday stresses and parenting, in *Handbook of Parenting: Applied and Practical Parenting*, vol. **4** (ed. M.H. Bomstein), Erlbaum, Mahwah, NJ, pp. 277–98.
37. Dearing, E., McCartney, K. and Taylor, B. (2004) Change in family income-to-needs matters more for children with less. In *Child Care and Child Development: Results from the NICHD Study of Early Child Care and Youth Development* (eds. NICHD Early Child Care Research Network), Guilford Publications, New York.
38. Cooper, P.J., Tomlinson, M., Swartz, L. *et al.* (1999) Postpartum depression and the mother-infant relationship in a South African peri-urban settlement. *British Journal of Psychiatry*, **175**, 554–58.
39. Tomlinson, M., Cooper, P. and Murray, L. (2005) The mother-infant relationship and infant attachment in a South African peri-urban settlement. *Child Development*, **76**, 1044–54.
40. Barbarin, O.A. and Richter, L.M. (2001) *Mandela's Children: Growing up in Post-Apartheid South Africa.* Routledge, New York.
41. Black, R.E., Allen, L.H. and Bhutta, Z.A. (2008) Maternal and child undernutrition: global and regional exposures and health consequences. *Lancet*, **371**, 243–60.
42. Skuse, D. and Bentovim, A. (1994) Physical and emotional maltreatment, in *Child and Adolescent Psychiatry: Modern Approaches* (eds M. Rutter, E. Taylor and L. Hersov), Blackwell Science, Oxford, pp. 209–29.
43. Frank, D.A. and Zeisel, S.H. (1988) Failure to thrive. *Pediatric Clinics of North America*, **35**, 1187–207.

44. Cravioto, J. and Delicardie, E.R. (1976) Malnutrition in early childhood and some of its later effects at individual and community levels. *Food Nutrition*, **2**, 2–11.

45. Valenzuela, M. (1990) Attachment in chronically underweight young children. *Child Development*, **61**, 1984–96.

46. Richter, L. and Griesel, L. (1994) Malnutrition, low birthweight and related influences on psychological development, in *Childhood and Adversity: Psychological Perspectives from South African Research* (eds M. Rutter, E. Taylor and L. Hersov), David Phillip, Cape Town, pp. 66–91.

47. Lester, B.M. (1979) A synergistic approach to the study of prenatal malnutrition. *International Journal of Behavioral Development*, **2**, 377–93.

31

Assessment of parenting

Marc H. Bornstein and Magdalen Toole

Eunice Kennedy Shriver National Institute of Child Health and Human Development, Bethesda MD, USA

31.1 Introduction

Theory and research have focused on assessing two broad domains of parenting infants. These are parenting cognitions and parenting practices. Both are significant because the ways that parents interact with their infants often, but not always, reflect their ideas about parenting [1]. Therefore, studying parenting beliefs allows researchers to gain insight into how and why parents behave as they do. Broadly construed, parental cognitions include parents' values, goals and attitudes as well as actual parenting knowledge of childrearing and child development. Cognitions serve many purposes, such as shaping parental expectations and practices and mediating the effectiveness of parenting [1, 2]. For example, research has shown that mothers who have more confidence in their parenting abilities are more empathic, less punitive and more appropriate in their developmental expectations [3].

Perhaps more obvious as influences in the lives of infants are the practices that parents exhibit and the experiences that they provide their infants. Five main categories of parenting practices during infancy have been identified. These are nurturant, social, didactic, material and language.

- *Nurturant caregiving* is concerned with meeting the infant's physical and survival needs.

- *Social caregiving* refers to the practices that parents employ to engage their infants in interpersonal exchange.

Parenthood and Mental Health: A Bridge between Infant and Adult Psychiatry   Sam Tyano, Miri Keren, Helen Herrman and John Cox
© 2010 John Wiley & Sons, Ltd

- *Didactic caregiving* includes various strategies parents use to orient and introduce their infants to the environment around them.

- *Material caregiving* consists of the ways in which parents supply and organize their infant's physical environment.

- *Language addressed* to infants is valuable in itself and crosses other categories of parenting practices [1].

Table 31.1 Assessments of parenting infants: major methods, advantages and disadvantages

Method	Advantages	Disadvantages
Reports	Helpful in early stages	Questionable relation to
Self-reports	Ecologically valid	performance
Questionnaires and	Only way to know about	Unsystematic, overgenerous,
Checklists	cognitions	biased
Interviews	Economical, labor-saving	Often retrospective
Focus groups	Best for frequent, concrete and	Conditioned by life circumstances
Others' reports	public issues	Worst for infrequent, abstract and private issues
Observations	Ecologically valid	Limited, constrained, incomplete
	Based on performance	Dependent on parameters of setting
	Direct, objective, reliable	Labor-intensive, time-consuming, expensive
		Requires coder reliability
Tests	Performance-based	Not (necessarily) ecologically valid
	Controlled, equal, fair	Labor-intensive

To assess parenting cognitions and practices, several methods are commonly employed (Table 31.1). One is to ask parents to report on their own parenting cognitions and practices, either through questionnaires or interviews of parents. Also, others who are close to the parent, possibly a spouse or an older child, can report about them. A second method is to observe and record the parent's behaviors, either in a natural setting or in an artificial one, such as a laboratory. Third, one can test parents experimentally to assay their cognitions and practices. Parenting cognitions are most easily studied through reports of some sort, whereas parenting practices are commonly studied through reports and observations. Each method holds unique advantages and disadvantages and offers distinct perspectives on parenting. Furthermore, the field is not dominated by one method; instead, researchers advocate the use of multiple methods of assessment when studying parenting [4]. For example, interviewing mothers, coupled with behavioral observations, allows researchers to reach a more complete understanding of parenting.

31.2 Self-report measures

One method used to collect information on parenting is to ask parents to report on their own cognitions and practices. If parental cognitions about their parenting are the focus of research, then self-reports are ideal forms of measurement. Historically, much research on parenting infants has consisted of reports. Parents kept detailed diaries on the progress of their infants' motor development and emotional and cognitive capacities as well as their own parenting [5]. This method is particularly helpful in the early stages of development where many practices are infrequent to observe and hard to test. Furthermore, young infants are not always willing participants in structured assessments, and therefore it may be difficult to observe all parenting situations. Because self-report data come directly from the parent, reports are also thought of as an accurate way to gather information. Parents are the only ones who know how they think about their role as a parent, and therefore self-reports are the only way to learn what a parent thinks or why a parent behaves as she or he does. Parents can also report on situations that experimenters would be unable to observe or test. Another advantage of this method is that it is economical and not labor-intensive.

However, several disadvantages attend the report method. First, data gathered by those who are not professional researchers may be unsystematic. Furthermore, because parents are not trained, they may either be overgenerous or miss important information because they do not know what to look for. Parent reports are also often retrospective, which could yield inaccurate data, as memory is faulty. An associated difficulty with parent reports is that, although parents may be relatively accurate when reporting about their current parenting, they may rely on generalized stereotypes [4]. In addition, life circumstances color parents' reports. For example, education, psychological functioning and expectations regarding parenting can all lead to inaccurate reporting [4]. While parents spend the most time with their infant, and therefore possess the most information about their own parenting, parents are also biased reporters. Because of this, they may distort their reports of their own cognitions and practices in relation to their infant. (One of the ways such reactivity is addressed in social psychology is by having the parent also complete a 'lie' or 'look good' scale.)

Two major variants of parental reports are questionnaires/checklists and interviews. Questionnaires and checklists can increase the validity of assessments of parenting because they do not rely as heavily on memory as do other types of self-reports. However, because they are structured they may miss information as well. An example is a questionnaire used to assess self-perceptions of competence, satisfaction, investment and role balance as a parent [6]. The questionnaire consists of a list of statements such as 'Some parents often can't figure out what their children need or want', but 'Other parents seem to have a knack for understanding what their children need or want.' The parent chooses which statement describes the parent best and then selects either *Sort of true for me* or *Really true for me.*

Structured interviews that ask specific questions in specific ways can also increase the reliability of parent reports. The Home Observation Measurement of the Environment (HOME) is an inventory that evaluates the quality and quantity of stimulation and support parents make available to a child in the home environment as well as aspects of family organization, routines, and involvement with extended family [7]. Focus groups, which are usually discussions centered on a set of structured but open-ended questions, are also used to gather report data about parenting [8]. However, coding interviews can be time-consuming; furthermore, group settings may discourage participants from explicitly stating much they might otherwise convey.

Parents are more reliable when reporting on certain types of activities compared to others. For example, when asked about frequent, concrete and public practices, parents report more accurately than when asked about practices that occur infrequently, are abstract, or private [4]. Thus, parents may be more reliable in reporting on actual practices, such as feeding, but may be less accurate when reporting on their feelings, such as how they think about discipline.

31.3   Reports by others

Another method for gathering information about parenting is to ask others who are close to or spend time with the parent and infant. For example, mothers may be asked to fill out questionnaires or report during interviews about the parenting of the infant's father [9]. Parents may also be asked about their relationship with each other as a means of determining the type of parenting environment in which the infant is growing up, and how the parents function as individuals as well as a co-parenting unit. The co-parenting relationship is an important aspect of parenting, as it concerns childrearing agreement, division of labor, support, and joint family management. Furthermore, the nature of the co-parenting relationship can impact the development of infants [10].

31.4   Observational methods

Observational methods are widely used when studying parenting infants. Observations are made either in a naturalistic setting, such as the family's home, or in a laboratory. When an observation takes place in a laboratory, researchers can exercise greater control over objects, people and the overall environment surrounding the participants [11]. However, an advantage of using naturalistic home observation is that, unlike experimental methods, it is thought to have sound ecological validity because data are gathered in a setting that the family normally encounters in their everyday lives. In general, observational methods are considered direct, objective and reliable [12].

Nonetheless, assessments obtained through observation are samples and so are necessarily constrained and incomplete. During an observation session, researchers are only able to evaluate a small percentage of the parent's everyday life, which limits the scope of data collected. Also, the situation in which parents are observed can impact the results. For example, observing a parent during free play will elicit a different set of parenting practices than will observing the same parent feeding an infant. In an observational situation different parenting practices may be missed because, for example, if an infant is content during an entire observation session then observers will not be able to see the parent soothe the infant. Likewise, if the infant is fussy then it may prove a challenge for the parent to play with the infant as she or he would normally. For that reason, the choice of parameters, such as location, objects, people available and activity presented, may alter the results obtained via observation. To make comparisons between different parents it is important to consider all aspects of observation situations. Another disadvantage of observational methods is that coding and transcribing data from observations can be labor-intensive, time-consuming and expensive. It can also be difficult to establish reliability between coders for some situations.

One study used observational methods along with questionnaires of parenting beliefs among Japanese American and South American mothers of infants [13]. Observers video-recorded mothers and infants in the dyad's home. Mothers were asked to ignore the observer and act as they naturally would during that time. Later, the observations were coded for social and didactic parenting behaviors, and the frequency and duration of those behaviors were calculated. Mothers also completed questionnaires about their parenting. This allowed the researchers to compare the amount of time that mothers actually engage in social and didactic behaviors with the amounts of time mothers say they engage in the same behaviors.

31.5 Experimental testing

Experimental testing is a third way that researchers assess parenting. Such tests might contain specific sets of activities or other items on which a parent receives a score that can be compared to other parents' scores on the same tasks. So imagine giving mothers pairings of play or language items and asking them to say which item of each pair is more advanced developmentally. Mothers' orderings of items can be matched to those established in the developmental literature [14]. Experimental testing methods are controlled and therefore considered equal and fair. However, it is always possible that a parent's performance is affected by the testing situation itself. Furthermore, results may be influenced in part by the parent's personality. Also, if tests highlight a parent's capacity, or lack thereof, for a particular activity, it is not clear whether results from tests apply to other situations. Additionally, testing methods are labor intensive.

31.6 Parental influence

Research has shown that parents influence infant development in many ways. For example, mothers who speak, prompt and respond with greater frequency during their infant's first year have 6-month-olds to 4-year-olds who score higher in standardized evaluations of language and cognition [15, 16]. In addition, the relationship between parents or with other caregivers can positively or negatively impact parenting as well as infant development. For example, parents who report greater marital satisfaction and lower levels of conflict are more competent and more sensitively responsive to their infants than parents whose relationships are unsupportive [17]. A spousal relationship full of conflict can detract from attentive parenting which may, in turn, cause infants to learn that parents are not reliable sources of caregiving. When confronted with an ambiguous stimulus, infants often look to a trusted adult for guidance, an act called social referencing. Infants socially reference their maritally satisfied fathers more than their maritally dissatisfied fathers [18].

Four key developmental characteristics distinguish the broad domains of parenting cognitions and practices with infants and so are often the subject of assessments of parenting. The first, *individual differences*, is that parents differ considerably in the ways that they parent, regardless of their cultural or economic group. For example, during the course of a fixed-duration home observation some mothers talked to their 4-month-olds 3% of the time whereas other mothers talked 97% of the time [19]. The second characteristic is the *consistency* with which parents parent. Parents tend to be relatively consistent in their cognitions and practices from day to day, but over longer periods of time, as infants grow and develop, parents alter their activities accordingly [1, 20].

The third feature relates to the relative *independence of parenting domains* from one another. Mothers engage in certain practices more than others, and although a mother may engage more frequently in one practice, such as face-to-face play, she will not necessarily engage more frequently in other practices, such as didactics [1]. Last, *relations between parenting cognitions and practices vary* [21]. Some researchers have found that parenting cognitions correspond with practices, others have not. For example, mothers' caregiving competence corresponds with their cognitions about the effectiveness of their parenting [21]. However, parents' cognitions about their parenting styles often do not correspond with their actual parenting practices. For example, Japanese American and South American mothers claimed to engage in more social than didactic interactions with their infants when, in actuality, both groups engaged in more didactic than social practices [12]. This suggests the importance of multimethod approaches that take into consideration both observations and self-reports.

31.7 Conclusion

Parents influence many aspects of infant growth and development through their cognitions and practices. To understand how, it is helpful to employ multiple methods of assessment. Self-reports, reports by others, observations and testing are often combined in research to yield the most comprehensive assessments of parenting.

31.8 References

1. Bornstein, M.H. (2002) Parenting infants, in *Handbook of Parenting*, Vol. 1, 2nd edn. (ed. M.H. Bornstein), Lawrence Erlbaum Associates, Mahwah, NJ, pp. 3–43.
2. Murphey, D.A. (1992) Constructing the child: relations between parents' beliefs and child outcomes. *Developmental Review*, **12**, 199–232.
3. East, P.L. and Felice, M.E. (1996) *Adolescent Pregnancy and Parenting: Findings from a Racially Diverse Sample*. Erlbaum, Mahwah, NJ.
4. Bornstein, M.H. (2008) Parents' reports about their children's lives, in *Handbook of Child Research* (eds A. Ben-Arieh, J. Cashmore, G. Goodman *et al.*), Sage, Thousand Oaks, CA, (in press).
5. Wallace, D.B., Franklin, M.B. and Keegan, R.T. (1994) The observing eye: a century of baby diaries. *Human Development*, **37**, 1–29.
6. Bornstein, M.H., Hendricks, C., Hahn, C.-S. *et al.* (2003) Contributors to self-perceived competence, satisfaction, investment, and role balance in maternal parenting: a multivariate ecological analysis. *Parenting: Science and Practice*, **3**, 285–326.
7. Bradley, R. (2009). The HOME environment, in *Handbook of Cultural Developmental Science* (ed. M.H. Bornstein), Taylor & Francis, New York, pp. 505–30.
8. Hughes, D. and DuMont, K. (1993) Using focus groups to facilitate culturally anchored research. *American Journal of Community Psychology*, **21**, 775–806.
9. Bornstein, M.H., Tamis-LeMonda, C.S., Pascual, L. *et al.* (1996) Ideas about parenting in Argentina, France, and the United States. *International Journal of Behavioral Development*, **19**, 347–67.
10. Feinberg, M.E. (2003) The internal structure and ecological context of coparenting: a framework for research and intervention. *Parenting: Science and Practice*, **3**, 95–131.

11. Lytton, H. (1971) Observation studies of parent-child interaction: a methodological review. *Child Development*, **42**, 651–84.

12. Bornstein, M.H. and Haynes, O.M. (1998) Vocabulary competence in early childhood: measurement, latent construct, and predictive validity. *Child Development*, **69**, 654–71.

13. Cote, L.R. and Bornstein, M.H. (2000) Social and didactic parenting behaviors and beliefs among Japanese American and South American mothers of infants. *Infancy*, **1**, 363–74.

14. Tamis-LeMonda, C.S., Chen, L.A. and Bornstein, M.H. (1998) Mothers' knowledge about children's play and language development: short-term stability and interrelations. *Developmental Psychology*, **34**, 115–24.

15. Bornstein, M.H. and Tamis-LeMonda, C.S. (1989) Maternal responsiveness and cognitive development in children, in *Maternal Responsiveness: Characteristics and Consequences* (ed. M.H. Bornstein), Jossey-Bass, San Francisco, pp. 49–61.

16. Nicely, P. Tamis-LeMonda, C.S. and Bornstein, M.H. (1999) Mothers' attuned responses to infant affect expressivity promote earlier achievement of language milestones. *Infant Behavior and Development*, **22**, 557–68.

17. Grych, J. (2002) Marital relationships and parenting, in *Handbook of Parenting*, Vol. 4: *Social Conditions and Applied Parenting*, 2nd edn (ed. M.H. Bornstein), Lawrence Erlbaum Associates, Mahwah, NJ, pp. 203–25.

18. Parke, R.D. (2002) Fathers and families, in *Handbook of Parenting, vol. 3, Status and Social Conditions of Parenting*, 2nd edn (ed. M.H. Bornstein), Lawrence Erlbaum Associates, Mahwah, NJ, pp. 27–73.

19. Bornstein, M.H. and Ruddy, M. (1984) Infant attention maternal stimulation: prediction of cognitive linguistic development in singletons and twins, in *Attention and Performance X* (eds H. Bouwhuis and D. Bouwhuis), Lawrence Erlbaum Associates, London, pp. 433–45.

20. Holden, G.W. and Miller, P.C. (1999) Enduring and different: a meta-analysis of the similarity in parents' child rearing. *Psychological Bulletin*, **125**, 223–54.

21. Ajzen, I. (2001) Nature and operation of attitudes. *Annual Review of Psychology*, **52**, 27–38.

22. Teti, D.M. and Gelfand, D.M. (1991) Behavioral competence among mothers of infants in the first year: the mediational role of maternal self-efficacy. *Child Development*, **62**, 918–29.

32

Principles of effective co-parenting and its assessment in infancy and early childhood

James P. McHale[1] and Elisabeth Fivaz-Depeursinge[2]

[1]University of South Florida St. Petersburg, USA
[2]Centre d'Etude de la Famille, Prilly, Switzerland

32.1 Introduction

This chapter addresses the assessment of parenting relationships between adults responsible for the care and socialization of infants and young children, relationships hereafter referred to as co-parenting alliances. The centrality of co-parenting alliances in families became a regular focus of family-oriented clinicians following the publication of S. Minuchin's structural family theory in 1974 [1], but did not fully penetrate the consciousness of other mental health professionals who work with parents, infants and very young children for another two decades. Since the mid-1990s, there has been an upsurge in both basic and applied research studies of co-parenting, though most published reports have involved two-parent Western nuclear families headed by children's mothers and fathers. This has been an unfortunate, unnecessarily limiting constraint, because co-parenting alliances exist in all families where more than just one person assumes responsibility for a child's care and upbringing [2]. The broad principles we describe in this chapter are relevant in assessing all kinds of co-parenting systems, at any age and in any form of family; however, for cases where special considerations or circumstances are known to bear meaningfully upon co-parenting assessments, we provide additional commentary concerning these considerations.

Parenthood and Mental Health: A Bridge between Infant and Adult Psychiatry   Sam Tyano, Miri Keren, Helen Herrman and John Cox
© 2010 John Wiley & Sons, Ltd

Why would co-parenting be a key aspect of adult mental health? Among the essential, existential motivations of human beings, including those suffering from mental illness, is the wish to be a good-enough mother or father. Co-parenting alliances are hence critically important because the odds of being good enough improve when the adult is supported by an effective co-parenting partnership. Helping patients to be good-enough parents therefore involves understanding and fortifying co-parenting relationships, too.

32.2   What is effective co-parenting?

McHale defined effective co-parenting partnerships as those in which adults agree about how the child should be raised, cooperate in carrying out shared objectives, and demonstrate mutual support and commitment in rearing their common child [3, 4, 5, 6]. As S. Minuchin outlined, in effectively functioning families an adaptive hierarchy exists with the two (or more) co-parenting adults at the helm, coordinating together in joint planning and decision-making and sharing executive power in the system [1]. The adults work collaboratively as a parenting team, consult each other so that each person has formative influence with no one individual exerting unilateral or dictatorial control, and resist overt or covert actions that co-opt children or triangulate them into positions of allying with one co-parenting adult against the other [4, 7, 8].

When assessing co-parenting alliances during infancy and early childhood, the essential facts clinicians must ascertain are:

- Have the adults reconciled ideological differences about how 'best' to parent sufficiently well so as to have established mutually agreed-upon, predictable routines for the child?

- To what extent do they provide (or fail to provide) mutual support and validation for one another's parenting efforts?

- And how well do they tend to children's emotional security within the family unit?

Parents' capacities to perspective-take and prioritize children's needs when co-constructing co-parenting alliances have been a prominent theme in the writings of Talbot and McHale [9, 10]; to be effective as co-parents, adults must take children's perspectives sufficiently well to recognize that:

- Children desire and profit from positive connections with each person who parents them; and that

- Oppositional parenting stances and covert denigration of the child's other parent or caregiver harm children [4].

32.3   Co-parenting as a triangular concept

Talbot and McHale's explicit focus on development of co-parenting alliances within a caregiver–caregiver–child *triangular* emotional system resonates with Fivaz-Depeursinge and Corboz-Warnery's work on the primacy of the family triangle during infancy [11], and stands as a key conceptual distinction setting co-parenting apart from marital systems in the family. Though marital and co-parenting subsystems show some overlap in families (effective co-parents successfully contain their own couple conflicts when actively tending to children [12, 13]), co-parenting is by definition a triadic or polyadic construct. To wit, McHale outlined how the same two parenting adults do not co-parent their different children in the same way [14], while Fivaz and her colleagues have shown how through their own contributions to the family process even very young babies meaningfully shape the dynamic that develops between their parents [15, 16].

32.4 Co-parenting and division of labor

In some conceptualizations of co-parenting in nuclear family systems, extensive attention is given to who does what in the childcare labor division [17]. While relevant to co-parenting dynamics in many families, labor division comes into play principally in situations where one caregiver feels overburdened and put upon and acts out her or his frustration by undermining the other parent. In many other families where one partner provides far more direct care than the other, co-parenting alliances function quite effectively as both partners agree on and are comfortable with the nature of their arrangement. What thus matters most is each parent's perceptions [18].

32.5 Co-parenting and children's adjustment

Why advocate investing substantial additional effort in evaluating the family's co-parenting alliance if evaluations of mothers and of the dyadic mother–child relationship system (and in many cases, even of the children individually) are already planned or available? Compelling evidence for the 'value added' of triangular assessments has come from dozens of empirical studies linking co-parenting dynamics during infancy and early childhood to central aspects of children's early social and emotional adjustment. This body of work was reviewed by McHale [14]; high co-parental antagonism and/or low co-parental mutuality and cohesion is tied to insecure attachment [22]; increases in child disinhibition across time [23]; externalizing and internalizing behavior problems [24, 25, 26]; and less well-developed pre-academic skills [14], academic competencies [27, 28] and peer competencies [29]. Speaking to the value-added issue, associations linking co-parental process to child adjustment typically remain in evidence even after statistically accounting for variability that can be traced to mother–child, father–child and marital relationship functioning [21, 23, 24, 30, 31, 32]. In other words, disruptions in the family's co-parenting alliance often explain why children's behavioral problems persist even though parent–child dyadic relationship systems appear to be functioning adequately.

The mechanisms by which co-parenting discord or detachment impairs infant and child development are likely both direct and indirect. Solidarity (or lack of it) in the co-parental alliance can indirectly affect children by influencing parents' engagement or sensitivity. Support between adults around childrearing challenges and dilemmas strengthens and enhances the parenting practices of each adult individually [6, 33, 34], and studies assessing marriages, parenting and co-parenting separately find that co-parental functioning is more proximally related to parenting than is marital quality [35, 36, 37]. A positive co-parenting alliance also supports fathering in families where parents are not married [38, 39]. Besides these indirect effects, there are likely also many direct ones. Chronic dissonance in caregivers' management of infants' feeding, crying, going-to-bed and night-time awakenings, and other regulatory demands and challenges undermine babies' quests to detect patterns of caregiving regularity and to attain stable internal rhythms. There are likely also attendant effects of caregiving dissonance on evolving physiological systems and processes, both cause and effect of early regulatory efforts [40, 41].

Infants become disorganized when parenting dissonance they encounter overwhelms them. Extreme cases of dissonance occur in families with parents suffering psychiatric disorders. In a study of triadic interactions in families of 9- to 18-week-old infants with mothers suffering from psychotic disorders, Gertsch *et al.* [42] found levels of triadic engagement in these families, compared to a non-clinical comparison group, to be far lower. Subsequently, Philipp, Fivaz-Depeursinge and colleagues [43] studied trilogue play in the context of therapeutic consultations with families of mothers who had suffered psychotic post-partum breakdowns, and found observable differences at all levels of interaction between the women, their young babies and the babies' fathers. As with dyadic pairs in this population, most of these families' interactions oscillated between disengagement and intrusion. Importantly, fathers' interactions appeared as, and sometimes even more, disturbed than those of mothers (often appearing quite controlling of babies). And almost inevitably, parents failed to support each other; ignoring signals or blatantly interfering with one another's interactions with the baby. Faced with paradoxical and very confusing stimulations the infants, even at this young age, adopted a hyper-vigilant stance. The impact on the child's emerging sense of self and development of defensive strategies appeared to be a powerful one.

More broadly, dissonant rule-setting and enforcement, mixed messages from parents about acceptability of anger and fear expression, denigrating portrayals of a parent by the other, chronic mis-coordination, and active interparental undermining confuses infants and young children, sabotages their internalization efforts, threatens felt security and assurance in the safety and integrity of the family unit, and may eventually entrain secrecy and disrupt moral development [2]. It is for these reasons that work with patients who parent young children must proceed from a *multi*-caregiver, at least triangular stance, so as to adequately address the context of the parent's socialization efforts. For unfortunately, the traditional two-person assessments clinicians are most accustomed to conducting with parenting adults (be they parent–child or husband–wife evaluations) overlook altogether the very potent socialization experiences and effects attributable to triangular co-parenting relationships.

32.6 What do mental health professionals need to know? The essentials

To be useful, an essential 'read' of the family's co-parenting alliance by clinicians must start by establishing identities and involvement of all the important parenting adults in the child's life, followed by evaluation of how the family's unique co-parental alliance functions with regard to:

- Mutual involvement/engagement by major co-parents;

- Presence/extent of active solidarity and collaboration between these individuals; and

- Presence/extent of co-parenting dissonance between them.

Establishing who is involved

In heterosexual two-parent family systems, the key co-parenting figures will be the child's mother and father. In gay and lesbian two-parent family systems, it is the two women or two men raising the child together. In some two-parent families, it will be sufficient simply to evaluate the co-parental alliance between these two people. If they are the ones providing the overwhelming preponderance of the child's care and socialization, then resolving problematic co-parental functioning between just the two of them will be the key to improving the child's adjustment.

However, in many other ostensibly two-parent family systems, there will be additional impactful co-parenting figures in the child's life. For example, grandparents and extended kin are co-resident and play active roles in caring for, regulating and socializing infants and young children in millions of households. Further, in industrialized countries where both parents work, daycare providers or other adults frequently spend as much or more waking time with infants and toddlers than do the child's parents. While these individuals are clearly not 'parents' in any literal sense, major child problems can and frequently do ensue if their socialization practices are incompatible with those of the child's parents. In short, even when children are parented in two-parent households, clinicians need a sense of who besides the parents might also be partners in co-parenting the referred child.

What of those families where only one biological parent is co-resident with the child? We have learned that co-parenting alliances operate in the majority of these families as well. In countless families where infants and young children reside alone with their mothers, non-resident fathers spend significant segments of time with the child and it is very important that they be involved in the clinician's co-parenting assessment. According to a major US study designed to better understand unmarried fragile families with both co-resident and non-co-resident fathers, positive co-parenting alliances during the early months and years after a baby's birth increase the odds of fathers remaining involved with their children into the school years; poor early co-parenting alliances, by contrast, are a risk factor for eventual father disengagement and disappearance from the child's life [39].

In Western countries, it is also common for women who may be 'single' mothers by census definitions to co-parent together with their mothers. Adaptive mother–grandmother co-parental alliances do evolve in such family systems, and grandmothers who co-parent can exert important 'gatekeeping' effects by enabling or blocking access of the child's non-co-resident father – thereby shaping children's emotional connections to their fathers, for good or ill. More broadly, in many cultures worldwide, relative caregiving and co-parenting in extended kinship systems is a normative family adaptation, though culturally informed conceptualizations of adaptive and problematic co-parenting among kinship family systems in non-Western cultures remains in short supply [6].

Co-parenting alliances also endure post-divorce, and so infants and young children will frequently have meaningful parent–child contact with not just their two biological parents but also with the new partners of their parents if the children share time between residences. Finally, in many situations where neither of the child's parents is able to care for children owing to abuse, neglect or other significant parenting problems, and kinship caregivers are not accessible to aid with co-parenting, children are ordered to be placed out-of-home for a period of time with a foster family before being reunited with their parents. In such instances, it is proper to consider the temporary foster family as co-parents and to carefully assess the degree of coordination or mis-coordination between their parenting efforts and those of the child's natal family. To reiterate: co-parenting alliances exist for virtually every parent and child; the responsibility of the clinician is to understand this, to ascertain who the relevant individuals are, and to gather as much information as possible about – if not from – each of these individuals.

Assessing co-parenting quality

Once the principals have been correctly identified, evaluation of how the family's co-parental alliance operates with respect to mutual involvement, solidarity and dissonance is completed. Ideally, both individually based and family group assessments would be completed, employing both interview and observation. The aim is to pinpoint the family's dynamics, assets and problems related to co-parenting. In approaching this process, it is useful to imagine how, from the child's perspective, the family functions along each dimension.

Mutual involvement/engagement

First, to assess the extent to which the different parenting adults are mutually involved/engaged with the child, a determination is made (usually from individual interviews) as to how well each parent manages to maintain active and ongoing involvement, provide input on major parenting issues and decisions, and increase level of participation in response to situations demanding heightened effort to best support the child. When ideal, the family ethic will be one of shared, open and mutual involvement with the child, and this should be so noted if it is already the case. In many other families, the judgement will be that periodic physical or emotional absenting by an important co-parent does occur, albeit episodically; in some cases such absenting will trigger (or be triggered by) another parent's over-involvement, while in other cases it will not. This is likewise noted. Finally, data from still other families will reveal either substantial exclusion of or disengagement by one of the child's important co-parents. Observations of the triad can be very useful in helping to substantiate parents' reports of levels of involvement, and in providing additional specific insights concerning the family's particular dynamics regarding co-parenting detachment and exclusion.

Active solidarity and collaboration

Second, a determination must be made about degree to which the central co-parenting adults trust, support, validate and cooperate with one another. In the ideal, the predominant impression would be that each co-parenting adult exhibits and experiences trust and support. In other families, however, the clinician will take note of feelings of distrust or of non-support expressed by one or more family members; even when not the interview's predominant theme, the presence of such sentiments does signal a theme worth pursuing. Finally, for a smaller subgroup of families, the clinician will take note of pervasive feelings of isolation, exclusion, invalidation and/or non-support articulated by one or more family members.

Co-parenting dissonance

Finally, a determination must be made about the extent to which there is major incompat-ibility in the viewpoints of at least one important caregiver about the nature of the child's difficulties and/or about how best to approach and handle the child. Degree of dissonance in any given family can be noted as being minimal, identifiable or substantial. It is important to note that, normatively, women are more likely than men to express discontent during initial interviews [14]; the absence of critical commentary about the co-parenting alliance during initial interviews with men cannot be taken as a reliable indicator that there are no underlying concerns. By contrast, voiced criticism by men is usually worthy of note and is of diagnostic value. We have also found that maternal grandmothers are prone to temper their criticism of their daughters' parenting during initial interviews, with criticisms tending to be more subtle and indirect. It is for these reasons that both the private survey responses provided by the two women and the use of observations to augment interview-based data are important. We will have more to add about mother–grandmother co-parenting alliances later.

32.7 Instruments of choice: observational, interview and self-report survey data

Observations

Because infant mental health clinicians have classically used observations of the mother–infant dyadic relationship and relied on maternal reports of marital co-parenting support to complement assessments of the parent's individual psychodynamics, the proposition that the clinician evaluate the entire family together during initial evaluations may seem excessive. Yet without seeing the entire family in action together, there is really no way to get a thorough and accurate read of the family's signature co-parenting dynamics.

Assessing trilogue play: the Lausanne Trilogue PlayTP

The clinician has at her disposal a powerful, brief, semi-structured assessment paradigm that can provide a read on both the co-parenting dynamics and on the infant or young child's contribution to the family process. The Lausanne Trilogue Play (LTP) [11] leads families through four distinct forms of interaction. In the first part, one parent plays with the baby while the second parent is instructed simply to be present. The parents then switch roles for the second part of the task. In the third part, all three family members play together and, finally, the adults interact while the baby is placed in the 'third party' position. Family members sit *en face* in a triangular configuration as they enact these four parts; even very young infants can participate if properly seated upright in an infant carrier or seat that gets placed on a table so that the infant's face and body rest at what would be chest height for the adults. Families should understand the purpose and set-up of the interaction in advance; detailed guidelines for proper employment of the clinical LTP assessment are detailed elsewhere [44].

Typically, interactions are videotaped and reviewed by clinicians after the assessment session ends and before the following session with the family. As with all assessments informed by family systems approaches, when evaluating the video footage special credence is given to the behavioral sequences and interactions revealed during the interaction. Such interactions belie much of what is necessary to know about structural and communication patterns and problems in the family; clinicians are looking for signs of co-parenting cooperation, interference and disengagement. The adults' behavior with one another and with the child will provide useful insights into family resources as well as problems; the family hierarchy (who takes charge, whether leadership is ultimately shared) and roles of the different adults and of the child in the family's dynamics can later be queried with the co-parenting adults as relevant footage is reviewed with them [45]. Of ultimate interest is identification of problematic coalitions and boundaries within the system so that these can be addressed during interventions with the family [7, 45].

Though initially designed as a three-person assessment, the LTP has been adapted to accommodate families with one or more siblings, in two versions: the Lausanne Family Play (LFP), structured in four parts as the LTP [11], and the Lausanne Pic-Nic, a free play situation where the family is asked to simulate a picnic [46]. Inclusion of all principals in family assessments is strongly recommended. As family therapists caution, observations are most useful when *all* of those individuals principally involved in the maintenance of the problematic patterns participate in the session. Impressions of family dynamics and communication patterns often shift significantly when a sibling participates in an assessment [14].

Especially pertinent to co-parenting assessments is how the co-parenting dynamics can change if a live-in grandparent who had been absent during earlier family sessions subsequently attends a session. In such cases, a different sequence pattern or alliance structure is often revealed [1]. Hence at minimum, the clinician must obtain but be sensitive to the limitations of triadic data alone in such families, for the entire point of taking the time to do an observational evaluation at all is to better understand the invisible family structures that may be maintaining the child's referral problem.

Semi-structured play/teaching observations

When there are several family members, the clinician can elect to use semi-structured observations (most typically some form of teaching and family play) to augment or substitute for the formal LTP or LFP assessment. Such data can be particularly revealing if compared with parallel dyadic (caregiver–child only) or triadic (co-parents and one child) assessments that employ an identical teaching/play format; distressed co-parents' parenting behavior deteriorates as they shift from dyadic to triadic settings, whereas the parenting of non-distressed adults stays more consistent across settings [47].

Another major advantage of use of semi-structured teaching and play tasks is that they would usually involve a wide variety of objects and games, allowing the family members to move freely about the room rather than remaining in one assigned place. These advantages are counterbalanced by several major disadvantages – that the crucial systematicity of the LTP or LFP assessment is lost, that family members can and often do wander out of camera view or get distracted by some peripheral object or event, and that the presence of subtle, often very meaningful, behaviors can more easily go undetected given the challenges in tracking multiple mobile people.

It is usually most ideal, especially with young children, to have the family seated for some interactions and mobile for others. This also often allows the clinician to establish whether a seemingly less-dominant partner becomes more active when constraints are removed, or whether the same partner structures and organizes things regardless of the nature of the task.

Assessing withdrawal during co-parenting discussions

An assessment paradigm especially useful for evaluating withdrawal from co-parenting is a staged 'who does what' dialogue between adults [48], using Cowan and Cowan's [17] Who Does What (WDW) instrument. Each parent individually completes the WDW, rating 24 childcare activities on a scale from 1 (she does it all) to 5 (we divide equally) to 9 (he does it all). After independently completing WDWs, partners are instructed to share their responses and reach consensus on each item; neither partner knows in advance they will be asked to share or adjust their original answers. Discussions are videotaped, so clinicians can take note of and later review with partners segments where each person broke off from active communication and collaboration by shutting down, participating minimally, showing little or no resistance when confronted with dissonant views, and/or allowing the partner to unilaterally determine the 'consensus' co-parenting ratings. In some families, no evidence of withdrawal or non-participation will be evident. In others, clinicians will see multiple instances of acceding to and distancing from the partner and little to no provision of input. These episodes are useful touch-points when pursuing later discourse between partners about what happens when they disagree.

Co-parenting interviews

Interviews with co-parents are indispensible in assessments of co-parenting. They provide succinct, relevant information about how the adults function, and reveal concerns harbored by parents not always accessible from observational data. A number of formal interview protocols have been published in the empirical literature, but there is no one favored instrument or protocol that has become a gold standard for clinical assessments. Most begin by establishing:

- Who the different co-parents are;
- How much time each adult ordinarily spends with the child in a typical week, when, and in what contexts (alone or as a family); and
- Which people get involved in which ways in looking after and socializing the child.

They then query individual parenting practices – what patients see as their own, and as each of their co-parents' strengths; and what they would want to change about both their own parenting and that of each co-parent. It is useful and revealing to ask what things patients believe their co-parents do especially well, for it can be diagnostic if someone is unable to name any of their co-parent's gifts or talents in parenting their shared child.

   Also queried is what has gone well in how parenting has been shared between the co-parenting adults, and what circumstances especially need to change if the adults are to provide a healthier parenting environment for the child. If pressed for time, clinicians can move straight to asking patients to name their major differences with their co-parent concerning what is best for the child, and the ways they believe these differences might be

Table 32.1 Interviews: questions parents can be asked

General

• Who are the major people involved in (child's) life as parents/caregivers?

• Tell me some things (co-parent) does that (child) responds really well to.

• What are the biggest differences of opinion that you and (each co-parent) have about what works best for your child?

• In what ways do you think these differences might be affecting your child?

More Specific

• Do you have trouble trusting (co-parent) to handle your child in certain situations in a way that allows you to feel comfortable? (Probe if yes)

• Does (co-parent) scrutinize your parenting far too closely? (Probe if yes)

• How often do you feel unsupported or not trusted as a parent by (co-parent)?

• When you are unhappy with how (co-parent) is handling the baby, how well are you able to say something to him or her about your feelings?

• When you do try to discuss parenting differences, how frequently do you get "stuck" without being able to come to a mutually agreeable decision?

• How often do you say things to (child) criticizing (co-parent's) parenting or demeaning them to the child? (Also probe answers to frequency questions)

affecting the child. Table 32.1 summarizes important general guidelines for interviews, and questions that can be posed about specific co-parenting processes and dynamics. Such details are helpful in planning co-parenting interventions.

Self-report questionnaire surveys

Finally, we wish to make brief mention of self-report surveys. Though used most often in research settings, the constructs these surveys assess are of interest and can be of some use in co-parenting assessments.

Surveys used to assess mother–father co-parenting alliances

Among the surveys used commonly with two-parent co-resident families are a 20-item Parenting Alliance Measure [22] that queries the degree of support adults feel from one another in their co-parenting alliance, and a 17-item Co-parenting Scale [14] on which parents rate behaviors they engage in that strengthen or undermine their co-parenting alliance. Alone, these surveys are of limited clinical utility but within the context of a more thorough evaluation designed to identify both co-parenting assets and co-parenting problems or liabilities, they can help crystallize problems for later follow-up.

Surveying co-parenting in multigenerational families

Though used most often with two-parent nuclear families, the themes the surveys described above address are also relevant for families where relative caregivers co-parent. Many core issues in parent–grandparent co-parenting alliances mirror those of nuclear families, despite unique distinctions in other ways. Lack of co-parenting support is an especially salient issue in families where parents must be separated from their young children for periods of time, such as when they serve jail or prison sentences for drug-related or other criminal offenses [49]. Particularly when the incarcerated parent is a young child's mother, a sense of disenfranchisement consolidates and often triggers maternal depression and despondency.

In such family situations, it is most often the children's maternal grandmother (and not the children's father) who takes on the primary co-parenting role though just as in nuclear families, the co-parenting adaptations that are made vary widely. Some grandmothers take pains to keep mothers' spirit and positive presence very much alive for the child while mother is away. Others berate the mother for her wrongdoings and inadequate parenting and instill dread in the children about the eventual return of the absent mother. Still others make no mention of mother at all during her absence. In these ways, the particular dynamics of promoting family integrity, of creating conflict and dissonance, and of exclusion that are captured by certain of the Co-parenting Scale items can be relevant in mother–relative kinship families. These items may also be useful in capturing dynamics relevant in 'fragile families' (where the child's mother and father do not marry and are not co-resident). Hence the Co-parenting Scale can be a useful tool when the aim is to heighten co-parents' sensitivity to positive and negative behaviors they may exhibit that serve to strengthen or cripple co-parenting solidarity, though it does not provide useful diagnostic guidelines or clinical cutoffs.

Surveying post-divorce family systems

Finally, because co-parenting relationships remain extremely important to the mental health of both parents and children in post-divorce families, Ahrons [50] designed a Quality of Co-parenting Communication Scale to assess both the quantity and quality of parents' ongoing communication about the child. Clinicians may find this survey useful in work with post-divorce couples, but they can also ask directly about key parent behaviors that telegraph how the co-parenting alliance is functioning. Parents' responses to these queries are of great aid in conceptualizing dynamics of the co-parenting relationship. Some examples of pertinent co-parenting dynamics to inquire about include:

- Can the co-parents speak to one another without hostility, arguments and criticism?
- Can they control anger when communicating with one another?
- Do they shield or fail to shield the shared child from conflict?
- Do they assure the child that they support and value the child's relationship with the co-parent(s)?
- Can they discuss/agree about child discipline; children's schedules/routines; TV/movies the child is allowed to watch, and other related issues?

- Do they interrogate the child about the co-parent's private life?

- Do they have the child keep secrets from the other parent?

- Do they pressure the child to align or take sides with them?

- Do they campaign to alienate the child from the other co-parent and to hate that person?

- Do they make unilateral decisions or fail to share information with the co-parent about the child's education, activities and medical issues?

In summary, self-report survey data can be useful in the context of a comprehensive, culturally informed co-parenting evaluation. Because a central aim of co-parenting assessments is to identify the degree of incompatibility in the co-parents' views of the child, and of what is best for the child, reports by each co-parent of child behavior on formal survey checklists can also be useful in helping to make this judgement. However, parents can also be asked directly how they perceive the child; how they feel about discipline, brokering children's peer relations, and the like; and whether their views resonate or clash with those of the co-parent.

In families exhibiting co-parenting distress, there are significant differences between the adults in whether or not they see their child as having problems of significance [15]. In other words, when there are co-parenting problems, the adults do not always even agree on whether their child is exhibiting problems that should be cause for concern. Knowing how each adult perceives the infant or young child is centrally important in conducting responsible co-parenting assessments, and self-report survey measures are one means of facilitating this conversation with families.

32.8 Conclusion

Our aim in this chapter has been to introduce mental health professionals to the importance of co-parenting alliances as part of their evaluation and conceptualization process in work with any patient who is a child or a parent. Such assessments augment in necessary ways, but do not replace, responsible assessments of parenting competency, risk and other core principles of ethical assessment practice [51]. It is essential to help establish functional co-parenting alliances between the individuals who share the parenting role, including and perhaps especially in those families where one or both of the parents are psychiatrically ill, if the adults are to overcome the almost inevitable difficulties in their families. Unfortunately, even the best designed of interventions often fails without the coordinated cooperation of all adults involved.

32.9 References

1. Minuchin, S. (1974) *Families and Family Therapy*. Harvard University Press, Cambridge, MA.
2. McHale, J. (2009) Shared child-rearing in nuclear, fragile, and kinship family systems: evolution, dilemmas, and promise of a coparenting framework, in *Strengthening Couple Relationships for Optimal Child Development: Lessons from Research and Intervention* (eds M. Schulz, M. Pruett, P. Kerig and R. Parke), American Psychological Association, Washington, DC.

3. McHale, J. (1995) Co-parenting and triadic interactions during infancy: the roles of marital distress and child gender. *Developmental Psychology*, **31**, 985–96.

4. McHale, J. (1997) Overt and covert coparenting processes in the family. *Family Process*, **36**, 183–210.

5. McHale, J., Lauretti, A., Talbot, J. and Pouquette, C. (2002) Retrospect and prospect in the psychological study of coparenting and family group process, in *Retrospect and Prospect in the Psychological Study of Families* (eds J. McHale and W. Grolnick), Erlbaum, New Jersey, pp. 127–65.

6. McHale, J., Khazan, I., Erera, P. *et al.* (2002) Coparenting in diverse family systems, in *Handbook of Parenting*, 2nd edn (ed. M. Bornstein), Erlbaum, New Jersey, pp. 75–107).

7. Fivaz-Depeursinge, E., Lopes, F., Python, M. and Favez, N. (in press) The toddler's role in family coalitions. *Family Process*.

8. Kerig, P. (2005) Revisiting the construct of boundary dissolution: a multidimensional perspective. *Journal of Emotional Abuse*, **5**, 5–42.

9. Talbot, J. and McHale, J. (2002) Family-level emotional climate and its impact on the flexibility of relationship representations, in *Attachment and Family Systems: Conceptual, Empirical and Therapeutic Relatedness* (eds P. Erdman, T. Caffery and J. Carlson), Taylor & Francis, New York, pp. 31–64.

10. Talbot, J. and McHale, J. (2004) Individual parental personality traits moderate the relationship between marital and coparenting quality. *Journal of Adult Development*, **11**, 191–205.

11. Fivaz-Depeursinge, E. and Corboz-Warnery, A. (1999) *A Primary Triangle: A Developmental Systems View of Mothers, Fathers, and Infants.* Basic Books, New York.

12. Cummings, E.M. and Davies, P. (1994) *Children and Marital Conflict: The Impact of Dispute and Family Resolution.* Guilford Press, New York.

13. Feinberg, M.E. (2003) The internal structure and ecological context of coparenting: a framework for research and intervention. *Parenting: Science and Practice*, **3**, 95–131.

14. McHale, J. (2007) *Charting the Bumpy Road of Coparenthood: Understanding the Challenges of Family Life.* Zero to Three Press, Washington, DC.

15. Fivaz-Depeursinge, E., Frascarolo, F., Lopes, F. *et al.* (2007) Parents-child role reversal in trilogue play. Case studies of trajectories from pregnancy to toddlerhood. *Journal of Attachment and Human Development*, **9**, 17–31.

16. McHale, J., Fivaz-Depeursinge, E., Dickstein, S. *et al.* (2008) New evidence for the social embeddedness of infants' early triangular capacities. *Family Process*, **47**, 445–63.

17. Cowan, P. and Cowan, C. (1992) When parents become partners: the big life change for couples. Basic Books, New York.

18. Khazan, I., McHale, J. and DeCourcey, W. (2008) Violated wishes concerning division of childcare labor predict early coparenting process during stressful and non-stressful family evaluations. *Infant Mental Health Journal*, **29**, 343–61.

19. Frosch, C., Mangelsdorf, S. and McHale, J. (2000) Marital behavior and security of preschooler-parent attachment relationships. *Journal of Family Psychology*, **14**, 144–61.

20. Caldera, M. and Lindsey, W. (2006) Coparenting, mother-infant interaction, and infant-parent attachment relationships in two-parent families. *Journal of Family Psychology*, **20**, 275–83.

21. McHale, J. Johnson, D. and Sinclair, R. (1999) Family-level dynamics, preschoolers' family representations, and playground adjustment. *Early Education and Development*, **10**, 373–401.

22. Abidin, R. and Brunner, J. (1995) Development of a parenting alliance inventory. *Journal of Clinical Child Psychology*, **24**, 31–40.
23. Belsky, J., Putnam, S. and Crnic, K. (1996) Coparenting, parenting, and early emotional development, in *Understanding How Family-Level Dynamics Affect Children's Development* (eds J. McHale and P. Cowan), Jossey-Bass, San Francisco, pp. 45–55.
24. McHale, J. and Rasmussen, J. (1998) Coparental and family group-level dynamics during infancy: early family precursors of child and family functioning during preschool. *Development and Psychopathology*, **10**, 39–58.
25. McConnell, M. and Kerig, P. (2002). Assessing coparenting in families of school-age children: validation of the Coparenting and Family Rating System. *Canadian Journal of Behavioural Science, 34*, 4–58.
26. Schoppe, S.J. Mangelsdorf, S.C. and Frosch, C.A. (2001) Coparenting, family process, and family structure: implications for preschoolers' externalizing behavior problems. *Journal of Family Psychology*, **15**, 526–45.
27. McHale, J., Rao, N., and Krasnow, A. (2000) Constructing family climates: Chinese mothers' reports of their coparenting behavior and preschoolers' adaptation. *International Journal of Behavioral Development*, **24**, 111–18.
28. Stright, A. and Neitzel, C. (2003) Beyond parenting: coparenting and children's classroom adjustment. *International Journal of Behavioral Development*, **27**, 31–39.
29. Leary, A. and Katz, L. (2004) Coparenting, family-level processes, and peer outcomes: moderating role of vagal tone. *Development and Psychopathology*, **16**, 593–608.
30. Feinberg, M., Kan, M. and Hetherington, E.M. (2007) The longitudinal influence of coparenting conflict on parental negativity and adolescent maladjustment. *Journal of Marriage and Family*, **69**, 687–702.
31. Katz, L.F. and Low, S.M. (2004) Marital violence, co-parenting, and family-level processes in relation to children's adjustment. *Journal of Family Psychology*, **18**, 372–82.
32. McHale, J., Kuersten, R. and Lauretti, A. (1996) New directions in the study of family-level dynamics during infancy and early childhood. *New Directions for Child Development*, **74**, 5–26.
33. Ehrensaft (1990)
34. McBride and Rane (1998)
35. Bonds, D. and Gondoli, D. (2007) Examining the process by which marital adjustment affects maternal warmth: the role of coparenting support as a mediator. *Journal of Family Psychology*, **21** (2), 288–96.
36. Margolin, G., Gordis, E. and John, R. (2001) Coparenting: a link between marital conflict and parenting in two-parent families. *Journal of Family Psychology*, **15**, 3–21.
37. Floyd, F., Gilliom, L. and Costigan, C. (1998) Marriage and the parenting alliance: longitudinal prediction of change in parenting perceptions and behaviors. *Child Development*, **69** (5) 1461–79.
38. Sobelweski, J. and King, V. (2005) The importance of the coparental relationship for non-residential fathers ties to children. *Journal of Marriage and Family*, **67**, 1196–212.
39. Carlson, M., McLanahan, S. and Brooks-Gunn, J. (2007) Co-parenting and nonresident fathers' involvement with young children after a nonmarital birth. Working Paper 910, Center for Research on Child Wellbeing, Princeton University.

40. Lewis, M. and Ramsey, D. (2005) Infant emotional and cortical responses to goal blockage. *Child Development*, **76**, 518–30.

41. Bornstein, M. and Suess, P. (2000) Child and mother cardiac and vagal tone: continuity, stability, and concordance across the first five years. *Developmental Psychology*, **36**, 54–65.

42. Gertsch Bettens, C., Favez, N., Corboz-Warnery, A. and Fivaz-Depeursinge, E. (1992). Les débuts de la communication à trois. Interactions visuelles triadiques entre père, mère et bébé. *Enfance*, **46**, 323–48.

43. Philipp, D., Fivaz-Depeursinge, E., Favez, N. and Corboz-Warnery, A. (in press) Young infants' triangular communication with their parents in the context of maternal post-partum breakdown. Case studies. *Infant Mental Health*.

44. Fivaz-Depeursinge, E., Corboz-Warnery, A. and Keren, M. (2004) The primary triangle: treating infants in their families, in *Treating Parent-Infant Problems: Strategies for Intervention* (eds A.J. Sameroff, S.C. McDonough and K.L. Rosenblum), Guilford Press, New York, pp. 123–51.

45. McHale, J. and Sullivan, M. (2008) Family systems, in *Handbook of Clinical Psychology, vol. II: Children and Adolescents* (eds M. Hersen and A. Gross), John Wiley & Sons, Inc., Hoboken, NJ, pp. 192–226.

46. Frascarolo, F., Favez, N., Dimitrova, N. and Lavanchy, C. (2006, July) Differences in a family picnic game at 5 years vary as a function of quality of transition to parenthood. Poster presented at the World Association of Infant Mental Health, Paris.

47. Lauretti, A. and McHale, J. (2009) Shifting patterns of parenting styles between dyadic and family settings: the role of marital distress, in *Psychology of Family Relationships* (eds M. Russo and A. de Luca), Nova Science Publishers, New York.

48. Elliston, D., McHale, J., Talbot, J. *et al.* (2008) Withdrawal from coparenting interactions during early infancy. *Family Process*, **47**, 481–98.

49. Cecil, D., McHale, J. and Strozier, A. (2008) Female inmates, family caregivers, and young children's adjustment: a research agenda and implications for corrections programming. *Journal of Criminal Justice*, **36**, 513–21.

50. Ahrons, C. (1981) The continuing coparental relationship between divorced spouses. *American Journal of Orthopsychiatry*, **59**, 415–27.

51. Gopfert, M., Webster, J. and Seiki, S. (2004) Formulation and assessment of parenting, in *Parental Psychiatric Disorder: Distressed Parents and Their Families*, 2nd edn (eds M. Gopfert, J. Webster and M. Seeman), Cambridge Press, pp. 93–111.

33
Legal assessment of parenting competency

Jean-Victor P. Wittenberg

The Hospital for Sick Children, Toronto, Canada

33.1 Introduction

This chapter explores the role of the infant mental health professional assessing the parenting competency of parents with infants or young children. Parenting competency, or parenting capacity, is a concept that straddles the fields of infant and adult psychiatry and also the medico-legal interface. Although inexactly defined in operational terms, it clearly refers to the degree of ability and motivation that parents have for rearing a particular child in a safe and supportive manner within a particular context. It becomes the salient question either when we encounter a child about whom we have child protection concerns or when the child protection system or the court system asks us to provide an opinion.

Infant mental health professionals are dedicated to improving the mental health of infants and young children. Thus we are committed to promoting the support of their families for those infants and of their communities for those families. To conduct a parenting capacity assessment we must address the needs and rights, vulnerabilities and strengths of both children and parents, and beyond that the vulnerabilities and strengths of our communities and society in general. As with many concepts that fall into the border-land of separate fields, controversies and compromises abound when we try to implement the principles and philosophies of any one. For example there are large cultural and religious differences between different parts of the world. These differences impact significantly on how babies, children and the responsibilities of parenting are conceptua-lized. Not all are in keeping with findings in scientific literature. Ideally when we intervene whether to provide therapeutic services or to conduct evaluations, our goal is to improve children's mental health. When we intervene with infants and toddlers to participate in decision-making for their futures, what we offer may have lifespan consequences. There is no one right way to conduct parenting competency assessments; there is no gold standard. All assessments must take notice of the context within which the assessment takes place. It is clear however, that much remains to be understood and there is much room for improvement.

33.2 Definitions of maltreatment

The question of parenting capacity arises in the context of possible child maltreatment. Child maltreatment is a legal concept, differently defined in different jurisdictions. Almost every country in the world however has signed the United Nations Convention on the Rights of the Child (1989) [1], which recognizes that families are the primary source of care and protection for children. Beyond that the Convention requires nations to provide special protection and assistance to children to enable them to reach their full potential as adults. Thus the Convention requires us to support families and also to protect children within families. Article 19 of the Convention requires governments to take all appropriate measures to protect children from abuse and neglect while in the care of the parent or legal guardian.

Each jurisdiction defines abuse somewhat differently. A review of legal definitions is beyond the scope of this chapter. Legal definitions are held within the context of cultural beliefs. There are wide variations: e.g. between secular and religiously observant cultures, between predominantly rural undeveloped and industrialized urban settings, between wealthy and deprived areas, etc. There may be differences between different countries and between different locales within the same countries, even within the same city. In order to make significant differences for infants and families, assessors have to be knowl-edgeable about the setting, the local beliefs and the scientific literature. Some parental behaviors that are seen as maladaptive in one setting might be adaptive in another. This chapter does not try to encompass the wide cultural variations that exist across the world except to caution that they must be taken into consideration when a parenting capacity assessment is carried out.

The Child and Family Services Act in Ontario, Canada, similar to laws in many other jurisdictions, states that:

1 The primary goal is to promote the best interests, protection and well-being of children.

2 In addition, support should be given to support the autonomy and integrity of the family unit and, wherever possible, should be provided on the basis of mutual consent.

3 It recognizes a child's need for continuity of care and for stable relationships within a family and cultural environment.

Thus our responsibility as a community and as a country is to support family functioning as well as to protect children from maltreatment and developmentally adverse experiences such as impermanence, instability and loss of cultural ties.

A Parenting Capacity Assessment (PCA) provides an opinion from an expert consultant as to whether a child should remain with particular caregivers or should be removed by force of law. Impermanence of caregivers has special significance for infants and toddlers who are in the process of forming attachments that optimally provide them with feelings of security. Decisions to remove infants and young children from their caregivers thus have implications for models of relationships that can persist for many years, even for a lifetime. Secure models of relationships are associated with significantly better outcomes in many areas of functioning. A decision to terminate a caregiver–child relationship or alternatively to leave a child in a compromised caregiver–child relationship is a life-altering decision. This is true for the child who is removed from parents and also for parents who lose a child.

A child is defined as being in need of protection when the child has suffered or is at risk of suffering physical harm, emotional harm or sexual abuse which is either inflicted by the person having charge of the child or caused by or resulting from that person's failure to protect the child. Thus maltreatment can occur either by acts of commission or by acts of omission. Neglect is as damaging as abuse [2]. Parents are also responsible to provide needed medical care for children and the care needed to protect their healthy development.

One difficulty in recognizing maltreatment lies in different perceptions of what maltreatment is. As early as 1992, Aganathos-Gorgopoulou wrote:

> International data suggest that child maltreatment is the product of a complex interaction of parental characteristics and the social and cultural conditions in which they exist. The value placed on children, on different categories of vulnerable children, on child-rearing practices (including views on physical punishment and the informal social sanctions regarding children and family organization and functioning) are central to the study of the phenomenon within each specific culture. [3]

More recent studies have supported that view. Many reports find that while extremes of maltreatment are recognized with similarity across cultures, other forms of maltreatment are overlooked and may be seen as normal within the culture (e.g. [4]). In other cases those who experienced particular forms of behavior that might be considered maltreatment tended to justify it [5]. Thus there are both cultural and individual factors which tend to create bias. The same biases can be at work and must be brought to their awareness in those who perform parenting capacity assessments.

Assessors must be aware of their power. In one review of British cases, 73% of dispositions followed the assessor's recommendations entirely [6]. Another study [7] found that many parenting capacity reports did not conform to guidelines recommended by the American Psychological Association. There is significant concern therefore, that parenting capacity reports are failing to provide the unbiased and informed opinions that the judicial system needs in order to make life-altering decisions for infants, children and youth as well as their parents.

33.3 Assessment is an intervention

Insofar as the purpose of infant mental health professionals who carry out parenting capacity assessments is to improve the overall mental health of individuals, attention must be paid to the impact of these assessments on children and families. Do the assessments protect those children who need protection? Do they lead to better alternatives for the children who are taken into care? Do the assessments lead to improvements in the mental health of families and children who are kept together by helping them access the help they need to function better? The data to answer these questions has yet to be collected. At present decisions are made in the absence of good outcome data [8].

Even when guidelines for parenting capacity assessments are followed there are major concerns about the effectiveness of the approaches that have been used not only by those carrying out the assessments but by social policy in general. Devaney and Spratt [9] wrote that there has been a perceived lack of progress in reducing the incidence of child abuse, and in improving the outcomes for children in both the short and longer term. Rather than trying to solve what they describe as a 'wicked problem', one that cannot be solved by directly applied solutions, they argue for earlier identification of and intervention with children who are experiencing multiple adversity, such as those living with parents misusing substances and those exposed to intimate partner violence. Theirs is more of a preventive approach that recognizes the failures of the present system.

Others have expressed concern about the present model for child protection. An alternative model called Therapeutic Jurisprudence has as its goal to turn judicial decisions to therapeutic goals [10]. At present the model has been much more developed within the criminal court systems (e.g. drug abuse courts, domestic violence courts) but it is also being developed in family courts (Canada) or juvenile courts (USA) where child custody issues are decided [11]. The power of the court is used to support respectful, open-minded relationships that recognize family strengths and potential, to coordinate child and family needs and resources, to track progress and provide accountability, to educate professionals about infant mental health, etc. [10].

At the same time, reports refer repeatedly to worsening trends in the mental and emotional life of families that appear in family courts in the USA [11]. Data collected by Wittenberg and Goodman (unpublished survey [12]) found that although referrals to child protection in one region had increased over the past three years, court involvement had decreased. This may seem to suggest that the severity of cases had decreased, however changes in government policy clearly affected case disposition. Whether cases were being handled with greater benefit to parents and children was unclear.

Reports based on studies from around the world identify maltreating families as more isolated and socially disconnected than others (e.g. [13]. Thus it may be that those cases which need it most are hardest to reach with offers of help.

Some interventions can be useful. For example, Zeanah *et al.* [14] found that some families could in fact be helped by a comprehensive preventive intervention in that rates of maltreatment for children who were taken into care decreased significantly subsequent to the intervention. However they also found that a greater number of infants and young children were not returned to their families of origin in the intervention group, probably because family functioning and degree of risk to the child were more closely scrutinized in those cases.

33.4 Infants and toddlers are a special group

There are concerns about the fate of all children and adolescents who experience maltreatment. Maltreatment is likely to have deleterious effects on children of all ages but there are particular concerns for children who are maltreated in their first years [15]. A large literature has found lifespan difficulties that include social problems, learning problems, self-esteem difficulties, mental health problems, physical disorders, etc. associated with adverse experiences in the first years. All of these are related to problems in infants' primary relationships.

Infants and toddlers from the child protection populations are over-represented in adult populations with high levels of pathology. They tend too to pass on their difficulties to their own children. This becomes an expanding, perpetuated social problem associated with many costs (financial, social, criminal, etc.) to our communities [16].

In part infants and toddlers are a group which is particularly vulnerable to lifespan consequences because of the nature of brain development in the early years. Children and youth who had experienced abuse were found to have smaller brains and larger ventricles, a finding that was more significant for those who experienced the abuse earlier in life [17]: 'Experience-based brain development *in utero* and the early years of life can set brain and biological pathways that affect health, competence and well-being' [16, 18]. Early experiences affect not only brain development but also the endocrine system (e.g. cortisol), the immune system and genetic expression through influences of the epigenetic systems.

33.5 Models of parenting capacity assessment

Caution must be exercised insofar as joining a mental health-care intervention with a judicial intervention. In order to provide a neutral and objective opinion, if that is ever possible, assessors should not be otherwise involved in the case. Previous involvement as a therapist or as a professional who made the referral to child protection services can bias the assessment. Even a professional who has carried out a clinical assessment of the child and parents may be biased because the focus of attention and model for interactions are significantly different in the two roles.

When accepting an undertaking to provide an opinion on parenting capacity, the professional needs to know beforehand, what specific questions are to be addressed. The relationship between the court or the child protection agency and the assessor must be clear and should be at arm's length. The assessor must be free to agree or disagree with the opinions of the referring agency, if that agency has expressed an opinion. The assessor's role is that of a consultant expert in some areas relevant to child development and parent–child relationships. The consultant can offer information and opinions within that area of expertise but not beyond it. The consultant must be as aware of what he does not know as of what he does know; of what is validated, empirically based information, the strength of that empirical base and its limitations. These guidelines are as relevant to the consultant's report as to any appearance to testify in court.

When being introduced to the family, the assessor must be sure that they understand his role. It is a role that is very different than that of health-care worker employed by the family for its own benefit. Parents do not have the right to use their discretion as to whether or not they will follow up on suggestions and recommendations made to them. They should be clear that confidentiality will not be maintained; all information they offer and all observations and opinions will be made available to the referring agent, which may be the child protection agency, the court, counsel for both sides, etc. At the same time it is important for parents to feel able to present themselves freely and in as good a light as possible. What parents and the assessor have in common, in almost all assessments, is what is in the best interests of the child or children involved. This can be made explicit and can help parents feel able to share a goal and help them find a way to engage in the assessment process.

There have been a number of approaches described for carrying out parenting capacity assessments. These vary as to the numbers of individuals involved, the frequency of assessment meetings, the use of standardized measures, etc. Some are done within the context of a therapeutic intervention such as a therapeutic access visits. A few have been described for specific application to infants and toddlers.

Steinhauer and his group [19] developed a manual that organized the collection of information into four areas: context, child, parent–child relationship and parent.

- *Context* including supports and stresses in the social environment; poverty; other relationships. This includes a careful assessment of the marital relationship if one exists. Some partners enhance a parent's functioning. Others compromise it and increase the risk to children.

- *Child* vulnerabilities, challenges and needs in the child; the child's history with these parents and how that history has affected her behavior, self-esteem and any medical, psychiatric, cognitive or social difficulties that make extraordinary demands on parents

- *Parent–child relationship* the predominant patterns in the parent–child relationship and the nature of the attachment between parent and child. Direct observations of parent–child interactions are called for in this assessment.

- *Parent* characteristics including impulse control, acceptance of responsibility, behaviors affecting parenting, manner of relating to society and use of clinical interventions. The parent's history from infancy to adulthood needs to be reviewed carefully. A history of being abused as a child does not mean the adult will be abusive as parent. If a parent shows reasonable parental functioning at one point in time, but a long-term pattern of better functioning and recurrent relapses into maladaptive functioning the assessor must consider the depth of the regressive drops in functioning and the risks and challenges it poses for a child. This can be the case for parents with serious psychiatric or substance abuse issues.

Many of the same categories are included in descriptions of other models. Almost all apply to parenting children and adolescents as well as infants; however, although attachment theory is often referred to, infants are almost a footnote in most guidelines.

Other authors cover the same territory with somewhat different emphases. Budd [20] and Azar *et al.* [21] comment on the need to focus on the parent's behaviors and skills as they relate to a parent–child relationship and to rearing a specific child. They also discuss parents needing to meet a minimal standard of parenting; however, this is very difficult to define. Donald and Jureidini [22] prioritize the parental ability to use reflective functioning in the context of the parent–child relationship. They write that parents must be able not only to accept their particular child but also to 'accept and be prepared to address their own intrinsic characteristics'. Schmidt *et al.* [23] provide guidelines from a perspective that emphasizes attachment findings. Each of these approaches clearly adds a useful perspective to the assessment work.

Some approaches emphasize the use of standardized measures and these may be useful for professionals trained in their application, scoring and interpretation. Some measures such as semi-structured interviews tend to be quite long and demand a high degree of training to achieve reliability in administration and scoring. Azar *et al.* [21] also makes the point that most measures assess individual characteristics and what is most relevant is the functioning of the parent and child together, of the relationship. In addition these instruments are not validated for use in this population [20].

There is a risk, when using measures, of creating an air of scientific truth but validity has yet to be demonstrated. Even when test outcomes have been shown to have significant associations with risks for maltreatment, it must be recalled that this data comes from comparisons of group scores and is usually retrospective rather than prospective; true from history but questionable when predicting future behavior. Parenting capacity is evaluated in a court room on an individual basis. Decisions must be based on assurances that are higher than the 5% level of confidence we accept for scientific validity. We would not want to remove 1 in 20 children from their parents without cause. We would not want to leave 1 in 20 children with maltreating parents. Caution must be applied before drawing conclusions of test results in individual cases. Nonetheless these measures can add useful information in the context of a more comprehensive assessment.

33.6 Core competencies for professionals doing parenting capacity assessments with infants

Some guidelines for PCAs have been written with infants and young children in mind. Harden [24] and the Michigan Association for Infant Mental Health [25] both cover much more than the PCA. Both emphasize the need for professionals who carry out PCAs that involve infants or toddlers to have taken special training in order to become expert in infant mental health. Professionals need to have knowledge about:

- How infants learn both cognitively and emotionally about the world and especially the world of relationships.

- Healthy and deviant development in all domains including gross and fine motor functioning, cognition, normal development from basic to complex emotions, emotional and behavioral regulation, social development. (This is crucial knowledge because of the high incidence of children with developmental delays in the child welfare population.)

- The development and presentation of secure and insecure attachment, with emphasis on disorganized attachment and attachment disorders.

- Psychopathology as it appears in infants and toddlers including specific syndromes such as post-traumatic stress disorders, pervasive developmental disorders, etc.

- Resources that are available in the community to support infants, toddlers and parents.

They need to have skills in assessing a parent's capacity and motivation to:

- Attend to an infant's physical needs, to protect an infant from harm and provide a safe environment.

- Attend supportively to an infant's normal development at different ages along all lines of development.

- Recognize illness or developmental difficulties in the baby and to seek help for them.

- Invest emotionally in the infant even when tired and stressed.

- Maintain a positive feeling for the baby and to understand the baby's behavior as informed by developmental understanding.

- Accurately read and effectively respond to an infant's cues and signals about physical and emotional experiences.

In addition these professionals need to be able to assess knowledge, skills and capacities that a parent of a child of any age must have to parent effectively and to be aware of disorders that may compromise parenting:

- Mental health and addiction or substance abuse problems and how they are likely to impact parenting and the parent–child relationship;

- Impulse control and frustration tolerance;

- The parental relationship, any degree of conflict and especially of domestic violence; the influence of parental partners (or other residents in the home) on each other as parents;

- The capacity to see the child as a separate being with a mind of her own when the parent is relaxed and also when stressed, especially when stressed by the child;

- The parental capacity to recognize areas in which they need to improve including those areas that may have led to maltreatment of the child; parent acceptance of their responsibility for the child;

- The capacity to recognize the workings of one's own mind and one's own foibles and vulnerabilities;

- The capacity to be involved in the community and to work with other parents, teachers, health-care workers and other professionals as the child needs them.

There are a few further important points made in descriptions of PCAs and the professionals who conduct them:

- Professionals must be able to recognize parental strengths as well as deficiencies. The possibility of bias in the assessor can blind them to parental strengths or deficiencies. Bias can arise from culturally determined beliefs. When the assessor is from a different culture, he may be more likely to be intolerant of unfamiliar behaviors in parents. When he is from the same culture he may not notice maladaptive parenting practices.

- Professionals must directly observe interactions between parents and children especially infants and toddlers. There are some calls for observations made in different locations at different times. It may be sufficient to make observations in a location familiar to the assessor who has seen many families interacting there and thus can make comparisons. Alternatively it may be sufficient to observe interactions in a location with which parents and child have become familiar, such as the parental home if visits occur there, or in a supervised child protection site if access visits have been occurring there. If the child is in foster care, observations of the child with the foster caregivers should be included. When there are two or more adults who will have responsibility for the child, all should be observed together and individually with the child. If there are more children in the home, it is useful to observe the parents with all the children to see how they cope with those added demands.

Assessors must seek to observe and understand the effects of parent or caregiver and child on each other. They must also assess to what degree the parent can make these observations of interacting influences themselves and can use these observations to guide their interactions with the children.

- Assessors must collect information from multiple sources. These include reports from foster caregivers, pediatricians or family doctors, psychiatrists, psychologists, physical or occupational therapists, individual or family therapists, etc. who provide health-care services to child and/or parents; daycare workers and teachers, access visit supervisors; child protection workers; etc. Interviews with other important informal sources of support in the family's social circle are also necessary if those supports are likely to provide what the parents need in order to function reasonably effectively.

Finally the assessor must come to conclusions about the following questions:

- Under what circumstances if any, are these parents capable of providing the support, stimulation, protection, treatment, education and recreation their child needs? Are they able to provide the constancy, stability and predictability that children need for security and healthy development?

- What are the challenges this particular child presents to these parents? What challenges would the child present to any parent?

- What will the child need in the way of support, stimulation, protection, treatment, education and recreation? In particular what extraordinary demands will this child make on parents? What will be the outcome for this child in the absence of those interventions as opposed to the outcome should those interventions be in place? Will parents be able to collaborate with community professionals and other parents to make those resources available to their children?

- What particular challenges do these parents present to this child? In some cases merely the presence of the parents causes disorganizing anxiety for children who have been maltreated.

- If parents need special education or treatment, will they avail themselves of those and are these likely to make a significant difference to their functioning as parents?

- Are the circumstances and supports available to parents sufficient to maintain their parental functioning?

33.7 Conclusions

1 The professional carrying out a parenting capacity assessment must integrate and apply knowledge of multiple systems and bodies of knowledge, to provide information and education to the child protection system or the judicial system with the goal of promoting the mental health and development of infants, young children and their parents.

2 Assessors must be aware of potential bias in themselves and others in the system.

3 Consultants providing PCAs that involve infants and toddlers need special training in infant mental health and development.

4 Outcomes in the child protection field are not yet well understood or supported by empirical data. Research is needed.

5 Parenting capacity is a functional, dynamic concept influenced by the nature of the parents, the child or children, and the circumstances and context within which they find themselves. Assessment must include observations and reports of functioning in different circumstances that include more and less stress and should include a review over long periods of time looking for significant fluctuations. These are in conflict with the degree of permanence that infants and young children need.

6 It may be that optimal outcomes will be fostered by more preventive, therapeutic approaches that include collaborations between mental health workers, child protection workers, providers of social services and the judicial system working within a model of therapeutic jurisprudence.

33.8 References

1. United Nations Convention on the Rights of the Child (1989) http://www.un.org/documents/ga/res/44/a44r025.htm.
2. Hildyard, K.L. and Wolfe, D.A. (2002) Child neglect: developmental issues and outcomes. *Child Abuse and Neglect*, **26**, 679–95.
3. Agathonos-Georgopoulou, H. (1992) Cross-cultural perspectives in child abuse and neglect. *Child Abuse Review*, **1**, 80–88.
4. Collier, A.F., McClure, F.H., Collier, J. *et al.* (1999) Culture-specific views of child maltreatment and parenting styles in a pacific-island community. *Child Abuse and Neglect*, **23**, 229–44.
5. Bensley, L., Ruggles, D., Simmons, K.W. *et al.* (2004) General population norms about child abuse and neglect and associations with childhood experiences. *Child Abuse and Neglect*, **28**, 1321–37.
6. Jamieson, N., Tranah, T. and Sheldrick, E.C. (1999) The impact of expert evidence on care proceedings. *Child Abuse Review*, **8**, 183–92.
7. Budd, K.S. (2001) Assessing parenting competence in child protection cases: a clinical practice model. *Clinical Child and Family Psychology Review*, **4**, 1–18.
8. Lennings, C. (2002) Decision making in care and protection: the expert assessment. *Australian e-Journal for the Advancement of Mental Health*, **1**, 2–13.
9. Devaney, J. and Spratt, T. (2009) Child abuse as a complex and wicked problem: reflecting on policy developments in the United Kingdom in working with children and families with multiple problems. *Children and Youth Services Review*, **31**, 635–41.
10. Goldberg, S. (2005) *Judging for the 21st Century: A Problem-solving Approach*. National Judicial Institute, Ottawa.
11. Lederman, C.S. and Osofsky, J.D. (2004) Infant mental health interventions in juvenile court: ameliorating the effects of maltreatment and deprivation. *Psychology, Public Policy, and Law*, **10**, 162–77.

12. Wittenberg, J. and Goodman, D. (2009) Survey of Infants and Toddlers in Family Court in the Peel Region. Unpublished data.

13. Gracia, E. and Musitu, G. (2003) Social isolation from communities and child maltreatment: a cross-cultural comparison. *Child Abuse and Neglect*, **27**, 153–68.

14. Zeanah, C.H., Larrieu, J.A., Scott Heller, S. *et al.* (2001) Evaluation of a preventive intervention for maltreated infants and toddlers in foster care. *Journal of American Academic Child and Adolescent Psychiatry*, **40**, 214–21.

15. Cicchetti, D. and Toth, S. (1995) Developmental psychopathology of child maltreatment. *Journal of American Academic Child and Adolescent Psychiatry*, **34**, 541–65.

16. Mustard, J.F. (2006) *Early Child Development and Experience-based Brain Development: The Scientific Underpinnings of the Importance of Early Child Development in a Globalized World*. The Founders' Network, The Canadian Institute for Advanced Research, Toronto.

17. DeBellis, M.D., Keshavan, M.S., Clark, D.B. *et al.* (1999) A.E. Bennett Research Award. Developmental traumatology. Part II: Brain development. *Biological Psychiatry*, **45**, 1271–84.

18. Shonkoff, J.P., Boyce, W.T. and McEwen, B.S. (2009) Neuroscience, molecular biology, and the childhood roots of health disparities: building a new framework for health promotion and disease prevention. *Journal of the American Medical Association*, **301**, 2252–59.

19. Steinhauer, P.D., Leitenberger, M., Manglicas, E. *et al.* (1995) *Assessing Parenting Capacity: Manual*. The Institute for the Prevention of Child Abuse, Toronto.

20. Budd, K.S. (2005) Assessing parenting capacity in a child welfare context. *Child and Youth Services Review*, **27**, 429–44.

21. Azar, S.T., Lauretti, A.F. and Loding, B.V. (1998) The evaluation of parental fitness in termination of parental rights cases: a functional-contextual perspective. *Clinical Child and Family Psychology Review*, **1**, 77–100.

22. Donald, T. and Jureidini, J. (2004) Parenting capacity. *Child Abuse Review*, **13**, 5–17.

23. Shmidt, F., Cuttress, L.J., Lang, J. *et al.* (2007) Assessing the parent-child relationship in parenting capacity evaluations: clinical applications of attachment research. *Family Court Review*, **45**, 247–59.

24. Harden, B.J. (2007) *Infants and Children in the Child Welfare System: A Developmental Framework for Policy and Practice*. Zero To Three, Washington, DC.

25. Michigan Association for Infant Mental Health (2005) *Guidelines for Comprehensive Assessment of Infant and Parents in the Child Welfare System*, 2nd edn. Michigan Association for Infant Mental Health, Southgate, Michigan.

34

Psychotropic drugs and lactation: to nurse or not to nurse

Zivanit Ergaz and Asher Ornoy

Institute of Medical Sciences, Jerusalem, Israel

34.1 Drug excretion into breast milk: general considerations

Human milk is the best nutrition for the newborn infant at least during the first few months of life. It is perfectly suited for the infant's gastrointestinal tract and also contains variable growth factors and protective factors against infection. It addition, nursing is an important factor in bonding and in maternal satisfaction with her growing child. Hence, breastfeeding is strongly advised and indeed the percentage of mothers nursing their infants is constantly rising [1, 2].

Nowadays, many women at childbearing age are on chronic medication including the period of pregnancy and lactation. Among the largest groups of drugs of chronic and continuous use are the various psychotropic drugs: i.e. sedatives, antidepressants, antipsychotic and antiepileptic drugs. These drugs are being used by more than 10% of lactating women [1, 2].

Most medications used by the nursing mother enter to some degree into breast milk, exposing the nursing infant to different levels of the drug (Tables 34.1 and 34.2). Its concentration in the milk is dependent on adult drug T½ (the time required for a drug

Parenthood and Mental Health: A Bridge between Infant and Adult Psychiatry   Sam Tyano, Miri Keren, Helen Herrman and John Cox
© 2010 John Wiley & Sons, Ltd

Table 34.1   Factors affecting drug concentration in breast milk

Maternal drug dosage ↑
Maternal plasma drug level ↑
Adult T ½ ↑
Proximity to the time of drug ingestion by the mother ↑
Drug pharmacokinetics
Drug molecular weight ↓
Drug protein binding ↓
Drug lipid solubility ↑
pKa ↑
First few days post-partum – large gaps between alveolar cells in milk buds ↑

Table 34.2   Factors affecting infant's drug brain level

Breast milk drug level ↑
Infant breast milk intake ↑
Drug oral availability ↑
Infant's plasma drug level ↑
Reduced infant's liver and kidney function during the first few months ↑
Drug binding to albumin ↓
Immature blood brain barrier during the first few months ↑

to be metabolized by half) maternal dose, mode of intake and type of drug. Usually, the doses entering breast milk are low and have sub-clinical effects and many of these drugs are undetectable in the serum of the nursing infant. In addition, the total dose reaching the nursing infant also depends on the amount of milk ingested by him. If the infant is fed on milk only, the daily intake is about one sixth of the infant's weight (i.e. about 150ml milk/kg body weight). Therefore even if the ratio of milk to maternal plasma concentrations is 1.0 or over, the nursing infant will ingest about one sixth of the maternal dose. For many drugs, the milk/plasma ratio is less than 1.0.

However, the susceptibility of the young infant to some drugs may be higher than that of the mother and therefore several drugs given to the nursing mother may cause definite clinical symptoms in the nursing infant. On the other hand, for a mother that is using psychotropic drugs, nursing might be a very important event that might contribute to her mental health. Hence, the treating physician should take into consideration the benefits of nursing to both the infant and mother before advising to refrain from nursing. It is also important to note that Teratogen Information Services in Israel, Europe and the USA are also qualified to advice as to the possible dangers imposed by specific drugs on the nursing infant, and they can always be contacted either by the treated mother or the treating physician.

Most psychotropic drugs enter human milk in relatively low concentrations and therefore only rarely induce clinical effects in the nursing infant. However, as these drugs are often used by nursing mothers we will refer to each one of these drugs separately, within the group of drugs it belongs.

34.2 Benzodiazepines

Benzodiazepines are used to control anxiety, panic attacks and seizures. The data concerning their use during lactation is based mainly on a small number of case reports.

According to the American Academy of Pediatrics (AAP) benzodiazepines, like other psychotropic drugs, have an unknown effect on these nursing infants and their use may be of concern [3]. On the other hand, the short-acting benzodiazepines: midazolam, clonazepam, clobazam and nitrazepam – are considered by the World Health Organization (WHO) group on human lactation safe for a short time if the maternal dose is low [3, 4]. Low passage was reported in lactating women supplemented with these drugs and no adverse effects were observed. Schaefer *et al.* [5] consider low doses of oxazepam and diazepam as the drugs of choice in this group for breastfeeding mothers, and put no limitations on the use of one or few doses of any of the benzodiazepines.

All benzodiazepines are distributed into human milk with peak concentrations in approximately 60 minutes. However, many of them are transferred in low concentrations.

The more commonly used benzodiazepines will be discussed here.

Clonazepam

Peak level: occurring within four hours of dosing. Adult T½: 18–50 hours; neonate T½: 140 hours; protein binding: 50–86%; milk/plasma concentration ratio: 0.33–0.37. Clonazepam was detected in only 1/10 infants exposed to the drug during pregnancy and the post-partum period, and not in the one whose mother was treated exclusively post-partum. No adverse effects were described in any of these infants. A female infant that was breastfed by a clonazepam-treated mother, who developed apnea, cyanosis and hypotonia within a few hours from birth, recovered, and the symptoms resolved within five days despite breastfeeding continuation.

Diazepam

Adult T½: 20–65 hours; neonate T½: 400 hours; protein binding: 99%; milk/plasma concentration ratio: 0.1–0.5. Diazepam has three active metabolites: desmethyldiazepam, temazepam and oxazepam. Although no adverse clinical effects were found in several breastfed neonates despite measurable drug levels, a case report of lethargy in a breastfed infant exposed to diazepam 10 mg t.i.d. and finding of the active metabolite oxazepam in the breast milk and infant's urine, led to a recommendation of lower drug dosage during lactation [6].

Midazolam

Adult T½: 2.5 hours; neonate T½: 7 hours; milk/plasma concentration ratio: 0.09–0.16. In several studies no measurable midazolam levels were detected in breast milk from mothers, 7 hours following 15 mg tablet intake but detectable concentrations were found in milk from one mother who accidentally took an additional tablet. In another two lactating women, breast milk concentrations of midazolam and its hydroxy metabolite gradually decreased, until four hours after drug intake, when it became undetectable [7]. Thus, in low doses nursing seems to be possible.

Nitrazepam

Adult T½: 27–30 hours; protein binding: 82%; milk/plasma concentration ratio: 0.18–0.53. Milk and maternal plasma concentration of nitrazepam was shown to increase by 60% from the first to the fifth day of treatment, but the milk/plasma ratio remained low and did not change during this time period.

In summary

It seems that breastfeeding is safe only with some of the benzodiazepines. Most adverse effects in breastfed infants were described in neonates that were exposed to benzodiazepines *in utero* and when the nursing mothers took relatively high doses. In women who take low doses, adverse effects are unlikely to occur, and nursing is possible. However, since there is insufficient information, the infants should be followed for signs of neurological depression, and caution should be taken if long treatment or high dose is necessary [8].

34.3 Phenothiazines

Phenothiazines are used in the treatment of psychosis, but also as anti-emetics and anti-allergic drugs. The data concerning their use during lactation is based mainly on a small number of case reports.

They are classified by the AAP as drugs of which the effect on infants is unknown but may be of concern [3]. The WHO workshop recommended that chlorpromazine and fluphenazine will be avoided if possible and, if used, the infant needs to be monitored for drowsiness [4]. Schaefer *et al.* [5] consider chlorpromazine, perphenazine and triflupromazine in low doses as the drugs of choice in this group for breastfeeding mothers.

Since women with schizophrenia suffer from increased risk of preterm birth and small for date infants, it is often difficult to differentiate the influence of drugs transferred during lactation from prenatal factors.

Phenothiazines are excreted into the milk. Their protein binding is about 90%.

The more commonly used phenothiazines will be discussed here.

Chlorpromazine

Adult T½ is 30 hours. In four nursing mothers no clear consistent milk/plasma relationship was found, but in two cases milk levels exceeded plasma levels. The metabolites were also found in some of the samples. Of two mothers who nursed their children, one infant of a mother whose milk level was 92 ng/ml was lethargic and drowsy compared to no adverse effects in the infant with maternal milk level of 7 ng/m [9]. While chlorpromazine was detected in the milk following a single oral dose of 1200 mg (20 mg/kg), it was not detected following a 600 mg oral dose.

Long-term adverse effects were found in three breastfed infants whose mothers were prescribed both halidol and chlorpromazine and showed a decline in their developmental scores from the first to the second assessment at 12 to18 months [10].

Normal development was reported in seven infants whose mothers received 50–150 mg/d chlorpromazine during pregnancy and postnatally, and in adopted infants in Papua New

Guinea whose foster mothers took chlorpromazine 100 mg/d, or metoclopramide 40 mg/d or both to induce lactation [11].

Chlorprothixene

Adult T½: 8–12 hours. Chlorprothixene and its metabolite chlorprothixene sulphoxide in milk exceeded plasma levels. The milk/plasma ratios were 1.2 and 2.6 respectively. The estimated infant dose of chlorprothixene was calculated to be 0.1% of the maternal dose/kg body weight.

Perphenazine

Adult T½: 8–20 hours. Milk/plasma ratio was evaluated in one lactating women during two drug regimens, and found a milk/plasma ratio 0.7–1. The infant's dose was 0.1% of that given to the mother. No adverse effects developed during three and a half months' lactation.

Trifluoperazine (trifluopromazine)

Adult T½: 15–28 hours. Milk and plasma drug levels were evaluated in two nursing women who suffered from schizophrenia. Milk/plasma ratio was inconsistent; one milk level was higher and one was lower than the plasma. Both infants were asymptomatic.

Zuclopenthixol

Adult T½: 12–28 hours. Zuclopenthixol decanoate peak serum concentration are obtained one week after intramuscular injection with clinical effect lasting two to four weeks. The milk/plasma ratio of zuclopenthixol levels from several schizophrenic women was found to be less than one, corresponding to very low drug dosage. No adverse effects were noticed and the infants were asymptomatic.

A relationship between sudden infant death syndrome and the use of phenothiazine-containing medications is suspected. Although chlorpromazine is structurally related to promethazine that is prescribed as antihistamine, and promethazine was related to apnea and sudden infant death syndrome [12], there are no reported cases of either of these adverse effects among nursing infants exposed to phenothiazines.

In summary

It is preferable to avoid the use of phenothiazines during lactation because there is insufficient data on their long-term effects. If nursing is necessary, mono-therapy and infant monitoring are recommended.

34.4 Butirophenones

The butirophenones are used in the treatment of schizophrenia and psychosis.

Haloperidol

Adult T½: 20 hours. Haloperidol, the most important drug in this group, is classified by the AAP as a drug which the effect on infants is unknown but may be of concern [3]. The WHO recommends avoiding using it in lactating mothers [4]. Schaefer *et al.* [5] consider haloperidol as compatible with breastfeeding.

Data considering breastfeeding during halidol treatment is sparse. The milk/plasma ratio is relatively high, and their concentrations in the nursing infant may be in the adult range. In most cases there are no behavioral changes.

Although developmental delay was demonstrated only in neonates under combined therapy it is recommended that in women who need haloperidol treatment, human milk will be given under strict supervision [10].

There is no data on milk concentration or usage during lactation of the other butirophenones.

34.5 Atypical neuroleptics

Atypical neuroleptics are used in the long-term management of schizophrenia because they have fewer side effects compared to the classical neuroleptics. The more common drugs are olanzapine (T½: 12–54 hours), clozapine (T½: 12 hours), risperidone (T½: 20 hours), quetiapine (T½: 6 hours), ziprasidone (T½: 7 hours), aripiprazole, sulpride (T½: 7 hours) and benzamide amisulpride (T½: 12 hours). There are no recommendations on the use of this drug group from either the AAP or the WHO. Schaefer *et al.* [5] consider several atypical neuroleptics, especially clozapine, olanzapine, quetiapine and risperidone, as acceptable for breastfeeding, while they advise to consider avoiding breastfeeding with other atypical neuroleptics.

Aripiprazole

Adult T½: 75 hours. Milk/plasma ratio in a lactating psychotic woman was 0.18 and 0.2.

Clozapine

Adult T½ is 12 hours. Milk/plasma ratio was found 4.3 and 2.8 at 1 and 7 days post-partum in a woman who was treated with clozapine from 9 weeks before the delivery [13]. Sleepiness in the breastfed babies of mothers using clozapine was reported in two case studies [5].

Olanzapine

A milk/plasma ratio of 0.5 without detectable infant plasma levels or adverse effects were found when a lactating woman developed psychosis 5 months after delivery. Milk/plasma ratio of 0.84 and no adverse effects on the infants (3 weeks to 6 months) was also found in 5 lactating women. Adverse effects were reported in several olanzapine-exposed infants. Gardiner *et al.* [6] found in 7 lactating women milk/plasma ratio of 0.1–0.6; no detectable infant plasma levels were found in the 6 neonates evaluated. Four had normal developmental evaluation and only one of the infants had drowsiness that vanished when the drug dosage was reduced [14].

Quetiapine

Adult T½: 6 hours. Milk/plasma ratio was 0.29 and no adverse effects were reported in a lactating women during quetiapine treatment. Maximal quetiapine milk level 1 hour after ingestion with pre-dosage level by 2 hours were found in a women whose infant showed no adverse effects at 4½ months while being breastfed. Among 6 women receiving combined drug therapy including quetiapine and either paroxetine, clonazepam or venlaxafine, only 2 had measurable milk levels with low estimated daily exposure below 0.01 and 0.1 mg/kg. Four had normal developmental score, one was in the lower range of normal development and one was one point of the normal in the mental score and in the normal range in the rest of the evaluation [15].

Risperidone

Adult T½ is 3 and 20 hours for risperidone and its metabolite 9-hydroxyrisperidone. Milk/plasma level was found to be 0.1–0.5 usually with very low plasma levels in the nursing infant and no adverse effects in the infant. Milk/plasma ratio was 0.42 and 0.24 for risperidone and 9-hydroxyrisperidone, respectively. Normal development at 9 months was described in another 2 breastfed infants.

Sulpiride

Adult T½: 7 hours. Sulpiride is an atypical antipsychotic that is also used for the initiation of puerperal lactation by increasing prolactin levels and thereby augmenting milk supply. There is no data on breastfed neonates.

Ziprasidone

Adult T½: 7 hours. Milk/plasma ratio was 0.06 in a schizophrenic mother treated with ziprasidone from the ninth day post-partum. Milk drug levels were undetectable during the first week of treatment and were considerably low later. The mother stopped breastfeeding at the beginning of the treatment.

There is no data on breastfeeding during ingestion of benzamide amisulpride, amisulpride and sertindole.

In summary

There is insufficient data on long-term effects of the atypical neuroleptics. Low drug levels were found in most milk samples studied and no certain developmental changes were found in breastfed infants. Hence, it is preferable not to nurse when treated with this group of drugs. If indicated, it is recommended to prefer mono-therapy and continue close monitoring of the infants.

34.6   Antimanic drugs

Lithium

Adult T½: 18–45 hours. The AAP consider lithium salts as drugs that have been associated with significant effects on some nursing infants and should be given to nursing mothers with caution [3]. The WHO recommends avoiding breastfeeding if possible [4]. Schaefer *et al.* [5] consider low doses of lithium as compatible with breastfeeding, but suggest follow-up of the nursing infant.

Milk/plasma ratio for lithium was around 0.5 in several studies with infants' sera levels about half the milk level and in 11 nursing neonates serum drug levels were up to one third of maternal serum level and no adverse effect were found in the infants. However, side effects were described in several infants including transient elevation of TSH, floppy infant, or other clinical signs. The infants recovered once nursing discontinued [16].

34.7   Anticonvulsants that are also mood-stabilizers

Carbamazepine, oxcarbazepine and valproic acid are anticonvulsing drugs used for the treatment of bipolar disorders. The AAP and WHO consider them as compatible with breastfeeding [3, 4]. The WHO recommends nursing but also monitoring the infants for side effects. Schaefer *et al.* [5] consider these drugs as compatible with breastfeeding.

Carbamazepine

Adult T½: 5–26 hours. Neonate T½: 8–37 hours. Milk/plasma ratio 0.07–1. Only few adverse effects were reported: Poor suckling in one infant [17], and transient jaundice in two infants who also had intrauterine exposure to carbamazepine [18].

Oxcarbazepine

Adult T½: 1–3 hours. Neonate T½: 22 hours. Milk/plasma ratio was 0.5 and 0.58. Normal development was found in an infant who had intrauterine exposure to carbamazepine from 20 weeks gestation, which was changed to oxcarbazepine a week before the delivery, and was breastfed for 18 months.

Valproic acid

Adult T½: 9 hours. Neonate T½: 9–49 hours. Milk/plasma ratio is very low, 0.01–0.1. The infant's blood levels are very low or undetectable. An infant who had intrauterine exposure to valproic acid developed at 11 weeks anemia and thrombocytopenia that persisted for a month and resolved only after breastfeeding was stopped [19].

34.8   Central nervous system stimulants

The AAP consider amphetamines as drugs of abuse for which adverse effects on the infant during breastfeeding have been reported; hence, nursing is not recommended [3]. A similar view is expressed by Schaefer *et al.* [5].

Dextroamphetamine

Adult T½: 10–28 hours. Milk/plasma ratio was 3.3 among four breastfeeding mothers whose 3.3–10 months infants had normal developments. Infants' drug levels were unde-tectable in one infant, 6% and 14% of the corresponding maternal plasma concentration in another two infants, and were not measured in the fourth infant.

Methylphenidate

Adult T½: 2–4 hours. Milk/plasma ratio was 0.8–1.6. In one mother suffering from attention deficit disorder milk/plasma ratio was 2.7. Her 6-month-old baby's drug levels were unde-tectable when taken 5.3 hours after the first maternal dose. The baby was breastfed for 5.5 weeks and supplemented during this time period with solid foods, without adverse effects.

34.9   Tricyclic antidepressants

Tricyclic antidepressants enter human milk, but no adverse effects were reported in most breastfed infants. Hence, nursing is possible [1]. The AAP and WHO consider most drugs of this group as drugs compatible with breastfeeding but they may be of concern as the effects are sometimes unknown [3, 4]. Schaefer *et al.* [5] also consider these drugs as compatible with breastfeeding except doxepin, which should be avoided.

Amitriptyline

Adult T½: 9–27 hours, and its active metabolite nortriptyline: adult T½: 37 hours. Similar serum and milk of amitriptyline and the active metabolite nortriptyline levels were found in a lactating woman receiving slow-release amitriptyline, with undetectable blood levels in the infant. Based on 6 reported cases in the literature of amitriptyline ingestion by lactating mothers, Weissman *et al.* calculated average milk/plasma ratio 0.8. They also analyzed 27 published cases of breastfeeding mothers taking nortriptyline and found no adverse effects [20]. Wisner *et al.* followed 12 infants in 2 published studies and found low levels of nortriptyline in one case and 10-hydroxynortriptyline in 3 cases but no adverse clinical effects were observed in the infants [21].

Clomipramine HCl

Adult T½: 20–30 hours. Milk/plasma ratio around 1 without adverse effects in the nursing infants were found in several cases. Among four nursing infants the parent drug and metabolites were undetectable. No adverse clinical effects were observed.

Desipramine

Adult T½: 7–60 hours. Milk/plasma ratio was 1–1.6 in several lactating women and no adverse effects were reported. Neither the drug nor its psychoactive metabolite level could be detected in the infant's serum and no adverse effects were found.

Lofepramine

Adult T½: 5 hours. One of its main metabolites is desipramine. No data was found on the possible transfer of this drug to milk. However, the drug leaflet states that it is excreted in human milk. If low doses are used, it seems possible to continue breastfeeding with close follow-up on the infant's behavior [5].

Doxepine HCl

Adult T½: 6–8 hours. Milk/plasma ratio was followed in a breastfed infant for doxepin and the active metabolite N-desmethyldoxepin and was found 0.51–1.44 and 0.54–1.45 respectively in the pre-fed condition and 0.79–2.39 and 0.85–1.8 in the post-fed condition. No detectable doxepin and very low levels of N-desmethyldoxepin were found in the infant plasma. Poor sucking, hypotonia and recurrent indirect hyperbilirubinemia were found in a 9-day-old infant who also had intrauterine exposure. Low doxepin and N-desmethyldoxepin levels were found in the infant serum. His medical condition improved at 14 days when breastfeeding was stopped [22]. There were several reports in infants with neurological disorders due to doxepin that disappeared after nursing was stopped. Almost undetectable doxepin infant plasma levels were found but accumulation of N-desmethyldoxepin was found reaching maternal plasma levels. Thus, it may be advisable not to nurse when the mother is taking this drug.

Imipramine

Adult T½: 6–18 hours. Milk/plasma ratio about 1.1–2 in 4 cases evaluated and undetectable infant drug levels were found in 2 cases in a literature survey by Weissman *et al.* [20]. Milk/plasma ratio was 1.2–2.3 in 5 women, normal neurological evaluation using the Bayley scales of infant development was found in the 4 infants that were breastfed.

No data was found on breastfeeding with trimeprimine and dibenzepin.

34.10   Tetracyclic antidepressants

Mianserin

Adult T½: 6–39 hours. Milk/plasma ratio was 3.3 and 0.8 in 2 infants evaluated 15 hours after last maternal dose. In the first case evaluated plasma and urine levels were undetectable, and in the second case plasma levels were not evaluated and only small amounts close to the limit of detection of the assay were found in the urine. No untoward effects were found.

Mirtazapine

Adult T½ is 37 hours. Milk/plasma ratio was above 1 but infants' serum levels were undetectable. Milk/plasma was 1.1 in 8 infants evaluated. None of several infants studied showed drug-related adverse effects and all were achieving developmental milestones.

As there is very little data on these drugs, a close follow of the nursing infants should be carried out if the treated mother prefers to nurse her baby.

34.11   Selective serotonin reuptake inhibitors

Short gestation and poor neonatal adaptation are associated with selective serotonin reuptake inhibitors (SSRI) treatment during pregnancy. An association between the maternal use of SSRIs in late pregnancy and persistent pulmonary hypertension of the neonate was also reported. Exposure to SSRI through breast milk was suspected to affect infant serotonin metabolism. Infants' 5-HT pre- and post-exposure to sertaline and fluoxetine experienced no significant change in platelet 5-HT levels except one infant with measurable plasma fluoxetine levels that had a decline in 5-HT levels that normalized when fluoxetine levels were undetectable and had no clinical adverse effects. It is generally accepted that nursing while the mother is exposed to SSRIs is possible [3, 5]. Schaefer *et al.* [5] consider sertaline, paroxetine, citalopram and fluvoxamine as the drugs of choice in this group for breastfeeding mothers. On the other hand, the AAP defines all SSRIs as drugs for which the effects on infants are unknown but may be of concern.

Citalopram

Adult T½ is 35 hours. Milk/plasma ratio was 1.1–1.8 in several women evaluated. Peak maternal level was found 3–9 hours post-dosage and milk/plasma ratio was 3 for both citalopram and its metabolite demethylcitalopram in a lactating woman. Infant plasma levels were at the limit of quantification for both citalopram and its metabolite, and no adverse effects were reported. Low citalopram and demethylcitalopram levels were measured in some of the infants. No adverse effects were noticed and all had normal Denver Evaluation. The neurodevelopment of all infants who also had intrauterine exposure was normal up to the age of one year.

Escitalopram

Adult T½: 27–31 hours. Milk/plasma ratio for escitalopram and its metabolite demethylescitalopram was found to be over 2.0 in several studies. However, drug blood levels in the infants were undetectable and all had normal developmental milestones. Post-delivery respiratory distress and necrotizing enterocolitis after intrauterine and breast-milk exposure to escitalopram was reported in a full-term baby [23].

Fluoxetine

Adult T½: 1–16 days for fluoxetine and 7 days for its active metabolite norfluoxetine. The National Toxicology Program, US Dept. of Health and Human Services, Center for the

Evaluation of Risks to Human Reproduction claimed that there is insufficient data to draw conclusions on how breast milk or therapeutic exposures to fluoxetine might affect development [24]. The AAP defines fluoxetine as a drug of which the effect on infants is unknown but may be of concern [3]. However, in most studies the infants' plasma levels were found to be very low and no infant had adverse effects. Normal neurological evaluation was also reported by several investigators . In several studies slight abnormal behavior or reduced weight gain were reported in some of the infants nursed while their mothers were exposed to fluoxetine however, no long-term adverse effects were reported among these nursing infants.

Paroxetine

Adult T½ is 21 hours. Although the milk/plasma ratio is around 1.0, generally infants' plasma drug levels were undetectable as evidenced by many studies. No adverse effects were reported. Normal pediatric examination was found in exposed infants at 6 weeks, 3 and 6 months. Normal weight gain and developmental milestones at 3, 6 and 12 months, among them including 1 infant that suffered from irritability, were reported in a questionnaire answered by 27 lactating women while taking paroxetine; 20 of them also during pregnancy. Combined drug therapy was evaluated in six women taking paroxetine of whom four also had quetiapine augmentation and one was also treated by clonazepam. Two infants whose mothers were taking quetiapine had slightly delayed mental and motor scores despite undetectable milk drug levels [15].

Sertaline

Adult T½ is approximately 26 hours. Maximal milk sertaline level was 5–9 hours after the dose in a lactating woman receiving sertaline and nortriptyline. Both drugs were undetectable in the infant's serum and no adverse effects were reported. Mean milk/plasma ratio for sertaline and its active metabolite desmethylsertaline was 2.3 and 1.4 respectively in 11 mothers. Drug levels doubled in hind-milk compared to fore-milk and maximized 7–10 hours after maternal dose. Low sertaline and desmethylsertaline plasma levels were detected in 3 and 6 infants respectively. No adverse effects were observed. Many other studies described mean milk/plasma ratio ranging from 0.4 to 4.8 for sertaline and its active metabolite desmethylsertaline. In most infants, blood drug levels were undetectable and all developed according to age and had no adverse effects. Highest drug levels were in hind-milk 8–9 hours after ingestion.

34.12 Serotonin and norepinephrine reuptake inhibitors

Duloxetine

Adult T½: 12 hours. Milk/plasma ratio was 0.116–0.4 among 4 women treated with duloxetine 40 mg/d twice daily for 3.5 days. Estimated infant dose was maximum 0.25% of weight-adjusted maternal dose. All women suffered from adverse effects and none of them breastfed their infants.

Fluvoxamine

Adult T½: 15 hours. Milk/plasma ratio was 0.3 in a breastfed infant and no adverse effects were found.

Venlafaxine

Adult T½ is 5–13 hours. Peak plasma level is achieved 2–4 hours from ingestion. Milk/plasma ratio was 3.26–5.18 and 2.93–3.19 for venlafaxine and O-desmethylvenlafaxine respectively. Undetectable venlafaxine and low O-desmethylvenlafaxine levels were found in 3 infants. Estimated weight adjusted infant dose was 7.6% of maternal dose. No adverse effects were noticed. Undetectable venlafaxine and low levels of its metabolite were found in the sera of other two breastfed infants, who had normal weight and development according to their age. Milk/plasma ratio was 2–3.2 and 2.3–3.2 for venlafaxine and its metabolite respectively in 6 lactating women. One of their 7 infants had detectable low venlafaxine levels and 4/7 had low O-desmethylvenlafaxine levels at an average 6.5 hours post-maternal dose. No adverse effects were noticed and all had age-appropriate Denver evaluation.

34.13   Noradrenaline reuptake inhibitors

Reboxetine

Adult T½ is 13 hours. Milk/plasma ratio was 0.05–0.08 for both fore-milk and hind-milk in 4 women. Calculated weight adjusted infant dose was 2% of maternal dose. Two of the mothers had additional drug treatment: one by escitalopram and the other by sertaline. Reboxetine was present in low levels in the serum of three infants and undetectable in the fourth. One of the infants had a history of poor neonatal adaptation that was related to intrauterine clomipramine exposure, and has developmental delay evident before reboxetine treatment was started [25].

Trazodone

Adult T½ is 7–8 hours. Trazodone is a triazolopyridine derivative with antidepressant activity unrelated to the other currently available psychoactive medications. The AAP consider trazodone as drug which the effect on infants is unknown but may be of concern [3]. Mean milk/plasma ratio was 0.142 in 4 healthy volunteers following ingestion of 50 mg trazodone. Peak maternal level was 2 hours after the dose. The child's adjusted dose was about 2% of the maternal dose. No other data is available.

34.14   Conclusions

Patients who are treated by psychotropic drugs during pregnancy must usually continue treatment also while they nurse their infants. Although most psychotropic drugs are known to be transferred into milk, their concentration in breast milk is often significantly lower than in the maternal serum. Moreover, taking into consideration that the infant's daily milk intake is about one sixth of his body weight, and that not all the drug is absorbed in his gut, it is not surprising that, in most studies, blood drug levels in the infant are very low or undetectable. This is the main reason why nursing is permitted with many of these drugs: SSRIs, tricyclic antidepressants, many of the phenothiazines and antiepileptic, mood-stabilizing drugs. On the other hand, women who are treated with benzodiazepines, tetracyclic antidepressants and lithium should, if possible, refrain from nursing or at least carefully follow up their infants for any change in behavior , feeding or sleep habits. It is generally advised, while nursing, to use the lowest effective drug dose to avoid polytherapy. It is not surprising that these rules are also advised for pregnant women.

34.15 References

1. Hale, T.W. (2004) Maternal medications during breastfeeding. *Clinical Obstetrics and Gynecology*, **47** (3), 696–711.
2. Ito, S. and Lee, A. (2003) Drug excretion into breast milk: overview. *Advanced Drug Delivery Reviews*, **55** (5), 617–27.
3. Ward, R.M., Bates, B.A. and Benitz, W.E. (2001) The transfer of drugs and other chemicals into human milk. *Pediatrics*, **108** (3), 776–89.
4. World Health Organization. Division of Diarrhoeal and Acute Respiratory Disease C, Section UN. Breastfeeding and maternal medication. Recommendations for drugs in the Eighth WHO Model List of Essential Drugs. Annex to Breastfeeding Counselling: a Training Course: WHO/CDR/95.11.
5. Schaefer, C., Peters, P. and Miller, R.K. (2007) *Drugs During Pregnancy and Lactation: Treatment Options and Risk Assessment*. Academic Press.
6. Patrick, M.J., Tilstone, W.J. and Reavey, P. (1972) Diazepam and breast-feeding. *Lancet*, **1** (7749), 542–43.
7. Matheson, I., Lunde, P.K. and Bredesen, J.E. (1990) Midazolam and nitrazepam in the maternity ward: milk concentrations and clinical effects. *British Journal of Clinical Pharmacology*, **30** (6), 787–93.
8. McElhatton, P.R. (1994) The effects of benzodiazepine use during pregnancy and lactation. *Reproductive Toxicology*, **8** (6), 461–75.
9. Wiles, D.H., Orr, M.W. and Kolakowska, T. (1978) Chlorpromazine levels in plasma and milk of nursing mothers. *British Journal of Clinical Pharmacology*, **5** (3), 272–73.
10. Yoshida, K., Smith, B., Craggs, M. and Kumar, R. (1998) Neuroleptic drugs in breast-milk: a study of pharmacokinetics and of possible adverse effects in breast-fed infants. *Psychological Medicine*, **28** (1), 81–91.
11. Kramer, P. (1995) Breast feeding of adopted infants. *British Medical Journal*, **311** (6998), 188–89.
12. Hickson, G.B., Altemeier, W.A. and Clayton, E.W. (1990) Should promethazine in liquid form be available without prescription? *Pediatrics*, **86** (2), 221–25.
13. Barnas, C., Bergant, A., Hummer, M. *et al.* (1994) Clozapine concentrations in maternal and fetal plasma, amniotic fluid, and breast milk. *American Journal of Psychiatry*, **151** (6), 945.

14. Gardiner, S.J., Kristensen, J.H., Begg, E.J. *et al.* (2003) Transfer of olanzapine into breast milk, calculation of infant drug dose, and effect on breast-fed infants. *American Journal of Psychiatry*, **160** (8), 1428–31.

15. Misri, S., Corral, M., Wardrop, A.A. and Kendrick, K. (2006) Quetiapine augmentation in lactation: a series of case reports. *Journal of Clinical Psychopharmacology*, **26** (5), 508–11.

16. Tunnessen, W.W. Jr and Hertz, C.G. (1972) Toxic effects of lithium in newborn infants: a commentary. *Journal of Pediatrics*, **81** (4), 804–7.

17. Froescher, W., Eichelbaum, M., Niesen, M. *et al.* (1984) Carbamazepine levels in breast milk. *Therapeutic Drug Monitoring*, **6** (3), 266–71.

18. Merlob, P., Mor, N. and Litwin, A. (1992) Transient hepatic dysfunction in an infant of an epileptic mother treated with carbamazepine during pregnancy and breastfeeding. *Annals of Pharmacotherapy*, **26** (12), 1563–65.

19. Stahl, M.M., Neiderud, J. and Vinge, E. (1997) Thrombocytopenic purpura and anemia in a breast-fed infant whose mother was treated with valproic acid. *Journal of Pediatrics*, **130** (6), 1001–3.

20. Weissman, A.M., Levy, B.T., Hartz, A.J. *et al.* (2004) Pooled analysis of antidepressant levels in lactating mothers, breast milk, and nursing infants. *American Journal of Psychiatry*, **161** (6), 1066–78.

21. Wisner, K.L., Perel, J.M., Findling, R.L. and Hinnes, R.L. (1997) Nortriptyline and its hydroxymetabolites in breastfeeding mothers and newborns. *Psychopharmacology Bulletin*, **33** (2), 249–51.

22. Frey, O.R., Scheidt, P. and von Brenndorff, A.I. (1999) Adverse effects in a newborn infant breast-fed by a mother treated with doxepin. *Annals of Pharmacotherapy*, **33** (6), 690–93.

23. Potts, A.L., Young, K.L., Carter, B.S. and Shenai, J.P. (2007) Necrotizing enterocolitis associated with in utero and breast milk exposure to the selective serotonin reuptake inhibitor, escitalopram. *Journal of Perinatal Medicine*, **27** (2), 120–22.

24. NTP-CERHR (2004) Monograph on the Potential Human Reproductive and Developmental Effects of Fluoxetine. *NTP Center for the Evaluation of Risks to Human Reproduction Monographs*, (13), i–III24.

25. Hackett, L.P., Ilett, K.F., Rampono, J. *et al.* (2006) Transfer of reboxetine into breast milk, its plasma concentrations and lack of adverse effects in the breastfed infant. *European Journal of Clinical Pharmacology*, **62** (8), 633–38.

35

Parent–infant psychotherapies and indications for inpatient versus outpatient treatments

Kaija Puura and Pälvi Kaukonen

Tampere University and University Hospital, Finland

35.1   Introduction

In previous chapters of this volume good-enough parenting and parenthood have been described, as well as risk factors affecting them. In short, even though the parents are sensitized and attuned to meet the needs of their newborn, psychological distress, mental illnesses and drug and alcohol abuse have been shown to impair their ability to engage and interact with their infants in a positive way. The infant may also have characteristics that make parenting more stressful, like great difficulties in regulating his physiological and emotional states, or chronic or recurrent illness or disability. For the child unsatisfying parent–infant interactions have long-term consequences, resulting in insecure or disorganized attachment and restricting the child's cognitive and socio-emotional development. Parenting is also a major developmental task in adulthood, and succeeding in this task can maintain psychological well-being of parents and give them sense of purpose even when they face adversities.

In infancy most emotional and behavioral problems can be seen as relational, occurring within interaction with the parent, and not being stable individual characteristics of the

Parenthood and Mental Health: A Bridge between Infant and Adult Psychiatry   Sam Tyano, Miri Keren, Helen Herrman and John Cox
© 2010 John Wiley & Sons, Ltd

child. In adulthood, individual problems and psychopathology of the parent can be seen affecting the interactions with the infant in a negative way. Even when the individual problems or illnesses of the parent are lifted, the quality of parent–infant interaction does not necessarily improve [1]. However, without experienced support, distressed or ill parents may not be able to focus on the infant and his needs [2]. Since parent–infant relationship experiences are of great importance to the mental health and personal development for both infants and parents, treating the relationship when problems occur seems not only reasonable but necessary. At the same time the parents' needs have to be sufficiently met.

35.2 Different forms of parent–infant psychotherapy

General principles

Parent–infant psychotherapy is a model of treatment that has been developing over the last 40 years. The focus of the treatment is the parent–infant relationship, not the infant nor the parent as individuals. The goal is to help the parent–infant dyad cooperate better in everyday life, and so increase its mutual adaptive capacity [3]. On the parent's side this means helping him or her to detect, understand and respond to the infant's needs appropriately and at the right time, e.g. to sensitize the parent to the infant's needs. This in term helps the infant to regulate his emotional and physiological states, and promotes his skills and capacity for initiating and sustaining interaction with the parent, both for learning purposes and for using the relationship as a secure base.

The ways for achieving this were named by Stern and Brushweiler-Stern [4] as 'ports of entry', including:

1 Working on the parents' representation of the infant;

2 Working on the level of interaction between the parent and the infant: and

3 Working on the infant's behavior.

The approaches used can be divided into:

1 Psychodynamically oriented parent–infant psychotherapies concentrating on the parent's representations;

2 More behaviorally oriented interactional parent–infant therapies; and

3 Parent–infant therapies integrating elements from both approaches.

In the behaviorally oriented parent–infant therapies and in psychotherapies integrating psychodynamic orientation and behavioral elements, some approaches also emphasize the third port of entry i.e. infant's active involvement and role as the initiator of interaction. These approaches can also be called infant-led therapies. The length of treatment in different approaches varies; in short interventions it can be from 1 to 20 visits carried out usually on a weekly basis. In some cases the duration of the treatment can extend to several years depending on the severity and complexity of factors affecting the parent–infant relationship. Each approach has its own supporters, and they have all been shown to have beneficial impact on parent–infant relationships [2, 5, 12]. There is some evidence showing that integrating both working on the representational and interaction level may produce results in shorter time.

Psychodynamically oriented parent–infant psychotherapy

The psychodynamically oriented approach is the oldest form of parent–infant therapy. It assumes that in therapy the parent's mental model of his or her relationship with the infant is modified by exploring the assumptions derived from parent's relationships with his or her own parents [6], named as 'ghosts in the nursery' by Selma Fraiberg [7]. The focus is on the parent gaining insight by making links between the problems emerging in the current relationship with the infant and with re-enactment or repetition of the parent's early and other past relationships. Increase in parental sensitivity and responsiveness is thought to result from parent's increasing capacity to differentiate the infant from him- or herself.

The infant is usually present in the therapy sessions, and the parent is instructed to interact with the infant while talking with the therapist. The therapist observes the interaction and listens to parent's description of his or her feeling and thoughts. In classical psychodynamic therapy the primary work is between the parent and the therapist. There are also psychodynamically oriented therapists who see the infant as a partner in the therapeutic process, and 'speak for the baby', constructing the baby's need for the infant and for the parent while the parent is still unable to do so [8].

Interactional approach in parent–infant psychotherapy

Interactional approaches in parent–infant psychotherapy intervene in specific behavioral transactions happening between the parent and the infant, who both are always present in the sessions. The therapist observes the interaction and guides the parent to detect and respond to infant cues. In many treatment models the therapist uses videotaped interaction as a tool both in the assessment and in treatment of the interaction. In both cases attention is given to pleasurable interactions between the parent and the infant, and the parent is always given positive feedback and encouragement. Examples of programs using interactional approach include Interactional Guidance [9] and Parent Consultation Model [10]. An example of infant-led interactional parent–infant therapy is Greenspan's 'floor time' [11], which focuses on specific developmental and relational goals. The therapist actively models and guides the parent in ways to interact with the infant in a sensitive and responsive manner to help the infant achieve the age-appropriate goals.

Multilevel infant–parent psychotherapy

In parent–infant psychotherapy working on both representational and interactional level has proven feasible and sometimes producing results quicker than other forms of parent–infant therapies. An example of this approach is the 'Watch, Wait and Wonder' program [12]. In the parent–infant sessions the therapist encourages the parent to observe the infant's self-initiated activity and to interact only at his or her initiative during the first half of the session. The second half of the session the parent is asked to talk about his or her feelings, thoughts, observations and interpretations of the interaction with the infant, while the therapist refrains from instructing or making interpretations. By talking together, the parent and the therapist attempt to understand the themes and relational issues that the infant is trying to learn with the help of problems emerging from the parent trying to follow the infant's lead. The discussion gives the parent an opportunity to explore issues with his or her previous relationship experiences, although the main aim is enable the parent to follow the infant's lead sensitively.

Attachment-oriented parent–infant psychotherapy

A parent–infant therapy technique based specifically on the attachment theory is the Theraplay [13]. In Theraplay the therapist is active and uses age-appropriate, familiar play to build playful interaction first between the therapist and the child, and then between the parent and the child. In a very problematic parent–child relationship it can be difficult for the child to accept any form of closeness with the parent; therefore the therapeutic work starts first with the therapist, who then gradually includes the parent in the interaction. Four aspects of parenting are emphasized: bonding, structuring of the situation, nurturing and challenging. The therapist communicates understanding for all actions the child may do, and gives constantly positive feedback on all initiatives the child does. The play session lasts for half an hour in accepting and playful ambience, with the element of surprise present. The play session is videotaped and afterwards the parent can watch the tape and discuss his or her experiences, thoughts and feelings concerning the session with the therapist. The aim is to increase the parent's reflective function, i.e. the capacity for understanding his or her own mental state and the infant's mental state [14].

Another example of therapy based on attachment theory is the Circle of Security intervention. It is a 20-week, group-based intervention containing both educational and therapeutic components [15]. It is designed to shift patterns of attachment–caregiving interactions in high-risk caregiver–child dyads to a more appropriate developmental pathway. In the first sessions the goal is to make the therapist and the group a 'secure base' for the parents from which they can explore their relationship with their child. The parents also get education on attachment behavior and its meaning with the help of discussion and a graphic image titled 'The Circle of Security'. In the sessions the therapists use edited videotapes of parents interacting with their children. Caregivers are encouraged to increase their sensitivity and responsiveness to the child's signals relevant to its moving away from them to explore, and its moving back for comfort and soothing, to increase their ability to reflect on their own and the child's behavior, thoughts and feelings regarding their attachment–caregiving interactions, and to reflect on experiences in their own histories that affect their current caregiving patterns.

Group therapy for parents and infants

In many places psychodynamically oriented parent–infant group therapy programs have been developed and executed successfully. In group therapy there are usually two therapists, so that in each session one therapist can focus more on observing and understanding the infants and the other on the parents. The parents are encouraged to talk about their experiences, thoughts and feelings about the infants and parenthood in the group. The therapists are responsible for creating a warm and accepting environment for this sharing, and also for helping the parents to use the peer group for gaining insight on their parenting and on their infants, and for getting support from the group.

Cognitive-behavioural approach

Parenting programs with cognitive-behavioral approach are often used in preventive programs. The cognitive-behavioral approach can also be used helping parents to deal with sleeping and eating problems, and with behavioral problems. Most of the cognitive-behavioral programs are targeted to preschool children and their parents, although elements of this approach have been included into other parent–infant therapies.

Family-oriented approaches

Ideas of involving both parents, and the whole family in mental health interventions for infants instead of focusing only on dyadic relationships have also emerged. The work of Fivaz-Depeursinge and Corboz-Warnery [16] with the Lausanne Trilogue Play has shown that parents interact with their infant in a different manner when they are alone with the infant compared to when they are together. While observation of mother–infant and father–infant dyads shows problematic issues in the parent–infant interaction, having the parents together with the infant and then together as a couple reveals issues that are burdening the family system and the marital relationship.

Crittenden and Dallos [1] have suggested integrating family system theory and attachment theory into the Dynamic-Maturational Model (DDM). They suggest using attachment relationship classification to understand interaction strategies and information-processing between family members. According to them there are three related topics to address in psychotherapy. They are the presenting problem; the underlying threat of survival, reproduction or survival of one's children; and finally the information-processing that transforms the experienced threat to maladaptive behavior. Since each family member will frame the presenting problem differently, and have a different personal history, creating understanding between family members may bring about positive, enduring changes. In the DDM model with infant and toddler families the goal is to work with the family unit to benefit the functioning of all family members.

Treating parent–infant dyads in adult in-patient unit

The hospitalization of the infant together with the parent, usually the mother, has been in use in adult psychiatric units from 1950s in connection with severe maternal mental illness, like post-partum depression, post-partum psychosis or other types of psychotic disorder. Traditionally the goal with having infants hospitalized with their mothers has been to support the mother–infant bonding and to avoid disruption of parent–infant relationship. This goal has best been achieved for mothers with post-partum psychosis, who usually recover completely. However, hospitalization without specific treatment focused on the parent–infant relationship may not be sufficient for improving parenting of mothers with affective disorders or schizophrenia [2], and there is a need for parenting interventions that aim to improve maternal sensitivity specifically for parents with psychotic disorders.

Residential mother–infant care

Recently residential mother–infant care has been used in pediatric units or in separate established units for treatment of problematic infant behavior, such as problems with feeding, settling down or sleeping. Among parents attending these units there are high levels of psychiatric morbidity, highlighting the importance of providing multifaceted interventions in order to address both infant and maternal psychological issues.

Treating parents and infants in child psychiatric units: the family day ward in Tampere

In many countries special units have been established for treating infant and toddlers and their families. In Tampere University Hospital in Finland the child psychiatric family ward was founded in 1993 for treating parent–child relationships and parenting problems in families with under school-aged children. In our model infant families are referred to the family day ward when the parents want help with parenting problems, the infant or toddler has emotional or behavioral problems, or special needs, or when staff in the primary health care, adult mental health services or social services is concerned about the parent–infant interaction. The whole family attends the day ward treatment daily for three weeks, coming to the ward in the morning and going back home in the afternoon.

Each family is treated by a child psychiatrist and a male–female pair of nurses. Services of a psychologist and a social worker are used when needed, and in case conferences led by the child psychiatrist the whole multidisciplinary team is present. The child psychiatrist interviews the family on arrival to the ward for their views on the presenting problem, and for their goals for the treatment. Individual assessment of the infant is done by the psychiatrist and psychologist. Observational assessment of the parent–infant interaction is used both for seeing problematic issues in the relationship, and also for therapeutic purposes. The nurse pair works with the family, engaging the family members in discussions of their needs and thoughts, the parents on their view of the infant and possible siblings, and on the parent–infant interaction that is constantly ongoing during the treatment. The nurses integrate techniques from family therapy, interactional guidance, cognitive-behavioral approach and attachment theory in their work. At the end of the treatment period the family is given open feedback and possible recommendations for further treatment.

Common factors in all approaches

Despite the differences between parent–infant therapy practices, all the approaches stress the importance of a trusting, accepting alliance between the parent and the therapist. This alliance shares features with an attachment relationship between a parent and an infant, and within it the previous experiences of parent's attachment relationships are often re-enacted [17]. Awareness of attachment theory and reaction patterns related to different attachment classifications can give the therapist a useful insight of what may be happening between the parent and the therapist. Nicole Guedeney has beautifully described ways of building the therapeutic alliance into a model of secure attachment relationship within health services (Personal communication, 2006). These include offering nurture (for example a cup of tea), acceptance, perseverance in keeping the parents within the program through actively contacting them when needed, and patience in building the shared trust.

Probably the most difficult issue in all parent–infant therapies is balancing the needs of the parent and the infant. This is particularly challenging in situations where there is concern for child neglect or abuse, and when parents are ambivalent about being treated. In these cases networking with relatives and friends of the family as well as social and other health-care services is essential. The first priority is that the infant is kept safe and well cared for. This may sometimes be achieved by ensuring concrete help and support for the parents with the help of their own social network or home visits from community nurses, home visitors, or other social welfare services. In cases where the infant is not safe with the parent, there is acute need either for child protection, or in case of mentally ill parents, hospitalization of the parent. In these situations the therapeutic alliance between the persons involved in treatment and the parents can be lost. This may be avoided by open discussion of the infant's needs and the purpose of the actions taken, which sometimes helps parents to recognize that they are incapable of caring for the infant. Parents may then consent to what we call 'shared parenting', where other caregivers take care of the everyday needs of the infant and parents can maintain positive contact with the infant.

35.3 Indications for inpatient versus outpatient treatment

The risks for dysfunctional parent–infant relationships described in this volume constituting the indications for parent–infant psychotherapy can be grouped into:

1 Difficulties in parent–infant relationship and parenting;

2 Special needs or problematic behavior of the infant or toddler; and

3 Problems with parental abilities caused by mental health problems, substance abuse or overburdened parenting.

Quite often there are several risk factors and several indications for treatment presenting concurrently, and it can be difficult to decide what form of treatment would be most effective for a particular parent and infant. Particularly with families with multiple risk factors, cooperation between several services is needed. In this chapter we will describe how infant families are treated in the Infant and Family Psychiatric Unit (IFPU) of the Tampere University Hospital. With this we hope to illustrate our thinking of the indications for various treatment forms.

The Infant and Family Psychiatric Unit in the Department of Child Psychiatry in Tampere University Hospital

In the IFPU we have an outpatient unit and an 'in-patient' unit, the family day ward described earlier in this chapter. Both have multidisciplinary teams consisting of a child psychiatrist, psychologist, social worker and nurses. The IFPU gets referrals from well-baby clinics, neonatal wards, adult psychiatric units, centers for drug- or alcohol-addicted parents and from family guidance clinics. The outpatient unit also does liaison work with the neonatal intensive care unit and other pediatric wards with infants and toddlers. Our treatment philosophy, integrative child psychiatry, was created under the lead of professor Tuula Tamminen and means a need-specific service in which different therapeutic approaches and techniques can be combined. In 60% of the referrals one or both parents have either mental health or addiction problems affecting the parenting; in 15% the main reason for referral is experienced problems in the parent–infant relationship, either difficulties in feeling affection for the infant or with managing child care; and in 15% of the referrals the infant has problematic behavior such as difficulties in feeding or sleeping, excessively anxiety or aggression, or other kind of special needs. After receiving the referral into the IFPU the child psychiatrists of both outpatient unit and the family day ward together with the head nurse of the unit decide upon the treatment plan for the family.

In cases where outpatient care is thought sufficient, the child psychiatrist and one other member of the outpatient team meet the family within one week. After the first session the child psychiatrist decides upon the assessment period, which serves also as the first, short intervention. The assessment consists of interviewing the parents, making videotaped assessment of the parent–infant interaction, a home visit, a case conference and feedback for the family. If the family is thought to benefit mainly from the day ward treatment, the child psychiatrist and the nurse pair designated to the case meet the family to plan the treatment period together with the parents. In cases where there are indicators of the need of more treatment (intensity and length), periods of both outpatient and day ward treatment are combined. The therapeutic process in these cases is supported with having a pair of therapists working with the family, with one therapist from the outpatient unit and one from the day ward. The family can then smoothly move between longer periods of outpatient treatment and shorter day ward periods focusing on some specific relationship problem and having the same people responsible for their care.

The responsibility for making and carrying out a treatment plan is considered for each individual case, but there are some general principles we apply. If the family is primarily referred to the IFPU for the first two reasons, then our unit takes the responsibility for designing and carrying out the treatment plan. If the reason for referral is parental mental illness or substance abuse, then the responsibility is shared with the adult psychiatric services and treatment plan designed in cooperation. With families in need for child protection or other social services, the treatment plan is designed in cooperation with them and responsibilities are clarified and shared.

Working mainly with parent–infant relationship problems

With cases where there are mostly relationship difficulties, such as the mother or the father or both having difficulties in learning to understand the infant's signals, or difficulties in feeling affection for the infant, and in milder feeding and sleeping problems, a period of weekly home visits for three to four months is started. The focus of the work is in the parent–infant relationship and the therapist uses a multilevel approach working on the experiences, feelings and thoughts of the parent while the parent is interacting with the infant in a free situation. When needed, the therapist openly wonders about what is happening in the interaction, bringing the infant's behavior and needs into the discussion with the parent. If the focus is mainly in the mother–infant relationship, the father is asked to attend one or two sessions. For some families this may be enough, and their care is then referred back to primary care services.

Particularly for families where parents have difficulties in dealing with the infant's or toddler's negative emotions like frustration or anger, or there are more severe of longer lasting problems with feeding or sleeping, a treatment period in the family day ward can be combined with the outpatient treatment. The day ward period can then be used for learning and practising sensitive and efficient parenting. For infants with feeding or sleeping problems the day ward setting provides several naturally occurring situations where parents can be supported and guided to succeed in difficult interactions, as the families are offered a meal and a snack each day and they also have their 'own room' to put the infant for a nap.

Working with infants with special needs or problematic behavior

For a proportion of the referrals, problems in infant behavior or special needs caused by illness or trauma are the main reason for entering our services. Infants and toddlers taken into custody because of neglect or abuse, and toddlers with problems in social development with suspicion for autism spectrum disorder are the most common examples.

For those traumatized infants and toddlers who have difficulties in forming an attachment relationship with their foster parents, either Theraplay treatment or family therapy focusing on attachment issues is offered in the outpatient setting. With infants and toddlers with excessive anger and violent outbursts, home-based family therapy in the outpatient unit is combined with intermittent treatment in the day ward. The focus of the family therapy is to help foster parents understand the behavior and needs of the child, while the day ward treatment is used for helping foster parents practise sensitive and effective ways of soothing and managing the child's anger and maladptive behavior.

Similarly for infants and toddlers diagnosed with an illness affecting their development or behavior, family therapy is offered as the first choice. In the family therapy the parents' thoughts and feelings concerning their child and the family situation are listened to for building a therapeutic relationship. Parents are also given education on child development and of the specific features of the child's illness. For some parents this may suffice to give them insight on how to change their interaction with the child to reduce problems. Usually parents need more help, particularly if the child is diagnosed with an autism spectrum disorder, attention deficit disorder, mood disorder or has severe problems of self-regulating behavior. Family therapy sessions focusing on how parents can practise sensitive, coherent parenting in the presence of the child's disorder are then continued. Here behavioral-cognitive techniques are often used within family sessions to teach parents ways of managing difficult situations with the child. Again day ward treatment is combined with the outpatient family therapy according to need.

Working with parents with mental health problems

For parents with mental health problems, the tailoring of adequate care of the parent–infant relationship is more complex. Current research points out that individual psychopathology of the parent and parent–infant relationship should both be treated, as individual therapy of the parent is unlikely in itself to benefit the parent–infant relationship and vice versa. Parents who are referred from adult psychiatric services usually have individual treatment and may have medication, and what is asked of the IFPU is the treatment of the parent–infant relationship. In these cases the parents are asked for permission for cooperation with the adult psychiatric services, and if possible the adult psychiatrist responsible for the parents' care attends some meetings where the parent–infant treatment is planned. This is needed for joint understanding of the family's situation, and for defining the goals and ways of treating the parent and the parent–infant relationship.

Even in those cases where the parent does not have any other treatment than perhaps medication and the parent–infant therapy provided by the IFPU, cooperation with the adult psychiatrist is helpful in situations when parents' mental health for some reason declines. The therapist from the IFPU can then discuss the treatment options with the parent and contact the adult psychiatric services for arranging the adult psychiatric care needed. Some of the families also need concrete support in managing household or childcare tasks for some period of time, and so social workers responsible for child and family services from the parents' hometown are invited to meetings with the IFPU and the family. Network meetings with the parents, their kin, adult psychiatry and social services at best reduce the fears or suspicions of the parents concerning different officials, and make it easier for them to accept offered help for their infants' sake.

In our unit parents with affective disorders are given parent–infant therapy that integrates psychodynamically oriented and interactional approaches. Depending on the severity of the symptoms the length of treatment can vary from three months to two years. For parents suffering from depression, parent–infant group therapy is also possible. The group therapy is psychodynamically oriented, but the therapists also give the mothers positive feedback of the mother–infant interaction seen in the group sessions.

When working with parents with personality disorders a huge task is to establish an alliance with the parents strong enough to prevent them from leaving the treatment when difficult issues are addressed. To accomplish this we try to make the relationship between the staff involved in the treatment to serve as a secure base for the parents, by giving the parents concrete nurture (coffee, tea, meals in the day ward) and positive feedback for their courage and willingness to seek help for their family.

In the therapeutic work the focus is more on the interactional level. This is motivated by the fact that the infants of parents with personality disorders are often experiencing unpredictable and disorganized parenting, and the need for improving the parent–infant interaction to more stable and coherent is imminent. Another reason for working mainly on the interactional level is the possibility of boosting parents' self-esteem with positive feedback given from good sequences seen in the interaction. After the relationship is formed, some parents with personality disorders are able to work on the representational level as well. Some parents with personality disorder need support in their parenting for many years, and many need help in concrete childcare and in managing daily life. For organizing these services and for avoiding confusion and conflicts between different officials and the family, networking in the form of joint meetings is often required.

Therapeutic work with parents with psychotic disorders in our experience requires close cooperation with adult psychiatric services, with the goal of lessening the reasoning biases, mental state attributional errors and other social cognitive impairments of the illness. In our unit, working with a parent with a psychotic disorder includes a network meeting during the assessment period with all officials already working with the family present together with the parents. This is needed for getting a picture of the situation of the family, of severity of the parent's illness, of the treatment and support the family is already receiving and of the possible concerns for the infant's health and safety. In most cases child protection services are already involved, usually helping the family with child and home care. If not, parents are usually asked for permission to involve their community social worker in the network. The actual parent–infant therapy is interaction-focused, emphasizing the positive aspects of the interaction with the use of video feedback.

Multi-risk and overburdened parenting

In families with multiple risk factors, parenting is often overburdened by parental mental health and substance abuse problems, low social support, unemployment and poverty. These families again need support on many levels: in managing their daily life, parents' own health, childcare and relationships between family members. With these families networking with other services such as social services, community health services, services for substance abusers, and adult psychiatric services is necessary. The first task is to assess what services are needed to make sure that the needs of the children are adequately met. This can mean for example organizing day care for the children to allow the parents to rest, or organizing treatment of either or both of the parents. The aim is to create some stability and predictability to the life of the family. When this is achieved, parents may be able to engage in working on their parenting. For multi-risk families we most often choose a home-based family-centered approach with focus on attachment and parent–child interactions, combined with intermittent treatment periods in the day ward.

Clinical vignette

Alice was referred to IFPU at the age of 6 months for anxiety, almost constant crying and eating problems. Her mother was depressed, and felt that Alice was too difficult for her to handle. Her father abused alcohol and, when drunk, was violent towards the mother. He was dissatisfied with Alice's refusal of food and felt she was undermining his authority. The mother was afraid of him and also afraid that he might hit Alice. On her request the father had moved out of their home three months earlier. During the assessment period in the outpatient unit both mother's and father's anxiety with Alice appeared to be immense and they were asked to come for an in-patient treatment period for three weeks. During the in-patient treatment both parents were supported to understand Alice's behavior and to respond to it. The nurses and the child psychiatrist from the outpatient unit had couple discussions with the parents, where they talked about attachment and the experiences the parents had had with their own parents. During the in-patient treatment Alice cried less, ate well and started to make contact with her father. The father was able to see how his drinking was affecting the family, and consented to see an adult psychiatrist. With the support of child protection services the family was united after the in-patient treatment and the parent–infant treatment was continued in the outpatient unit.

35.4 When parents reject treatment

For various reasons some families and parents cannot accept treatment offered to them. Some families agree to a follow-up session, where we can discuss their situation again and sometimes they are able to continue working with us after a pause. Those families that do not want our services are referred back to the primary care level with a request that they will follow up the infant. The primary health care nurse is also asked to work with the parents to make it easier for them to accept a new referral if it is still needed. In cases where there is a serious concern and possible need for child protection services, we tell the parents that we have to inform their community social worker of their needs. The child protection services then work with the family, making sure that the infant's needs for safety and care are met. Quite often this results in re-engagement of the treatment in our unit, either with the parents or, if there has been a need for taking the infant into custody, both with biological and foster parents.

35.5 Conclusions

In this chapter we have attempted to give an overview of different types of parent–infant psychotherapies and to give an example of how they can be used in clinical practice. The overview is not exhaustive, and no doubt there are other equally good or better ways of treating parents and infants than those suggested here, including those that are not recorded in the internationally accessible literature. What we wish to emphasize, however, is the need for specialists in infant and adult mental health to work together to create more comprehensive and efficient treatment models for families with infants and toddlers. It is also important to evaluate and report the methods and findings. Knowing how dire the consequences of dysfunctional parenting can be, this could be one efficient way for improving the well-being of all humankind.

35.6 References

1. Crittenden, P. and Dallos, R. (2009) All in the family: integrating attachment and family systems theories. *Clinical Child Psychology and Psychiatry*, **14**, 389–409.
2. Wan, M.W., Moulton, S. and Abel, K.M. (2008) A review of mother-child relational interventions and their usefulness for mothers with schizophrenia. *Archives of Women's Mental Health*, **11**, 171–79.
3. Mäntymaa, M. (2006) Early mother-infant interaction: determinants and predictivity. Academic dissertation. Acta Universitatis Tamperensis 1144. Tampere: Tampereen yliopis-topaino Oy Juvenes Print. Electronic version: Acta Electronica Universitatis Tamperensis 519, http://acta.uta.fi.
4. Stern-Bruschweiler, N. and Stern, D. (1989) A model for conceptualising the role of mother's representational role in various mother-infant therapies. *Infant Mental Health Journal*, **10**, 142–56.
5. Cicchetti, D., Rogosh, F.A. and Toth S.L. (2006) Fostering secure attachment in infants in maltreating families through preventive interventions. *Development and Psychopathology*, **18**, 623–49.

6. Cramer, B. (1998) Mother-infant psychotherapies: a widening scope in technique. *Infant Mental Health Journal*, **19**, 151–67.

7. Fraiberg, S. (1980) *Clinical Studies in Infant Mental Health; The First Year of Life.* Basic Books, New York.

8. Binet, E. and Dolto, F. (1999) *Prospects: the Quarterly Review of Comparative Education*, Vol. **29** (3). UNESCO: International Bureau of Education, Paris, pp. 445–54.

9. McDonough, S.C. (1993) Interaction guidance: understanding and treating early infant-caregiver relationship disturbances, in *Handbook of Infant Mental Health* (ed. C. Zeanah), Guilford Press, New York.

10. Harrison, A. (2005) Herding animals into the barn: a parent consultation model. *Psychoanalytic Study of the Child*, **60**, 128–53.

11. Greenspan, S. Floortime. http://www.icdl.com/dirFloortime/overview/index.shtml.

12. Cohen, N.J., Muir, E., Parker, C.J. *et al.* (1999) Watch, Wait, and Wonder: testing the effectiveness of new approach to mother-infant psychotherapy. *Infant Mental Health Journal*, **20**, 429–51.

13. Jernberg, A.M. and Booth, P.B. (1998) *Theraplay: Helping Parents and Children Build Better Relationships through Attachment-Based Play.* Jossey-Bass, San Francisco.

14. Fonagy, P. and Bateman, A. (2000) Effectiveness of psychotherapeutic treatment of personality disorders. *British Journal of Psychiatry*, **177**, 138–43.

15. Marvin, R.S., Cooper, G., Hoffman, K. and Powell, B. (2002) The Circle of Security Project: attachment-based intervention with caregiver-preschool child dyads. *Attachment and Human Development*, **4**, 107–24.

16. Fivaz-Depeursinge, E. and Corboz-Warnery, A. (1999) *The Primary Triangle: a Developmental Systems View of Mothers, Fathers and Infants.* Basic Books, New York.

17. Schmitt, F., Lahti, I. and Piha, J. (2008) Does attachment theory offer new resources to the treatment of schizoaffective patients? *American Journal of Psychotherapy*, **62**, 1–15.

36

The symptomatology of a dysfunctional parent–infant relationship

Campbell Paul

Royal Children's Hospital, Melbourne, Australia

36.1 Introduction

The human infant at the outset is a person whose literal survival depends on the quality of the reciprocal relationships with her caregivers. Parents provide, and the baby stimulates, an intricate process of finely attuned, orchestrated and contingent interpersonal behaviors which are essential for the development of a healthy maturing development [1]. At all levels of mind and brain activity, from the creative cortical functions to the brainstem regulation of attention and consciousness, the unfolding of the individual's optimal epigenetic program is dependent on a sensitive infant–parent relationship.

Parental mental illness has the capacity to profoundly disrupt the developing relationship between a baby and her troubled parents. The communicative dance between an infant and her parents is subtle and mutually powerful. Recent decades have seen an immense development in our understanding of and intervention with women's mental health problems in the perinatal period. We are also beginning to understand more about the experience of fathers and their babies and their roles and dyadic and triadic relationships.

Parenthood and Mental Health: A Bridge between Infant and Adult Psychiatry   Sam Tyano, Miri Keren, Helen Herrman and John Cox
© 2010 John Wiley & Sons, Ltd

Clinical vignette 1

Cassie was a young woman of 27 years, a music teacher, hospitalized because of a severe manic illness precipitated by the birth of her first son, Henry. When he was aged 5 months, they were referred to an infant mental health program because of his increasingly severe withdrawal. He was emotionally flat, avoidant and his body was very hypotonic with his chin crumpled down to the floor as he sat unsupported. Cassie's manic depressive illness followed the death of her maternal aunt who had cared for her since her mother had died. Cassie was aware of the problems facing an infant whose mother was depressed, and she was determined not to deprive her son. She was desperately 'stimulating' him. She sang, talked, jiggled and held him constantly, pushing her face into his line of sight, fearing that he would really suffer otherwise. This driven, well-intentioned but highly intrusive parenting of Henry appeared to drive him to despair. His 'good-enough' mother was absent, because his mother was unable to interact with him in an attuned way. Her parenting behavior, even when it came to feeding, changing and bathing him was totally non-contingent. So paradoxically, Henry was alone in the very intense presence of the other.

36.2 'Good-enough' parenting

A baby cannot exist alone: it is essentially part of relationship. [2]

The nature of the relationship between the baby and his mother is crucial for the development of a sense of who he is as a person. According to Winnicott [2], the *ordinary devoted mother* provides care for and holds and handles her baby in a way that allows him to develop the idea that initially he was omnipotent. Gradually by a process of manageable frustrations and hence some 'disillusionment' he comes to be at one with himself and his environment. This 'handling' is enacted time after time, for example when the baby is being fed by his parent: 'the baby feeds, and the baby's experience includes the idea that the mother knows what it is like to be fed'[2]. In ordinary circumstances, the *good-enough mother* acts as an alive mirror, reflecting back to the baby an awareness of his own bodily actions, his affects and emotions and later on perhaps his own thoughts and hence he acquires an integrated sense of self. Winnicott said: 'the mother's ego support facilitates the ego organization of the baby. Eventually the baby becomes able to assert his own individuality and even feel a sense of identity.'[2]

It has become increasingly important for us to understand more about the experience of parenthood in the context of serious mental illness, and from an infant mental health point of view to understand more about the baby's own experience of having a parent with a major mental illness.

36.3 Parenting in the context of mental illness

Especially since the revolutionary move away from institutional to community care of adults with major mental illness, a person with such an illness is as likely to become a parent as others in the broader community. The arrival of the baby for parents in this context presents a series of major challenges as well as a potential for a joyful new identity. There may be a conflict between the best interests of the baby and of her parents.

Parents with less severe illness such as depression and disorders of personality development often also experience difficulties in the process of meeting the social and emotional and physical needs of their babies [3].

For depressed parents the impact of the distortions of 'good-enough' parenting behavior upon the child seems to be especially dependent on the presence of other additional risk factors such as a lack of partner or family support, low educational or economic status or neonatal risk factors [3]. In this context children may display higher rates of insecure attachment, higher rates of anxiety at school age, conduct and behavioral difficulties for boys and some variable cognitive difficulties. Murray concludes that the later child cognitive difficulties may be accounted for by lack of parental contingency, insensitive or unresponsive parental behavior, hostile or intrusive behaviors and a reduced parental imitation when with the baby [3].

Children of parents with a psychotic disorder have heightened risk of developing a wide range of severe mental disorders. The Helsinki High-Risk Study [4] demonstrated that in the long term the offspring of mothers to serious psychotic disorders have a greatly increased risk of schizophrenia spectrum disorder, in addition to an increased risk for any mental disorder. The studies also demonstrated that the negative symptoms of schizophrenia in the mother appeared to be related with a worse outcome for her child in the long term [5]. Serious mental illnesses such as schizophrenia and bipolar affective disorder have significant heritability. Studies using current understandings of the role of epigenetics upon social and emotional and psychopathological development will help clarify the relative impact of genetic endowment and early infant–parent relationship upon later psychopathology.

Although parents with florid positive symptoms may not be able to care for their babies alone in the short term, Snellen [6], in a study of mothers with their infants in a mother and baby psychiatric unit, found that those with persistent treatment-resistant negative symptoms were more likely to have a significantly disturbed infant–parent relationship.

36.4 Qualities of infant–parent interaction

Parental depression

Postnatal depression is a very prevalent phenomenon affecting from 10% to 15% of women and their infants in the community. Studies have shown [3] that mothers with postnatal depression may find it hard to focus on the baby's experience, miss infant cues, fail to recognize the baby's immediate need for comfort and demonstrate intrusive and over-stimulating behavior. There is an associated reduction in the mother's sensitivity to her baby, a reduced *emotional availability*, with consequent high rates of insecure attachment in their children compared to those of non-depressed mothers. Similar findings, although from far fewer studies, have been found with fathers [7] who may also experience depression in the postnatal period [perhaps 3% to 6% of new fathers).

Clinical vignette 2

Fiona had brought her 4-year-old son to be seen because of his emotional and developmental delay. She was very tearful as she explained what the world between her and her son had been like when she had been depressed. She said for the first two years of his life when she spoke to him it was as if 'I was always just reciting a shopping list'. For Fiona the relationship with her son meant 'always just going through the motions'. She fed him, changed his nappy and put him to bed but she was unable to play with him or be with him in any lively sort of way. She said she felt that she had hated him, but no one except Fiona herself and her son knew about it. Looking back she said with poignancy that 'he must have been as lonely and as desperate as I was'.

36.5   Assessing infant–parent interaction

A large number of methods have now been developed to assess the nature of an infant–caregiver relationship [8]. Assessment methods include those which are based on direct observation and analysis of parent–infant interactions in various contexts [9], and also those that employ narrative interviewing to assess the parent's internal working models [10, 11]. Recent developments include the systematic assessment of the mother–infant–father triad [8, 12].

The relationship between an infant and her parents is an exquisitely sensitive one and, being a dynamic system, even small distortions can lead to an increasingly disordered relationship. One method of describing perturbations in the development of infant–caregiver relationships is contained in DC: 0-3R, the diagnostic classification of mental health and developmental disorders of infancy and early childhood [13]. This classification system provides categories with which to describe the infant's characteristic behavioral quality and the affective tone and the psychological involvement between caregiver and infant. The Parent–Infant Relationship Global Assessment Scale (PIR-GAS) gives a clinical indication of the overall quality of the relationship.

Characteristics of interaction between parents with major mental illness and their infants

Parents with borderline personality disorder

The impact upon the infant–caregiver relationship when parents have borderline personality disorder can be profound. Such parents have often experienced extremely disrupted, ambivalent and frightening relationships in their own childhood, and their own consequent impulsivity, poor control of anger, volatile relationships and unstable sense of self can make it very difficult to provide an emotionally containing environment for their own infant.

Newman and her colleagues [14] worked with a group of mothers with borderline personality disorder and their babies. Their study explored the interactional patterns between mothers and babies and the mothers' parenting perceptions. From this and other studies they report that mothers with borderline personality disorder were generally *less sensitive, poorly attuned, more intrusive, lacked responsivity and provided less structure* in the interactions with their babies. The infants seemed less well socially and emotionally organized. In one reported study half of the infant–mother dyads demonstrated a *disorganized attachment* classification using the Strange Situation paradigm.

Targeting the infant–parent relationship difficulties, they have implemented a trial using two relevant therapeutic intervention models; Watch Wait and Wonder, and Interactional Guidance [14].

Impact of parental mental illness on the infant–parent relationship

Factors which may influence the outcome of the infant–parent relationship:

- Overall severity and temporal pattern of the maternal illness
- Pattern of the mother's disturbance:
- Onset: before pregnancy, during pregnancy, after pregnancy
- Onset: with the first or subsequent pregnancies
- Duration of illness: brief, prolonged, intermittent.

Nature of the of mother's psychotic symptoms [15]:

- The meaning of the infant to the mother, in relation to the baby's father and mother's own family and other meaningful connections
- The capacity of the mother to understand her infant's thoughts and feelings, and to hold her baby in mind: capacity for reflective functioning [11]
- Predominantly negative symptoms
- Psychotic symptoms which see the incorporation of the infant in parents delusional ideation
- Chronicity of the psychotic symptoms.

Other factors:

- Supportive partner and family relationships
- Impact of co-morbid illness on the mother's long-term social and emotional adjustment
- Housing, poverty, physical health.

Using attachment theory to understand the impact of parental mental illness upon the infant

Children of parents with serious mental illness are at risk later of significant psychopathology in a number of developmental areas. There is some evidence that demonstrates that infants in a dyadic relationship that is characterized as insecure or disorganized are likely to experience high risk for subsequent psychopathology.

It is likely that the nature of the infant–parent relationship accounts for much of this problematic trajectory, although considerable research still needs to be done. Wan, Abel and Green [16] reviewed the literature around the relationship between maternal psychopathology and the child's attachment to his mother and how this may influence the unfolding of developmental and clinical risk. They produced a model for the transmission of risk, and reviewed the level of evidence provided by research studies. The model is a developmental psychopathological one which seeks to integrate a number of factors such as *non-genetic mechanisms* (stressful environment, exposure to maladaptive parenting), *vulnerabilities and developmental outcomes of the child*, with *moderators* (child characteristics, characteristics of the mother's disorder and of her partner) and how they interact with each other to affect the outcome for the child of the mother with schizophrenia, and later for the child as an adult [16, 17].

In another review of studies looking at the impact of maternal psychopathology on the attachment status of the child and mother, Wan and Green [18] concluded that, from the available evidence, it seems that children may develop vulnerable attachments (insecure or disorganized) when cared for in the context of prolonged or severe maternal psychopathology and especially in conjunction with other risk factors such as trauma, loss or parental attachment problems indicated by parental 'unresolved' attachment status. Most children exposed to mothers with mental health problems in the absence of these other factors seem not to develop lasting attachment disorders.

Parental reflective functioning

Slade and colleagues [11] have described how the quality of infant–caregiver attachment may influence the infant's own development. They suggest that the mother who is able to understand the nature and function of her own mental states, as well as those of her child, is better able to provide for the child an experience of physical and psychological comfort or safety. Building on the work of Fonagy and others [10] with the concept of reflective functioning, the Parent Development Interview was developed in order to assess the mother's representations of her infant, of her relationship with her infant as well as how she sees herself as a mother. This parental reflective functioning capacity is predictive of the quality of the infant's attachment at later stages and development. Higher levels of maternal reflective functioning are indicative of secure infant–caregiver attachment status later on.

This is consistent with the Winnicott's [2] description that the 'good-enough mother', in her moment-to-moment interactions, was able to help the infant feel safe and contained. This has implications for intervention since it may be that helping mothers (and fathers) to think more sensitively about behavior and relationships may lead to more sustained change in their own caregiving behavior, consequently the infant feeling more held and connected. Several parent reflective functioning-based interventions with high-risk families have been commenced [18].

Fathers and psychotic illness

Fatherhood is a biological fact although with new reproductive technologies an increasingly complex state. Most research on parenthood and mental illness is focused on the mother–infant relationship but there always is a relationship of some kind with the father or father representation. The role of the father for infants whose mother has a serious mental illness may range from being totally absent or of unknown identity, to living apart with regular contact, to being the effective primary carer. Increasingly there are enduring relationships between men and women with serious mental illness. In assessing the quality of parental care experienced by an infant it is common to omit the contribution of the father who may also have a significant mental health problem. Few studies have looked at the effect of mental illness or substance abuse upon fathering with infants. The direct effects (upon infant caregiving) and indirect effects (upon the mother's own adjustment and social circumstances) may be profound. There is some association between depression in the father and a higher risk of behavior problems in his children, especially boys [7].

Triadic assessment

How does the baby experience being part of *triad in relationship* with both parents, one of whom has a major mental illness and how does she experience the process of interacting with both parents? Philip [12] used the Lausanne Trilogue Play paradigm in assessing four families where the mother had a post-partum psychotic illness. The families studied experienced an 'absence of a sense of true intersubjectivity' and seemed to find it very difficult to recognize the emotional experience and the communications of the other, including the infant. The parents seemed to be more controlling towards their babies and they failed to be supportive of one another in being with their baby. They seemed to show contradictory signals, for example softly talking while at the same time shaking the baby roughly. The babies however seemed to demonstrate a sort of paradoxical lack of connection and pseudomutuality in their interactions. These babies seem to show something like role reversal seen in older children. It is as if in trying to manage contradictory affective information from their primary carers they needed to develop a degree of hyper-vigilance, looking at their parents, but with a vacant gaze. Philipp and her colleagues note the similarity between these babies' behaviors and the sorts of pathological defenses described by Selma Fraiberg, such as gaze aversion, shutting down and falling asleep [19].

36.6   The infant response in the context of a dysfunctional relationship

In the face of a dysfunctional caregiver relationship, the infant may respond in a number of ways. The baby's behavior can be conceptualized initially as part of a defensive response to perturbations in otherwise normal genetically guided developmental pathways. Babies are in a state of developmental flux and change. If these defensive responses are persistent or the underlying stress or trauma is severe or persistent enough, these responses may develop into an ongoing disorder [13].

The infant's response to significant stress or trauma may be to follow one of two broad pathways: to withdraw and conserve or to be hyper-vigilant and responsive.

Infant defenses

Fraiberg [19], in working with high-risk families, observed a group of infant defenses, which she called pathological, in infants aged between 3 and 18 months. These babies had experienced danger and deprivation. She described five pathological psychological defenses:

1 *Avoidance*: at times total avoidance

2 *Freezing*: immobilization, frozen posture

3 *Fighting*: from fear, against helplessness

4 *Transformation of affect*: painful affect is transformed into apparent pleasure

5 *Reversal*: of aggression against the self.

The latter behaviors were more evident in the older toddlers, but it seems that all the observed behaviors occurred in response to profound psychic trauma.

Understanding the baby's own experience within the context of the relationship with the caregiver is critical in making decisions about therapeutic interventions. Understanding the experience of the infant is necessary to fully understand the parent's experience.

Methods for assessing the infant's state include:

- Direct observation of the baby's behavior to build a picture of the inner world of the infant. Trevarthen [20] emphasizes the need to meet the baby directly: 'To know what a baby feels and thinks, we must engage with her, allowing ourselves to feel the sympathetic response that the other's actions and feelings invite.'

- Guedeney [21] has developed an assessment scale (the Alarm Distress Baby Scale – ADBB) based on an evaluation of video-recorded assessment of the infant in the course of a routine health check. The scale provides a measure of infant withdrawal and capacity to engage with the examiner.

- In evaluating an infant's attachment status in a particular dyad, the child's response to separation and reunion is assessed using the Strange Situation procedure. The younger infant's response to the Still Face procedure provides some similar information about the nature of the infant's quality of relationship attachment [18].

- A series of Story Stem narrative analytic procedures provide access to the inner world of the preschool and older child [22].

- Careful and reflective use of our own responses to the infant and his troubled parents. How do I think the baby is feeling? How does this baby's behavior leave me feeling? This requires active consideration since we may otherwise be blind to the inner world and avoid experiencing the distress or helplessness of the infant [23].

Clinical vignette 3

Wendy, aged 5 months, and her mother, Sarah, aged 22, were referred to an infant mental health clinician by Sarah's mental health case manager because of concern about the relationship between Sarah and Wendy. Sarah had a history of several acute psychiatric hospital admissions when she was profoundly depressed and had suicidal ideation and persecutory and sexual delusions with frightening auditory and visual hallucinations. As a young child and adolescent she was the victim of significant emotional and sexual abuse from persons within her family. Sarah became pregnant to a young man who was admitted to the same acute psychiatric ward, but she did not continue a relationship with him after they were each discharged. Sarah delivered Wendy when she was very isolated and recovering from her most recent bout of depression and psychosis.

Sarah was very excited about the birth of Wendy but she seemed overwhelmed in the immediate period after the birth. Sarah and Wendy stayed in the obstetric hospital for 10 days post-delivery to enable Sarah to get to know her baby. She breastfed during this period but she started bottle-feeding when she left hospital. Sarah and her clinicians were anxious about antipsychotic medication in her milk.

A number of intensive home-based support services became involved. This included three-times-a-week home visits to help Sarah get to know her baby and manage the practicalities of feeding, bathing and other aspects of baby care. Sarah was keen to learn, but it seemed that she found it difficult to retain information provided to her and to anticipate Wendy's emotional needs.

Wendy herself appeared sad, with an empty affect and little capacity to engage with her mother or the infant mental health clinician. It was difficult to obtain any mutual gaze with her, her body tone was very low, she made no vocalizations and the clinician was left feeling very perturbed by Wendy's state. The likelihood of a depressive state was confirmed during a formal assessment of Wendy using the ADBB. An independent rater found Wendy to be in the range of likely clinical depression (score: 12).

Infant depression

Infant withdrawal is consistent with the development of a depressive disorder in infancy, but may occur and arrange other situations, for example severe attachment disorders, post-traumatic stress disorder and some medical conditions. Guedeney [21], in discussing the connection between infant withdrawal, depression and attachment difficulties, emphasizes that 'infant withdrawal is an emergency' and can become a persisting state which is very costly for the infant's development.

'Anybody's child'

Kumar [24] in an important paper, ' "Anybody's child": severe disorders of mother-to-infant bonding', reported on a group of women who described an 'unexpected and often catastrophic failure to love one or more of their babies'. What was the baby's experience of this lack of love, which was sometimes intensified into hate or feelings of rejection or a wish to harm? In the presence of good physical care, can the baby detect an absence of love? Can the baby detect an absence of emotional holding and containment?

'Disorganized' infant and toddler behavior

Parents with serious mental illness may find it difficult to shield their child from the sometimes chaotic and frightening internal world they experience themselves. The infant may be presented with a disturbed parent who is both the caregiver and the one who is frightening or threatening. The baby may be either hyper-vigilant or withdrawn.

Schuder and Lyons-Ruth [25] discussed fearful arousal of infants and young children exposed to confusing and contradictory messages from their caregivers. The classification of *disorganized attachment* is characterized by a number of types of disrupted emotional communications from mother to infant.

Some of the strong infant contradictory and confusing behavior patterns described include: approach followed by avoidance; freezing; stilling slowed movements; a dazed look; simultaneous contradictory behaviors; moving towards but then turning away; the child who cries as she seeks physical comfort; incomplete or interrupted sequences of behavior; suddenly stops or changes; stereotypies; or who stumbles for no apparent reason.

Young children may show fear of their parent: hunched shoulders, fearful face expression, strange distorted facial expressions, multiple changes in mood, seem disorganized or confused [25].

For the very young infant, the lack of an attuned responsive carer constitutes a trauma in itself [25]. If the caregiver is not available to regulate the infant's physiological response to arousal and stress, both internal and external, the infant can feel equally distressed and disorganized. The caregiver's unavailability means the infant experiences *interactive dysregulation*. As a consequence the neuro-endocrine stress response system may then be out of control. This may not be as obvious as with trauma in the older child. Schuder and Lyons-Ruth [25] stress how the experience of trauma experienced in infancy is different from later stages of life. The parent who is emotionally unavailable is likely to be unable to help the infant with his own constant task of emotional and physiological self-regulation. These are described as the 'hidden traumas' of early dysregulation: 'In human infancy, however, experienced threat is closely related to the caregiver's affects and availability rather than the actual degree of physical or survival threat inherent in the event itself' [25].

A significant number of infants who are in relatively low-risk situations, that is not subject to direct maltreatment, may still demonstrate disorganized attachment patterns with their primary carer. Parents may have significant mental illness and are not directly abusive, yet they may still parent their infant in such a way that to the infant their behavior appears confusing or frightening and leaves them feeling uncontained.

It may be that the infant's current and future capacity to develop an awareness of the inner world of the other, her capacity for intersubjectivity, is also diminished when an infant grows with a persistent disorganized attachment style. Psychobiological dysregulation may follow persistent insensitive caregiving, with the infant and young child showing deviations in the way their hypothalamic axis and biological stress system operate.

Trevarthen and Aitken [1] argue that significant developmental psychopathology may occur when the baby's intrinsic potentiality for 'intersubjectivity' is disrupted. Intersubjectivity is a capacity which is critical for the development of dynamic 'motive states' necessary for learning.

In their research looking at ordinary human infant development, Trevarthen and Reddy [20], engaged directly at an emotional level with infants and have opened up an awareness of some of the baby's other *complex infant organized feeling states* and relationships. For example they have been able to demonstrate the development of coyness, shyness and teasing in typically developing babies in the first six months of life. We do not know the impact upon these creative capacities of the baby when their primary carer suffers from mental illness. It may be that there is an impingement upon the baby's essential desire and capacity to be a social organism.

It is likely that these manifestations of the infant's complex inner emotional world are important in eliciting an emotional response from important adults around them.

The baby who is not able to elicit an enlightened response from her troubled mother also finds that her mother is deprived of her baby's lively engagement. The baby, when becoming depressed, is likely to intensify the mother's own feeling of depression or emotional flatness, which results in her feeling even more miserable, angry, self-blaming or seemingly devoid of emotion.

Clinical vignette 4

Jeremy was born to a very vulnerable young couple. Jeremy's 20-year-old father had a history of some psychotic symptoms in his teens and heroin use but, despite this, with the announcement of the pregnancy the couple determined to stay together. At the end of Jeremy's first three months of life it was clear however he had a serious degenerative neurological disorder. Both parents became increasingly depressed, despondent and described soulless mechanical care of their baby. Tearfully Jeremy's mother said she could not bear to look at her baby and said that she had actively considered suicide.

In the course of a family assessment the therapist, in an almost involuntary way, started to mirror some of Jeremy's spontaneous hand movements. The therapist and the baby gazed upon each other and upon each other's hands. The therapist started to clap, the baby made a clapping movement as well. The parents saw this, and in doing so seemed to become aware that there was a person residing in their baby's floppy body. They felt relieved because they felt that the baby could not, would not, communicate and connect with them. They now felt that there was an emotional connection and that they could do something. Jeremy's clapping became more and more organized and he used it as a way of indicating to his parents that he needed them. It was as if the baby was helping the family stay together and providing the parents with a sense of purpose. After this 'moment of meeting' [26] his parents seemed much more able to offer him lively contingent parenting.

36.7 Implications for prevention and intervention

The process of deciding what is in the best interests of the child, the infant, remains a complex and difficult task. Our services need to work with families to balance the rights of the infant and the needs of the family to ensure the best outcome for the child.

Preventive intervention needs to work on a number of levels [27]: the improvement of the general health and well-being of parents with mental illness including obstetric, medical and mental health, early identification and treatment of emerging depressive or psychotic symptoms, the development of collaborative community supports and the opportunity for parents to develop their parenting skills.

Comprehensive assessment of each individual infant and family should lead to the selection of an appropriate therapeutic intervention [27]. For those families where a parent has a serious mental illness a close and ongoing collaboration is needed between a range of agencies including the adult mental health service, infant mental health, family support agencies, child protective agencies and early childhood health. A number of integrated perinatal and infant mental health services have been developed. Some mental health services have developed specific programs for supporting professionals working directly with infants in families with a serious mental illness in order to keep the baby in mind.

Understanding how we feel: countertransference in working with infants whose parents have major mental illness

The infant mental health clinician may feel in an invidious position as she tries to identify with both the baby and his troubled parents. For example when a seriously depressed mother says she feels like driving her car with her baby aboard into a lamppost we take notice. We also may feel confused and professionally impotent since we realize that this advocating for the infant may produce major distress for the parent. In this context, close collaboration between the extended family, infant and adult mental health as well child welfare services is important.

Gubler Gochman [28] discusses the difficulty of working in infant–parent psychotherapy with seemingly conflicting therapeutic aims when one works from the conventional social value that 'mothers should take care of their children'. The usual treatment objective is the prevention of psychopathology in the child through improving the infant–caregiver attachment process. At times however, the therapist must be able to step back and acknowledge the presence of various conflicting goals, one of which is to acknowledge that the very troubled mother may not be able to provide the quality of care which her baby really needs. She notes that some women with major mental illness, although functioning well in other areas of their lives, may, because of persistence of 'negative symptoms', remain too psychologically defended to allow for the process of empathy towards their children. She argues it is possible to change the therapeutic objective to one whereby the mother allows the infant to develop a relationship with a different carer and that this is consistent with the mothers' general wish for their child 'to have a good life'.

Fraiberg emphasized the need to include the baby in work with extremely vulnerable families. Engaging the baby enhanced engagement with the family: 'the importance of the baby being present for therapy . . . we need the privilege of entering their intimate lives' [23].

36.8 Conclusion

Living with a serious mental illness can be a frightening and disorganizing journey. Becoming a parent during this journey presents a number of issues for each of the parents, the infant and family and also for the therapeutic personnel. For such parents the arrival of a new baby is an opportunity for real personal growth and can offer a new meaning for living. However we know that mental illness can directly impair a parent's capacity to provide the baby with the necessary sensitive and attuned parenting. The indirect effects of serious mental illness can be disabling as parents are often isolated socially and economically.

The nature of parenting in the context of mental illness is complex: the consequences for the baby and her development depend on many factors. The problems facing parents range from more common depression in the postnatal period to much less common, more severe illnesses such as schizophrenia and bipolar affective disorder. It is clear that the more severe the illness, and the greater the number of vulnerabilities, the more at risk is the infant's development. Considerable further research is needed in this area, but a good understanding of the baby and her own inner world is important in understanding the nature of the relationship with her parents and what support and intervention is most appropriate.

36.9 Acknowledgements

I wish to thank the families and colleagues with whom I have been privileged to work, and I acknowledge that I have changed clinical details in order to protect their identities.

36.10 References

1. Trevarthen, C., Aitken, K.J. (1994) Brain development, infant communication, and empathy disorders: intrinsic factors in child mental health. *Development and Psychopathology*, **6** (4) 597–633.
2. Winnicott, D.W. (1965) The theory of the parent-infant relationship, in *The Maturational Processes and the Facilitating Environment: Studies in the Theory of Emotional Development.* The Hogarth Press and the Institute of Psycho-Analysis, London, p. 37.
3. Murray, L., Cooper, P. and Hipwell, A. (2003) Mental health of parents caring for infants. *Archives of Women's Mental Health*, **6** (Suppl.2), s71–s7.
4. Niemi, L., Suvisaari, J.M., Haukka, J.K. *et al.* (2005) Cumulative incidence of mental disorders among offspring of mothers with psychotic disorder: results from the Helsinki High-Risk Study. *British Journal of Psychiatry*, **186**, 355–56.
5. Niemi, L.T., Suvisaari, J.M., Haukka, J.K. and Lonnqvist, J.K. (2005) Childhood predictors of future psychiatric morbidity in offspring of mothers with psychotic disorder: results from the Helsinki High-Risk Study. *British Journal of Psychiatry*, **186** (2), 1 February, 108–14.
6. Snellen, M., Mack, K. and Trauer, T. (1999) Schizophrenia, mental state, and mother and infant interaction: examining the relationship. *Australian and New Zealand Journal of Psychiatry*, **33** (6), 902–11.
7. Ramchandani, P. and Psychogiou, L. (2009) Paternal psychiatric disorders and children's psychosocial development. *Lancet*, **374** (9690), 28. August, 646–53.
8. Feldman, R., Granat, A.D.I., Pariente, C. *et al.* (2009) Maternal depression and anxiety across the postpartum year and infant social engagement, fear regulation, and stress reactivity. *Journal of the American Academy of Child and Adolescent Psychiatry*, **48** (9), 919–27.
9. Hipwell, A.E. and Kumar, R. (1996) Maternal psychopathology and prediction of outcome based on mother-infant interaction ratings (BMIS). *British Journal of Psychiatry*, **169** (5), 1 November, 655–61.
10. Fonagy, P., Gergely, G. and Target, M. (2007) The parent-infant dyad and the construction of the subjective self. *Journal of Child Psychology and Psychiatry*, **48** (3/4), 288–328.
11. Slade, A., Grienenberger, J., Bernbach, E. *et al.* (2005) Maternal reflective functioning, attachment, and the transmission gap: a preliminary study. *Attachment and Human Development*, **7** (3), 283–98.
12. Philipp, D., Fivaz-Depeursinge, E., Corboz-Warnery, A. and Favez, N. (2009) Young infants' triangular communication with their parents in the context of maternal postpartum psychosis: four case studies. *Infant Mental Health Journal*, **30** (4), 341–65.

13. Zero to Three (2005) *Diagnostic Classification of Mental Health and Developmental Disorders of Infancy and Early Childhood*, revised edn (DC: 0-3R). Zero to Three Press, Washington, DC.

14. Newman, L. and Stevenson, C. (2008) Issues in infant–parent psychotherapy for mothers with borderline personality disorder. *Clinical Child Psychology and Psychiatry*, **13** (4), October, 505–14.

15. Hipwell, A.E. and Kumar, R. (1997) The impact of postpartum affective psychosis on the child, in *Postpartum Depression and Child Development* (eds L. Murray and P. Cooper), Guilford Press, New York and London, pp. 265–94.

16. Wan, M.W., Abel, K.M. and Green, J. (2008) The transmission of risk to children from mothers with schizophrenia: a developmental psychopathology model. *Clinical Psychology Review*, **28** (4), 613–37.

17. Wan, M.W., Salmon, M.P., Riordan, D.M. *et al.* (2007) What predicts poor mother-infant interaction in schizophrenia? *Psychological Medicine*, **37** (4), 537–46.

18. Wan, M.W. and Green, J. (2009) The impact of maternal psychopathology on child-mother attachment. *Archives of Women's Mental Health*, **12**, 123–34.

19. Fraiberg, S. (1982) Pathological defenses in infancy. *Psychoanalytical Quarterly*, **51**, 612–35.

20. Reddy, V. and Trevarthen, C. (2004) What we learn about babies from engaging with their emotions. *Zero to Three*, January, 9–15.

21. Guedeney, A. (2007) Withdrawal behavior and depression in infancy. *Infant Mental Health Journal*, **28** (4), 393–408.

22. Robinson, J.L. (2007) Story stem narratives with young children: moving to clinical research and practice. *Attachment and Human Development and Psychopathology*, **9** (3), 179–85.

23. Fraiberg, S., Adelson, E. and Shapiro, V. (1975) Ghosts in the nursery: a psychoanalytic approach to the problems of impaired infant-mother relationships. *Journal of the American Academy of Child and Adolescent Psychiatry*, **14** (3), 387–421.

24. Kumar, R.C. (1997) 'Anybody's child': severe disorders of mother-to-infant bonding. *British Journal of Psychiatry*, **171** (2), 1 August, 175–81.

25. Schuder, M.R. and Lyons-Ruth, K. (2004) 'Hidden trauma' in infancy: attachment, fearful arousal, and early dysfunction of the stress response system, in *Young Children and Trauma: Intervention and Treatment* (ed. J.D. Osofsky), Guilford Press, New York.

26. Stern, D.N. (1998) The process of therapeutic change involving implicit knowledge: some implications of developmental observations for adult psychotherapy. *Infant Mental Health Journal*, **19** (3), Fall, 300–8.

27. Zeanah, P.D., Stafford, B. and Zeanah, C.H. (2005) Clinical interventions to enhance infant mental health: a selective review. Journal [serial on the Internet]. Available from: http://www.healthychild.ucla.edu.

28. Grubler Gochman, E.R. (1992) A note on deep-seated social values social values and countertransference in mother-infant dyadic psychotherapy. *Psychoanalytic Psychology*, **9**, 405–8.

37

Mental health of parents and infant health and development in resource-constrained settings: evidence gaps and implications for facilitating 'good-enough parenting' in the twenty-first-century world

Jane Fisher,[1] Atif Rahman,[2] Meena Cabral de Mello,[3] Prabha S. Chandra[4] and Helen Herrman[1]

[1]University of Melbourne, Australia
[2]University of Liverpool, UK
[3]World Health Organization, Geneva, Switzerland
[4]National Institute of Mental Health and Neurosciences, Bangalore, India

37.1 Introduction

All infants and young children require skilled parenting in order to thrive and develop optimally. The essential elements are: competent caretaking; sensitivity, responsiveness, emotional warmth and cognitive stimulation. 'Good-enough parenting' is closely related to the health and survival and the mental health and well-being of mothers, fathers and

Parenthood and Mental Health: A Bridge between Infant and Adult Psychiatry   Sam Tyano, Miri Keren, Helen Herrman and John Cox
© 2010 John Wiley & Sons, Ltd

families. These in turn are linked in all countries and communities to the prevailing social, economic and cultural living conditions. While parents and families in most places can benefit from direct assistance and support in the important task of parenting, in many resource-constrained parts of the world structural and social change is also essential to allow a chance for parenting in adequate conditions. The capacity of mothers and fathers to provide good parenting in conditions of social and economic deprivation vary across countries and neighborhoods with the complex interaction of socio-cultural, community, family and individual factors (see Chapter 30). However whether poverty is absolute or relative the barriers to good parenting it creates are likely to be higher overall in poorly resourced countries. The lessons learned from research in high-income countries have rarely been applied in these settings. Conversely new research from low-income settings revealing the importance of gender and social equity to parenting capacity is likely to be applicable to the wider world including wealthier countries.

The mental health and well-being of mothers and fathers is of central importance to the health and development of children and is a focus of substantial research attention in the high-income countries of the world. In resource-constrained settings, evidence has become available in recent years for the influence of social conditions on the health and behaviour of mothers. To date there has been no research about fathers or the way that parenting is shared in these contexts and this is an international research priority. In the meantime we will discuss in this chapter the research evidence about the mental health of mothers and how this reflects women's social position, rights and consequent capacity to parent, in the world's low- and lower-middle-income countries. On this basis and by extension from knowledge of fathering gained from research in high-income countries we will discuss the importance of social conditions and the potential of interventions to provide support where required for mothers, fathers and families.

Safe motherhood is now assured and pregnancy-related deaths are rare in women living in the world's high-income countries. However, most women live in the world's 112 resource-constrained low- and lower-middle-income countries [1], where they have less access to family planning services, skilled birth attendants, health-care facilities in which to give birth, and basic and emergency obstetric care, than women have in high-income countries. They are less likely to have completed primary schooling, to be able to generate an adequate and secure income; and to have had the sexual and reproductive health education that is essential to being able to make autonomous choices about when and how many children they wish to have. They are more likely to live in crowded circumstances and to be poorly nourished and carrying a coincidental burden of infectious diseases including the substantial burden of HIV and AIDS. Their lives are more likely to be constrained by rigid gender stereotypes about appropriate roles and responsibilities for women. Gender-based violence is prevalent in all contexts, but especially in cultures in which girl children and women are devalued and their rights ignored. In these contexts women are at greater risk of dying from pregnancy-related causes, to experience the maternal morbidities of hemorrhage and infection, to give birth to babies who are underweight and not to have access to the health care they need in these circumstances. Their babies are more likely to die and less likely to thrive than babies born in industrialized countries [2].

It is in the context of assured maternal and infant survival and health that consciousness of the psychological aspects of pregnancy, childbirth and early parenthood has been able to grow in the clinical, research and human development communities. In the past 50 years there has been copious and increasingly sophisticated research into the psychological aspects, social needs and nature and determinants of mental health problems during reproductive life [3]. The research has focused predominantly on the experiences of women during pregnancy and after childbirth, and on the consequences of their sensitivity, responsiveness and caretaking skills for the health and development of and later emotional attachments formed by their infants.

It was once asserted that women living in traditional settings in resource-constrained countries did not experience post-partum mental health problems because they experience 'confinement': a prescribed period of dedicated care after birth, an honored status, relief from normal tasks and responsibilities and social seclusion [4, 5]. However recent research suggests that this is an oversimplified view and that the ethnographic research on which it was based detected cultural beliefs and firmly held opinions, but did not assess women's experiences systematically or directly [6]. Confinement comprises both social – increased recognition and practical support – and cultural elements – observation of traditional rituals and behaviors. For women everywhere it appears to be the social: warm, non-judgemental help rather than the cultural dimension that is protective [10]. It is inaccurate to presume that confinement is available to all women or always experienced as supportive.

There remain gross disparities in the quantity of evidence available: almost all high- and upper-middle-income countries have comprehensive data on which to base policy and prac-tice, but only 10% of low- and middle-income countries have any data [7]. A series of studies in the last decade have found that the rates of depression in women after childbirth are two to three times higher than those in resource-rich countries: including 23% in Goa, India [8]; 34.7% in a poor South African township [9]; 32.7% in the south of Viet Nam [10]; 40.4% in Edirne, Turkey [11] and 40% in Rawalpindi, Pakistan [12]. Much less research evidence about mental health during pregnancy in these settings is available, but in Tamil Nadu, India 16% [13]; and in rural Pakistan 25% [14] of women attending antenatal services were depressed.

The effects of maternal depression are amplified when families are living with poverty and chronic social adversity [15]. The environment in resource-constrained settings is usually more difficult than in the industrialized world and the social capital that once characterized rural communities is being eroded in many places through globalization and increased movement of people seeking income and relief from poverty. A mother's competence in childcare is thought to play a greater role in her infant's chance of survival and health in low-and middle-income countries. In these settings maternal depression has been linked directly to higher rates of diarrhoeal diseases, infectious illness and hospital admission, reduced completion of recommended schedules of immunization and worse physical, cognitive, social, behavioral and emotional development in children, and may lead to reduced child survival [12, 15, 16, 17]. Maternal and child health are global priorities, but pregnancy-related mortality and morbidity in women and infants in many resource-constrained countries have been resistant to amelioration [2]. There is as yet no consideration of mental health in international initiatives to reduce pregnancy-related deaths and maternal morbidity and improve infant survival and development.

In contrast to the available literature on the parenting of mothers with mental health problems, including the emerging literature described above, that on the parenting of fathers with mental health problems is meager even in wealthy parts of the world (Chapter 21). The existing work indicates that across the lifespan from infancy through adolescence, depressed fathers give suboptimal parenting. The way that this affects the social and emotional development of their children, the effects of other disorders and the possibility of new parenting interventions to assist fathers are so far unknown.

Extensive work in the USA and Europe has also defined the importance of the alliance between mothers and fathers to children's early social and emotional adjustment (see Chapter 32). Observational, interview and self-report studies have been conducted. Alliances between the parents or parental figures including extended family members or other central caretakers exist in all families where more than one person assumes responsibility for a child's care and upbringing. Mutual involvement and solidarity of the involved parental figures are central to the child's adjustment. Discord and detachment impair infant and child development through direct and indirect mechanisms. We are unaware of studies on these topics in low-and middle-income countries despite their evident relevance to good-enough parenting.

We now have substantial expert knowledge about women's psychological functioning during reproductive life and while working as mothers of infants. The importance of the family environment and the father's role is evident in general experience and an emerging area of research in high-income countries. One of the challenges in facilitating 'good-enough parenting' in the communities of the twenty-first century is to find ways to translate this knowledge into accessible, available and suitable programs and social changes to meet the needs of the majority of parents who live beyond its current reach.

37.2 Social model of mental health

Mental health is related inextricably to an individual's life circumstances and personal experiences and also to wider contextual factors. These include a society's concern for gender, ethnicity and the human rights to education, equal social and economic participation, safety, individual autonomy and freedom from discrimination [18]. A social model of health takes all these factors into account and presumes that an individual's state of health or experience of illness is determined by personal experiences, social circumstances, culture and political environment in addition to inherited or biological factors. Reflecting this social model of health, the World Health Organization defines mental health in broad terms as:

> the capacity of the individual, the group and the environment to interact with one another in ways that promote subjective well-being, the optimal development and use of mental abilities (cognitive, affective and relational), the achievement of individual and collective goals consistent with justice and the attainment and preservation of conditions of fundamental equality. [19]

This definition makes it clear that day-to-day opportunities to use individual abilities and skills, to experience personal achievement and a sense of effectiveness are fundamental to experiencing an inner, subjective sense of well-being that is in turn the basis of effective functioning. The definition also emphasizes the importance of development over the whole course of life. Early experiences and opportunities influence later capacities for participation. Relationships with other people are centrally important to individuals, allowing trust, intimacy and the giving and receiving of affection, support and care, as well as the opportunity for shared experiences. The social, cultural, economic and political living environment is crucial and mental health cannot be realized without justice and equality of human rights; through inclusion of all and fairness of opportunity and access to adequate resources on which to live [18]. These are intrinsically gendered.

37.3 Parenting and mothers' social position

Even in the contemporary world, women's rights to equality of access to education, personal safety, reproductive choice and freedom from discrimination are not recognized universally. They are particularly important to mental health and mothering. The relative contributions of biological, psychological and social factors to depression in mothers were assessed in a recent [20] multilevel analysis in 50 US states. Self-reported depression symptoms were collected from more than 7700 women together with publicly available data from the 50 states in which they lived. Women who lived in states in which female political participation was high, reproductive rights recognized and employment and economic autonomy assured had significantly lower average levels of depressive symptoms than others. As there is no basis to presume that women in general are biologically or psychologically different between states, it was concluded that that social determinants outweigh both intrinsic biological and individual psychological factors in explaining the prevalence of depression in women.

The lower social position occupied by women in most societies is amplified during the years of mothering little children when social and economic participation are reduced and the unpaid workload increased. This is integral to both the higher level of risk factors for poor mental health that they face and the lower levels of protective factors to which they have access. In the studies of maternal mental health from resource-constrained settings the risk factors for poor mental health were consistent with this social model. They include:

- Poverty and chronic social adversity, including limited education and opportunities for income generation, and crowded living conditions [10, 14, 21];

- Gender-based violence, including emotional, physical and sexual abuse during childhood, and family violence, including by intimate partners [8, 22];

- Lack of autonomy to make sexual and reproductive decisions [23];

- Unintended pregnancy, especially among adolescent women who have not had access to family planning services [10, 21];

- Lack of empathy from partners and gendered stereotypes about the division of household work and infant care [10, 21, 23, 24, 25];

- Excessive workloads and severe occupational fatigue [13];

- Lack of emotional and practical support or criticism from her own mother or mother-in-law, or peer group [10, 13, 14, 22];

- Gender discrimination and devaluing of women; [23]

- Cultural preference for male children [8].

Overall it is estimated that about 1 in 10 pregnant women and mothers of newborns in high-income countries have significant mental health problems, but 1 in 3 to 1 in 5 in the resource-constrained countries from which evidence is available [8, 10, 14]. Pregnancy and childbirth-related conditions were ranked first and depression fourth as contributors to the burden of disease experienced by women globally in 2003 [26]. When these conditions co-occur, the human suffering can be extreme and the consequences for infant health and development severe.

37.4 Human rights, mental health and child health and development

In September 2000, 189 member states ratified the United Nations Millennium Declaration that every woman, man and child has the right to development and freedom from want and that progress has to be measurable and demonstrable. In order to ensure this aim, it defines goals, targets and indicators for combating poverty, hunger, disease, illiteracy, environmental degradation and discrimination against women as central to development. There is growing recognition that maternal mental health is fundamental to attaining the Millennium Development Goals of improving maternal health, reducing child mortality, promoting gender equality and empowering women, achieving universal primary education and eradicating extreme poverty and hunger.

In 2005 the World Health Organization (WHO) established the Commission on the Social Determinants of Health (CSDH) [27] to 'marshal the evidence on effective strategies to promote health equity'. It reported in 2008 that in all contexts there are social gradients in health, with the poorest having much worse health than those who are socio-economically advantaged. These disparities reflect diverse factors, not just health services and systems, but are indicators of social injustice. The CSDH recognizes in particular the importance of early childhood development (ECD) to social equity and adult health, well-being and productivity. It concludes that 'the process of development is influenced not only by a child's nutrition and health status, but also by the kind of interactions, beginning in utero [that] infants and children develop with caregivers'. The environments in which children live in the earliest years of life, and the quality of emotional security, intellectual stimulation and sensitive care they receive during the early years set a critical foundation for their entire life course. 'Early childhood development influences health and development status, basic learning, school success, economic participation, and social citizenry' [28]. Opportunities provided to infants and young children are crucial in shaping lifelong health and developmental status.

37.5 Promotion of infant health and development and prevention of maternal mental health problems

The health sector has a unique role to play in supporting young children's growth and development. This includes promoting all aspects of child development with systematic and well-implemented education of and support for parents, and identifying children in need of increased intervention. In all settings there is some provision for pregnancy-related health care and assessment of the health of newborns and young children, including for vaccination.

Interventions for promoting ECD are optimally located within regular primary health care. Integrating health and nutritional interventions with home or facility-based psychosocial interventions is a cost-effective approach which can have lasting benefits on children's competence. There are effective and mostly low-cost actions that can be taken to prevent the damage and remedy the deficiencies. While delivery of ECD services depends on the local context, there are case studies which illustrate that successful programs can be implemented at all income levels. The WHO in collaboration with UNICEF, the World Bank and other partners has developed the Care for Child Development package that provides age-appropriate recommendations for all children on play, communication, nutrition and responsive feeding, and includes intervention strategies when problems are identified. The package has a checklist for health-care providers to use to identify and manage problems. It covers the age range from newborn through 36 months. It also includes recommendations for care during pregnancy and the mental health of mothers.

These recommendations can be given to caregivers by health workers, nutrition workers or community health workers. The package provides an evidence-based, theoretically sound and tested method for supporting ECD. It incorporates all WHO principles including equity, child rights, integration of services, life course approach and community participation and is a synthesis of the most effective approaches that have worked in the context of developing countries.

The feasibility of delivering the Care for Child Development in resource-poor settings has been demonstrated in Brazil and South Africa. In Turkey investigators found an effect on the quality of the home environment one month after a single health centre visit. Incorporating developmental counseling within primary care may improve family satisfaction, quality of care and parenting practices, greater parenting confidence, and fewer concerns about the child's development.

To date, most investigations in this field have presumed that infants' behavior reflects parenting factors, and that for example poor developmental outcomes are a direct consequence of maternal depression. However, there is growing recognition that the relationship might be reciprocal and that infant behavior, especially prolonged inconsolable crying and sleeping and feeding difficulties, are likely to exert an adverse effect on a mother's confidence and affect. In high-income settings, there is increasing evidence that effective parenting education benefits maternal mental health through enhancing maternal efficacy with flow on benefits for self-confidence [29]. Universal strategies to promote skilled care of infants like the Care for Development package are therefore likely to contribute to the prevention of maternal mental health problems in low-income settings.

There is debate about whether the most effective approach to improving maternal mental health and the capacity for parenting is to use indicated interventions for women with current clinically significant depressive symptoms or other illness, selective interventions for women at risk of developing illness, or universal preventive interventions to be offered to all women to reduce population prevalence [30]. However all of these approaches are required to improve population mental health and reduce the burden of illness and its consequences for child development. The need to address specific 'upstream' and 'downstream' factors will differ across countries, communities and families as described in Chapter 30, and a situation assessment is warranted in most countries and regions.

37.6 Preventing and ameliorating maternal mental health problems and potential benefits for infant health and development

Even when effective prevention strategies are available, there is a need for interventions to assist mothers with mental health problems. In high-income countries there are diverse approaches to treatment. There is evidence that both psychotherapeutic interventions including cognitive behavioral therapy, interpersonal therapy and pharmacotherapy can be effective in reducing maternal depression. However these depend on availability of and access to highly skilled mental health professionals. Few low- and lower-middle income countries have sufficient mental health professionals available to meet the population's needs. Further, in order to be incorporated into existing health care, interventions have to be acceptable, affordable, accessible and based on local evidence. The challenge is to develop and demonstrate the effectiveness of interventions to address: women's psychological needs in the work of mothering; children's developmental needs; the mother–infant relationship; and the social determinants of poor maternal and infant health in resource-constrained settings. Interventions to ameliorate mental health problems are required in all settings. In time it is essential to develop and implement cross-sectoral and multifaceted strategies to prevent them.

Interventions to address maternal mental health problems have been studied recently in low- and lower-middle-income countries. Some focus on the mother directly. Rahman *et al.*'s Thinking Healthy Program (THP) [32], is a manualized intervention incorporating cognitive and behavioral techniques of active listening, collaboration with the family, non-threatening enquiry into the family's health beliefs and challenging and substitution of alternative information when required, and inter-session practice activities. Rojas *et al.* [33] used eight, weekly, structured psycho-educational groups comprising information about symptoms and treatments, problem-solving and behavioral activation strategies and cognitive techniques with examples illustrative of the postnatal period and free antidepressant pharmacotherapy.

Others targeted the child, with assistance to the mother being offered opportunistically. Baker-Henningham *et al.* [31] in Jamaica tested a half-hour weekly home-visiting intervention which aimed to improve mothers' knowledge and childrearing practices and parenting self-esteem through the use of home-made toys, books and household items to demonstrate age-appropriate activities for the child by involving mother and child in play and provide experiences of mastery and success for mother and child. The importance of praise, responsiveness, nutrition, appropriate discipline and promotion of play and learning were emphasized in a friendly empathic approach, but there was no specific focus on problem solving or addressing maternal concerns.

Rahman *et al.*'s Learning Through Play (LTP) [34] program was developed for use by lay home visitors in Canada and has been adapted for use in resource-constrained countries. It includes images demonstrating infant development, parent–child play activities and other activities to promote skilled parental caretaking to promote cognitive and social-emotional development. The images are accompanied by simple text suitable for groups with low literacy and together these are presented as a calendar demonstrating developmental progress. The intervention group received a half-day session on LTP in late pregnancy, with a calendar for take-home use. Subsequently each mother received 15- to 20-minute home visits once a fortnight at which her infant's development was discussed using the calendar as a reference point until her baby was 12 weeks old. Participants were encouraged to meet informally in groups to apply the techniques in the calendar and provide mutual support to each other.

Cooper and his international team [9] sought to improve mother–infant relationship using a local adaptation of the Health Visitor Intervention Program incorporating principles of the WHO's Improving the Psychosocial Development of Children program that aims to enhance maternal sensitivity and responsiveness to and interactions with her baby. The health visitors used items from the Neonatal Behavioral Assessment Scale to sensitize the mother to her infant's abilities and needs in hour-long home visits antenatally and at scheduled intervals post-partum.

These interventions were all assessed in settings with very few specialist mental health professionals and, apart from Rojas *et al.*'s [33] study, were implemented by local non-specialist community health workers, under the supervision of trained and experienced health professionals or health researchers. All studies included comparisons with women who did not receive the intervention and measured maternal distress or depression by diagnostic or self-report measures as an outcome.

Mothers who received the Thinking Healthy Program in Pakistan were less likely to be depressed, less disabled, and had better overall functioning and perceived social support at 6 and 12 months post-intervention than mothers who received usual standard care [32]. Rojas *et al.* [33] in the trial from Chile reported that the crude mean Edinburgh Postnatal Depression Scale (EPDS) score was lower for the intervention group than for the usual care group at 3-month follow up, but by 6 months this difference was no longer evident. Mothers who received the multi-component group therapy were more compliant with antidepressant use, attended their primary care provider more frequently and had better social functioning at 3 months than those in the standard care group.

In Baker-Henningham *et al.*'s [31] study from Jamaica, mothers who received the home-visiting intervention but not mothers in the control group had a significant reduction in depressive symptoms. Mothers receiving 40–50 home visits had the greatest decline in depressive symptoms and those who received fewer than 24 visits had no improvement compared to the control group. Mothers in Pakistan who received the Learning Through Play program had more knowledge about infancy than those in the comparison group, though there were no differences in self-rated emotional distress [34].

In the randomized controlled trial of the intervention from Khayelitsha, South Africa [35], self-rated maternal depressive symptoms were lower in the intervention group at both assessments than those for the control group, but were significant only at 6 months follow-up [35]. Mothers in the intervention group were however significantly more sensitive and less intrusive in their interactions with their infants at both 6 and 12-month follow-up. More infants in the intervention than the control group were securely attached and there were higher rates of anxious-avoidant attachment in control than intervention group.

37.7 Addressing the social determinants of compromised early childhood development and maternal mental health problems

The social determinants of compromised early childhood development were an explicit focus of the Commission for Social Determinants of Health Development's Report; and their contribution to depression in mothers was recognized explicitly in the theoretical rationales for some of the treatment studies described above.

In order to achieve the Millennium Development Goals related to reduction of poverty and malnutrition and realization of gender equality, and primary education for all, investments in the earliest years of life are essential. Early opportunities for learning in combination with improved nutrition increase the chances that a child will attend and stay in school, will learn effectively while in school, and will be able to use the learning for becoming a more productive worker and caregiver of the next generation in adulthood. The combined impact of gender discrimination, poverty, depression and social exclusion place children at great risk and their combined impact is even more severe [28]. Investments for child development include but go beyond those required for survival; rather, they are a set of evidence-based, recognized interventions to improve the child's development and the quality of the child's environment.

Cooper *et al.* [9, 35] acknowledge that chronic social and economic adversity and exposure to violence compromise infant health and development, and that maternal depression amplifies these effects. Given the difficulties in altering the environment they proposed that an approach which aimed to improve mothering capacity might reduce maternal depression and ameliorate poor outcomes for infants. In the report of their recent randomized controlled trial [35], they note that the lower prevalence of maternal depression in Khyalitsha, the peri-urban research site, compared with that found in their earlier prevalence survey and pilot studies [9] was likely to be attributed to the general improvement in economic and social circumstances that had occurred in the interim.

In the theoretical rationale for the Thinking Healthy Program [32], the authors acknowledged that women in Pakistan occupy a lower social position than other family and community members and in this situation can feel defeated, hopeless and unable to exert agency. The need to improve women's social status in order to promote their mental health was recognized, but also that this requires a subtle and staged approach. Recognizing that there was potential for the intervention to be perceived as a challenge to traditional cultural beliefs about women's roles and responsibilities, the need to minimize resistance by engaging family members was explicit. The intervention had therefore to be culturally and socially acceptable not only to individual women, but also to members of her extended family. Mental illness is highly stigmatized in many low-income countries, including Pakistan. Formative research revealed that women with depression did not regard their state of mind as an illness, but rather as a reflection of their social and economic circumstances and of pejorative gender stereotypes. There was potential to worsen women's predicaments by applying explicit diagnostic labels and describing the program as being about depression. Stigma was reduced and acceptability increased by presenting the intervention as one to promote the health and development of babies, and that healthy strong mothers were best able to achieve this. It was also reflected in the integration of the THP in the standard community-based maternal and child health education program rather than being stand-alone.

The choice of language reflected this: the intervention was presented as 'training' and not 'therapy', the providers as 'trainers' not mental health workers, and the term 'depression' was not used. In addition to careful choice of constructs and language, comprehensibility was maximized through the development of visual materials appropriate for non-literate participants. While each step of the intervention was documented in the THP manual, it was multimodal and providers were permitted to use independent judgement to make pragmatic adjustments, for example to seek external assistance to reduce gender-based violence.

37.8 Implications for facilitating 'good-enough parenting' in the communities of the twenty-first century

Overall, this body of evidence, generated in diverse countries and settings, provides promising guidance for strategies to facilitating 'good-enough parenting' through assisting mothers and very young children in all countries, including the world's many resource-constrained communities.

First it is clear that women are responsive to programs which recognize the value of their work as mothers and provide them with the skills and knowledge they need to care well for their infants. Structured psycho-educational approaches which teach them how to undertake these tasks are of more value to them than empathic support alone. These approaches require tailoring to differences in literacy including emotional literacy and to the social, economic and political contexts of their lives.

There is increasing evidence from the industrialized world that although there are some flow-on benefits, interventions need to attend explicitly to the needs of the mother, the infant and to mother–infant interaction. The outcomes of the trials described suggest that this also applies in resource-constrained settings. Interventions for maternal mental health can have a positive impact on infant health and development, but the effect is stronger if the infant health component is a direct, rather than an incidental focus of the intervention. The South African and Pakistani trials where the focus was placed on mother–infant interaction improved the quality of interaction and maternal knowledge of infant development respectively, but had weaker or no effects on maternal mental health.

This last observation has important implications for helping mothers parent better in an atmosphere of trust, sharing and support. Most mothers (even in the most resource-poor settings) will do all they can for their infant, sometimes at the cost of their own physical and mental health. Women with young children often have role strain because of the multiple demands made on them. They not only have to look after the infant and other young children, they also have to fulfill other social, economic and physical demands of the family. If women are to be more effective parents they need their own mental health and physical health needs to be looked after. Communities need to find ways of supporting young mothers, such as young mum's clubs and groups and ways of helping mothers to find time to exercise, eat and have their leisure needs fulfilled.

Considering culturally appropriate ways that fathers and other parental figures may be included or influenced to provide support for these initiatives is important and relevant to their success, based on the evidence from high income countries as well as common sense. With rapid urbanization and more mothers being involved in income-generating work, the role of fathers needs to be defined better in all societies and they need to share the work of parental caretaking. There remains a serious lack of evidence about the work of fathering in resource-constrained settings including the impact of gender stereotypes on men's capacity to provide infant caretaking and to participate fully in domestic life, and the contributions that fathers make to the optimal health and development of their infants and the healthy functioning of their families.

Finally, all the intervention trials were the products of collaborations between high-income and low-income countries, with expert technical and local knowledge being applied together to generate evidence of value to the country and to the wider international community.

37.9 Conclusion

Good-enough parenting is essential to realizing the Millennium Development Goals and requires direct attention to the social determinants of health. Multi-sectoral strategies are required to address parenting and mental health, including poverty alleviation and violence prevention. However these are long-term goals. Immediate responses are required that value the work of mothering and the costs that it imposes on women's lives, and the cooperative role of fathers. The particular challenge to resource-constrained countries, with their international partners, is to capitalize on available knowledge and develop and implement accessible, affordable, non-stigmatizing, gender-informed, evidence-based psycho-educational programs to address the needs of parents and infants as they grow in the context of poverty and social adversity. Good-enough parenting in the twenty-first century will require more active involvement of societies, communities and families in support of parents and parenting.

37.10 References

1. World Health Organization Statistical Information System (2008) *World Health Statistics 2008*. World Health Organization, Geneva.
2. Lissner, C. (2001) *Safe Motherhood Needs Assessment version 1.1*. World Health Organization, Geneva.
3. Fisher, J. and Cabral de Mello, M.T.I. (2009) Pregnancy, childbirth and the postpartum year, in *Mental Health Aspects of Women's Reproductive Health. A Global Review of the Literature* (eds J. Fisher, J. Astbury, M. Cabral de Mello and S. Saxena), World Health Organization and United Nations Population Fund, Geneva, pp. 8–43.
4. Stern, G. and Kruckman, L. (1983) Multi-disciplinary perspectives on post-partum depression: an anthropological critique. *Social Science and Medicine*, **17**, 1027–41.
5. Howard, R. (1993) Transcultural issues in puerperal mental illness. *International Review of Psychiatry*, **5**, 253–60.
6. Wong, J. and Fisher, J. (2009) The role of traditional confinement practices in determining postpartum depression in women in Chinese cultures: a systematic review of the English language evidence. *Journal of Affective Disorders*, **116** (3), 161–69.
7. Fisher, J., Cabral de Mello, M., Tran, T. and Izutsu, T. (in press) Maternal mental health and child survival, health and development in resource-constrained settings: essential for achieving the Millennium Development Goals. Statement from the UNFPA – WHO International Expert Meeting: The interface between reproductive health and mental health. Maternal mental health and child health and development in resource constrained settings Hanoi, June, 2007. WHO, Geneva.
8. Patel, V., Rodrigues, M. and de Souza, N. (2002) Gender, poverty, and postnatal depression: a study of mothers in Goa, India. *American Journal of Psychiatry*, **159**, (1) 43–47.
9. Cooper, P., Landman, M., Tomlinson, M. *et al.* (2002) Impact of a mother-infant intervention in an indigent peri-urban South African context. *British Journal of Psychiatry*, **180**, 76–81.
10. Fisher, J., Morrow, M., Ngoc, N. and Anh, L. (2004) Prevalence, nature, severity and correlates of postpartum depressive symptoms in Vietnam. *British Journal of Obstetric and Gynaecology*, **111**, 1353–60.
11. Ekuklu, G., Tokuc, B., Eskiocak, M. *et al.* (2004) Prevalence of postpartum depression in Edirne, Turkey, and related factors. *Journal of Reproductive Medicine*, **49** (11), 908–14.
12. Rahman, A., Lovel, H., Bunn, J. et al. (2003) Mothers' mental health and infant growth: a case-control study from Rawalpindi, Pakistan. *Child: Care, Health and Development*, **30**, 21–27.

13. Chandran, M., Prathap, T., Muliyil, J. and Abraham, S. (2002) Post-partum depression in a cohort of women from a rural area of Tamil Nadu, India. *British Journal of Psychiatry*, **181**, 491–504.

14. Rahman, A., Iqbal, Z. and Harrington, R. (2003) Life events, social support and depression in childbirth: perspectives from a rural community in the developing world. *Psychological Medicine*, **33**, 1161–67.

15. Walker, S., Wachs, T., Meeks Gardner, J. *et al.* (2007) Child development: risk factors for adverse outcomes in developing countries. *Lancet*, **369**, 145–57.

16. Patel, V., de Souza, N. and Rodrigues, M. (2003) Postnatal depression and infant growth and development in low income countries: a cohort study from Goa, India. *Archives of Disease in Childhood*, **88** (1), 34–37.

17. Rahman, A., Bunn, J., Lovel, H. and Creed, F. (2007) Maternal depression increases infant risk of diarrhoeal illness: a cohort study. *Archives of the Diseases of Childhood*, **92**, 24–28.

18. Herrman, H. and Jané-Llopis, E. (2005) Mental health promotion in public health. *Promotion and Education: ProQuest Education Journals*, Supplement 2.

19. World Health Organization (1981) *Social Dimensions of Mental Health*. World Health Organization, Geneva.

20. Chen, Y.-Y., Subramanian, S.V., Acevedo-Garcia, D. and Kawachi, I. (2005) Women's status and depressive symptoms: a multilevel analysis. *Social Science and Medicine*, **60**, 49–60.

21. Owoeye, A., Aina, O. and Morakinyo, O. (2006) Risk factors of postpartum depression and EPDS scores in a group of Nigerian women. *Tropical Doctor*, **36**, 100–3.

22. Hussain, N., Beve, I., Hussain, M. et al. (2006) Prevalence and social correlates of postnatal depression in a low income country. *Archives of Women's Mental Health*, **9**, 197–202.

23. Rodrigues, M., Patel, V., Surinder, J. and de Souza, N. (2003) Listening to mothers: qualitative studies on motherhood and depression from Goa, India. *Social Science and Medicine*, **57**, 1797–1806.

24. Agoub, M., Moussaoui, D. and Battas, O. (2005) Prevalence of postpartum depression in a Moroccan sample. *Archives of Women's Mental Health*, **8**, 37–43.

25. Aydin, N., Inandi, T. and Karabulut, N. (2005) Depression and associated factors among women within their first postnatal year in Erzurum province in eastern Turkey. *Women and Health*, **41** (2), 12.

26. Mathers, C.D., Bernard, C., Moesgaard Iburg, K. *et al.* (2003) *Global Burden of Disease in 2002: Data Sources, Methods and Results*. World Health Organization, Geneva.

27. CSDH (2008). Closing the gap in a generation: health equity through action on the social determinants of health. Final Report of the Commission on Social Determinants of Health. World Health Organization, Geneva.

28. Irwin, L., Siddiqi, A. and Hertzman, C. (2007) Early Child Development: A Powerful Equalizer. Final Report for the World Health Organization's Commission on the Social Determinants of Health. World Health Organization, Geneva.

29. Barlow, J., Coren, E. and Stewart-Brown, S. (2005) Parent-training programmes for improving maternal psychosocial health. *Cochrane Database of Systematic Reviews*.

30. Lumley, J., Austin, M.-P. and Mitchell, C. (2004) Intervening to reduce depression after birth: a systematic review of the randomized trials. *International Journal of Technology Assessment in Health Care*, **20** (2), 128–44.

31. Baker-Henningham, H., Powell, C., Walker, S. *et al.* (2005) The effect of early stimulation on maternal depression: a cluster randomised controlled trial. *Archives of the Diseases of Childhood*, **90**, 1230–34.

32. Rahman, A., Malik, A., Sikander, S. *et al.* (2008) Cognitive behaviour therapy-based intervention by community health workers for mothers with depression and their infants in rural Pakistan: a cluster-randomized controlled trial. *Lancet*, **372**, 902–9.

33. Rojas, G., Fritsch R., Solis, J. *et al.* (2007) Treatment of postnatal depression in low-income mothers in primary-care centers Santiago, Chile: a randomised controlled trial. *Lancet*, **370**, 1629–37.

34. Rahman, A., Iqbal, Z., Roberts, C. and Husain, N. (2009) Cluster randomized trial of a parent-based intervention to support early development of children in a low income country. *Child: Care, Health and Development*, **35**, 56–62.

35. Cooper, P., Tomlinson, M., Swartz, L. *et al.* (2009) Improving the quality of the mother-infant relationship and infant attachment in a socio-economically deprived community in a South African context: a randomised controlled trial. *British Medical Journal*, **338**.

Index

Parenthood and Mental Health: A Bridge between Infant and Adult Psychiatry Sam Tyano, Miri Keren, Helen Herrman and John Cox
© 2010 John Wiley & Sons, Ltd

This index was prepared by Neil Manley

Printed and bound by CPI Group (UK) Ltd, Croydon, CR0 4YY

09/06/2025

14685994-0001